CW00766326

Gynaecological Ultrasound in Clinical Practice

Gynaecological Ultrasound in Clinical Practice

Ultrasound imaging in the management of gynaecological conditions

Edited by Davor Jurkovic, Lil Valentin and Sanjay Vyas

Contents

About the authors

Harm-Gerd Karl Blaas
National Centre for Fetal Medicine, Department of Obstetrics and Gynaecology, University Hospital of Trondheim, Norway

Charlotte Chaliha MRCOG
Consultant Obstetrician and Gynaecologist, Royal London Hospital, Whitechapel, London, UK

Sturla Eik-Nes MD PhD
Professor, National Centre for Fetal Medicine, St Olav's Hospital, University of Trondheim, Norway

Timothy Hillard DM FRCOG
Consultant Gynaecologist, Department of Obstetrics and Gynaecology, St Mary's Maternity Unit, Poole Hospital, Poole, UK

Davor Jurkovic MD FRCOG
Consultant Gynaecologist, Department of Obstetrics and Gynaecology, University College Hospital, London, UK

Vikram Khullar MRCOG
Consultant Obstetrician and Gynaecologist, Department of Obstetrics and Gynaecology, St Mary's Hospital, London, UK

Christopher Lee MRCOG
Research Fellow, Early Pregnancy and Gynaecology Assessment Unit, King's College Hospital, London, UK

Louise Melson MRCOG
Specialist Registrar, Department of Obstetrics and Gynaecology, St Mary's Maternity Unit, Poole Hospital, Poole, UK

Amanda J O'Leary MRCOG
Specialist Registrar, Llandough Hospital, Penarth, Wales, UK

Rehan Salim MD MRCOG
Consultant Gynaecologist, Department of Obstetrics and Gynaecology, University College Hospital, London, UK

Emma Sawyer MB BS
Research Fellow, Early Pregnancy and Gynaecology Assessment Unit,
King's College Hospital, London, UK

Povilas Sladkevicius MD PhD
Consultant, Department of Obstetrics and Gynecology, Malmö
University Hospital, Lund University, Malmö, Sweden

Abdul H Sultan MD FRCOG
Consultant Obstetrician and Gynaecologist, Department of Obstetrics
and Gynaecology, Mayday University Hospital, Croydon, Surrey, UK

Harsit R Tejura MRCOG
Specialist Registrar, Neville Hall Hospital, Abergavenny, Wales, UK

Ranee Thakar MD MRCOG
Consultant Obstetrician and Urogynaecologist, Department of
Obstetrics and Gynaecology, Mayday University Hospital, Croydon,
Surrey, UK

Johanna Trinder MRCOG
Consultant Obstetrician, Department of Obstetrics and Gynaecology,
St Michael's Hospital, Bristol, UK

Lil Valentin MD PhD
Professor of Obstetrics and Gynaecology, Lund University, University
Hospital, Malmö, Sweden

Sanjay Vyas MD FRCOG
Consultant Obstetrician and Gynaecologist, Southmead Hospital,
Bristol, UK

Michael John Weston MRCP FRCR
Consultant, Department of Ultrasound, St James' University Hospital,
Leeds, UK

Joseph Yazbek MB BS
Research Fellow, Early Pregnancy and Gynaecology Assessment Unit,
King's College Hospital, London, UK

Abbreviations

A&E	accident and emergency
AP	anterior–posterior
BPD	biparietal diameter
CI	confidence interval
CNS	central nervous system
CO2	carbon dioxide
COMS	cerebro-oculomuscular syndrome
CRL	crown–rump length
CSM	Committee on Safety of Medicines
CT	computed tomography
D&C	dilatation and curettage
DPMA	depot medroxyprogesterone acetate
EED	early embryonic demise
ERPC	evacuation of retained products of conception
ET	endometrial thickness
FSH	follicle-stimulating hormone
GnRH	gonadotrophin-releasing hormone
hCG	human chorionic gonadotrophin
HRT	hormone replacement therapy
HSG	hysterosalpingography
HyCoSy	hystero-contrast sonography
Hz	hertz
IUCD	intrauterine contraceptive devices
IUI	intrauterine insemination
IVF	*in vitro* fertilisation
LBWC	limb–body wall complex
LH	luteinising hormone
LMP	last menstrual period
MHz	megahertz
MRI	magnetic resonance imaging
MSD	mean gestational sac diameter
MVA	manual vacuum aspiration
OHSS	ovarian hyperstimulation syndrome
OIES	omphalocele, exstrophy, imperforate anus, spinal defects
OR	odds ratio
PCOS	polycystic ovary syndrome
PMB	post-menopausal bleeding
RCOG	Royal College of Obstetricians and Gynaecologists

RCR   Royal College of Radiologists
Rh   rhesus
RR   relative risk
SD   standard deviation from the mean
SERM   selective estrogen receptor modulator
SIS   saline infusion sonohysterography
TVS   transvaginal ultrasound
TVT   tension-free vaginal tape
VEGF   vascular endothelial growth factor
WHI   Women's Health Initiative

Preface

This book came about because the Royal College of Obstetricians and Gynaecologists took a decision to integrate gynaecological ultrasound imaging into gynaecological practice and set up a Special Skills Module in gynaecological ultrasound. The theoretical content for this module was delivered at regular meetings in September for seven consecutive years. These meetings were always over-subscribed and enormously popular. We had put together the contents of the meeting and the lectures were delivered by leaders in the field, most of whom are authors in this book.

We would like to think that our efforts led to the next change, which was integration of ultrasound into gynaecology training. This change has now taken place and, thus, the need for a separate training module has disappeared. However, the need for a reference source remains, and this was our driving force in producing this book.

It is clear to us that the use of ultrasound imaging in gynaecology goes well beyond simple picture recognition. A skilful gynaecological sonographer will bring together scan findings and the clinical scenario to enhance patient care. We believe this leads to targeted investigations and, just as importantly, to strategies for non-intervention. We have included chapters on clinical gynaecology, which we believe are essential for making best use of gynaecological ultrasound, and we make no apology for doing so in what some may see as an ultrasound textbook.

Just as one could never imagine a cardiologist without a stethoscope, we find it impossible to imagine a gynaecologist without an ultrasound scanner. We celebrate this evolution in our clinical practice and hope that this book helps many others to follow.

Davor Jurkovic
Lil Valentin
Sanjay Vyas

1 Ultrasound imaging in gynaecological practice

Amanda J O'Leary, Harsit R Tejura, Sanjay K Vyas

Introduction

Diagnostic medical ultrasound was first developed in the 1960s but it did not become part of routine clinical practice until the late 1970s. Transvaginal ultrasound scanning was introduced in the 1980s and it has expanded rapidly because of the improved quality of pelvic imaging provided by high frequency (5–7 Hz) transducers. Although the transvaginal view of the pelvis is more limited in comparison with transabdominal scans, in most cases it is sufficient for a thorough evaluation of the uterus and adnexa. This advantage is particularly apparent in women who are overweight and in those with a retroverted uterus.

It is important that, before commencing a scan, a complete medical history is taken. Ultrasound examination should complement rather than replace clinical assessment, which ensures the appropriate interpretation of the scan findings. Use of gynaecological scan without an appropriate history or indication will almost certainly yield a multiplicity of abnormal scan findings, which may be clinically irrelevant and which may result in inappropriate management. Ultrasound examination follows the principles of clinical palpation. This combined examination is often helpful when trying to identify the source of pelvic pain or assessing mobility and tenderness of a pelvic mass. It can also be valuable in establishing the presence or absence of a lesion. This is particularly important in patients who are difficult to examine clinically (because of obesity, lack of relaxation or involuntary guarding) or where there is a conflict between the findings at clinical pelvic examination and the patient's symptoms.

This chapter provides an overview of the contribution of ultrasound examination to the evaluation of gynaecological conditions. Additional details will be covered in the following chapters.

Pelvic pain

Ultrasound imaging can be used to assess women with a history of acute or chronic pelvic pain. It allows a quick non-invasive assessment of the pelvis and abdomen and it may be used as the first line investigation of patients with pelvic pain to confirm or exclude the provisional diagnosis based on clinical history.

During the scan, as well as looking for morphological abnormalities, an attempt to identify areas of pain or discomfort may help to achieve the correct diagnosis. Most patients who present with acute abdominal pain and who have a normal ultrasound scan experience a spontaneous resolution of their symptoms.[1]

Ultrasound imaging is useful in determining the extent of ovarian and adnexal involvement in women with pelvic inflammatory disease (Figures 1.1, 1.2). With inflammation, the organs are not freely mobile against each other and this can be detected on scan. In the presence of inflammation, the bowel is sometimes seen to be adherent to the tubes, uterus and ovaries. The most severe form of pelvic inflammatory disease leads to a tubo-ovarian abscess (Figure 1.3). Ultrasound is helpful both in diagnosis and treatment of pelvic abscesses. Ultrasound-guided transvaginal drainage of an abscess is a safe and effective alternative to surgical drainage.

Abnormal vaginal bleeding

Ultrasound is an effective tool for investigating women with a history of abnormal vaginal bleeding. It provides a clear view of the myometrium and endometrium and enables detection of clinically significant lesions such as uterine fibroids and endometrial polyps. Diagnosis of focal endometrial lesions can be further improved by saline infusion sonography, which increases both the sensitivity and specificity of ultrasound diagnosis (Figure 1.4).

Ultrasound is particularly helpful in assessing women with a history of postmenopausal bleeding and it can distinguish between women with postmenopausal bleeding who need to undergo invasive testing, with either endometrial sampling or hysteroscopy, from those who do not require any intervention.[2] However, it should not be forgotten that cervical and vaginal lesions could also cause bleeding and a speculum examination before the scan is mandatory in all women with bleeding disturbances.

Pelvic masses

Ultrasound imaging is the method of choice for the evaluation of women with either a palpable or clinically suspected pelvic mass. It enables a detailed characterisation of most ovarian lesions and it can reliably discriminate between benign and malignant masses. In the

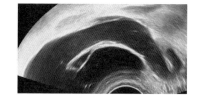

FIGURE 1.1 A typical ultrasound image of a hydrosalpinx, which is characterised by the irregular shape of the cyst, incomplete septations and hypoechoic fluid

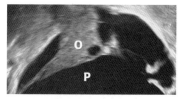

FIGURE 1.2 A case of severe pelvic adhesions resulting in the formation of a peritoneal pseudocyst (P). Healthy ovaries (O) are suspended within anechoic fluid, which occupies most of the lesser pelvis. An incomplete septation is also seen

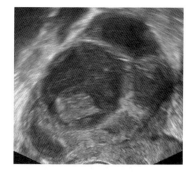

FIGURE 1.3 A tubo-ovarian abscess is recognised by the presence of a multilocular echogenic mass with thick septations in a woman with clinical features of pelvic infection

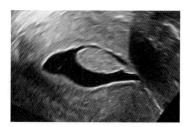

FIGURE 1.4 Longitudinal section of the uterus showing the uterine cavity distended with fluid. An endometrial polyp is clearly demonstrated arising from the anterior wall of the uterus

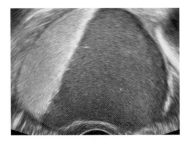

FIGURE 1.5 A large ovarian cyst containing fluid levels and hyperechogenic material. These are typical features of a dermoid cyst

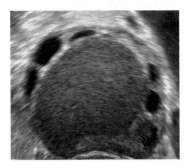

FIGURE 1.6 An endometrioma typically presents as a hyperechoic cyst, which is located in the centre of the ovary and is surrounded by healthy ovarian tissue

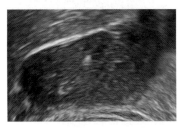

FIGURE 1.7 A solid hypoechoic tumour located separate from the uterus is a typical appearance of an ovarian fibroma

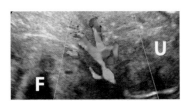

FIGURE 1.8 A large vascular pedicle connecting the uterus (U), with a large pedunculated subserous fibroid (F) on the right

diagnosis of malignancy, the reported sensitivity of the subjective evaluation of the greyscale image varies from 82% to 100%.[3] Moreover, a correct specific histological diagnosis, such as dermoid, endometrioma, fibroma or hydrosalpinx, can be made in up to 50% of benign masses (Figures 1.5–1.7).[4]

The most common pelvic masses are uterine fibroids. They are typically hypoechoic and may be intramural, subserosal or submucosal. Scan is helpful in documenting size, position and change with medical therapy. It may be difficult in some cases to differentiate a solid ovarian tumour from a pedunculated subserosal fibroid. In these cases, the pedicle between the mass and the uterus can be demonstrated if pressure is applied with the probe between the uterus and the mass (Figure 1.8). Tubal masses can usually be differentiated from ovarian masses by recognising the ovary as a separate and movable structure.

It is important to be aware of other masses, particularly those that arise from the bowel, which may present as pelvic masses. Typically, bowel segments have a central echogenic area surrounded by a hypoechoic wall and they may demonstrate peristalsis.

The advantage of ultrasound imaging in the management of pelvic masses is that it is widely available, non-invasive, relatively cheap, does not use ionising radiation and is able to provide definitive diagnostic information in a large variety of clinical settings and so enable optimal treatments to be planned.

Early pregnancy assessment

The development of ultrasound has been a major advance in the management of early pregnancy problems. A transvaginal scan can detect a normal intrauterine pregnancy as early as 4 weeks and 3 days after the last menstrual period in women with regular 28-day cycles (Figure 1.9).[5,6] Ultrasound is used to determine both the pregnancy location and viability. In approximately 90% of cases of suspected early pregnancy complications, a single scan can provide all the information necessary to plan further management. Multiple pregnancies can also be detected at an early stage and the chorionicity can be determined (Figure 1.10).

Transvaginal scan is also important in the evaluation of women with gestational trophoblastic disease.[7] Although it may be difficult to differentiate the various pathological types of gestational trophoblastic disease by their scan findings alone, the combination of clinical, laboratory and sonographic findings can usually specify the type and extent of the trophoblastic disease that is present (Figure 1.11).

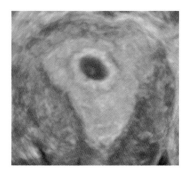

FIGURE 1.9 A three-dimensional scan through the uterus showing a small 4-week pregnancy, located in the centre of the uterine cavity

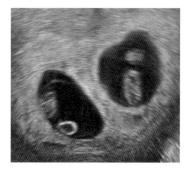

FIGURE 1.10 An example of dichorionic, diamniotic twin pregnancy at 7 weeks of gestation. The ability to visualise two separate chorionic cavities facilitates assessment in early pregnancy of less than 10 weeks of gestation

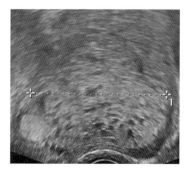

FIGURE 1.11 An example of complete hydatidiform mole diagnosed in an asymptomatic young woman. The uterine cavity is distended with a large tumour, which is shows microcystic structure typical of molar pregnancy

Fertility assessment

Transvaginal ultrasound also has an important role in the study of female fertility. It can be used to document both normal physiology and pathological situations. Ultrasound assessment of the uterus can exclude congenital uterine malformations and submucous fibroids, which may have an effect on fertility. Healthy fallopian tubes cannot be seen on the scan. However, in women with tubal damage, hydrosalpinges may be seen as sausage-shaped cystic structures.[8] In some cases where adhesions have formed in the pelvis, the organs are not freely mobile against each other and this can be detected on transvaginal scan.

Tubal patency can be assessed by the procedure hysterocontrast sonography. Ultrasound is also used to monitor follicular development and ovulation in spontaneous and stimulated cycles (Figures 1.12, 1.13).

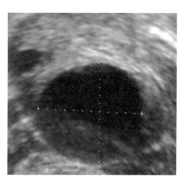

FIGURE 1.12 A preovulatory follicle visualised on day 12 of menstrual cycle is seen as a small hypoechoic cyst with a thin and smooth inner wall

Conclusions

Information from ultrasound imaging combined with that from the bimanual pelvic examination allows for a more complete assessment of the patient. However, ultrasound imaging should not be relied on as a sole diagnostic method but rather considered an adjunct to physical examination to confirm the diagnosis.

It reduces the need for surgery and favours the use of more conservative approach, such as expectant and medical management. In women who do require surgery it also helps in selecting the optimal operation and the most suitably skilled operating surgeon.

Gynaecological ultrasound imaging can be helpful only if it results in a correct diagnosis being made. This, in turn, is highly dependent upon

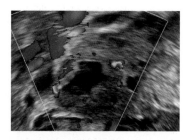

FIGURE 1.13 A follow-up scan 2 days later shows that the follicle has collapsed and there is an irregular vascular structure in its place typical of a corpus luteum

the competence of the examiner. An examiner who lacks the theoretical knowledge and practical skills risks making an incorrect diagnosis that may harm the patient. Therefore, both proper training and sound clinical knowledge of the subject are essential.

The role of ultrasound alongside clinical history and examination led to the development of gynaecology assessment clinics. The advantages of this approach to both clinical management and patient satisfaction are clearly demonstrated in the successful model of early pregnancy assessment clinics. 'One-stop' clinics for the assessment of postmenopausal bleeding, pelvic masses and menstrual problems are being introduced.[9] These clinics allow a diagnosis to be made and a management plan to be formulated and discussed at a single visit, which has a great appeal to both patients and health providers.

REFERENCES

1. HARRIS R D, HOLTZMAN S R, POPPE A M. Clinical outcome in female patients with pelvic pain and no pelvic ultrasound scan findings. *Radiology* 2000; **216**: 440–3.

2. AKANDE V A, VYAS S K. Questioning the ubiquity of outpatient endometrial sampling in the management of menstrual disorders. *BJOG* 2003; **110**: 971–4.

3. TIMMERMAN D, SCHWARZLER P, COLLINS W P, CLAERHOUT F, COENEN M, AMANT F, *et al*. Subjective assessment of adnexal masses using ultrasonography: analysis of variability and experience. *Ultrasound Obstet Gynecol* 1999; **13**: 11–6.

4. BUY J N, GHOSSAIN M A, HUGOL D, HASSEN K, SCIOT C, TRUC J B, *et al*. Characterization of adnexal masses: combination of color Doppler and conventional sonography compared with spectral Doppler analysis alone and conventional sonography alone. *AJR Am J Roentgenol* 1996; **166**: 385–93.

5. PENNELL R G, BALTAROWICH O H, KURTZ A B, VILARO M M, RIFKIN M D, NEEDLEMAN L, *et al*. Complicated first trimester pregnancies: evaluation with endovaginal us versus transabdominal technique. *Radiology* 1987; **165**: 79–83.

6. TIMOR-TRITSCH I E, ROTTEM S, THALER I. Review of transvaginal ultrasonography: a description with clinical application. *Ultrasound Q* 1988; **6**: 1–34.

7. FLEISCHER A C, JAMES A E JR, KRAUSE D A, MILLIS J B. Sonographic patterns in trophoblastic disease. *Radiology* 1978; **126**: 215–20.

8. TESSLER F N, PERRELLA R R, FLEISCHER A C, GRANT E G. Endovaginal sonographic diagnosis of dilated fallopian tubes. *AJR Am J Roentgenol* 1989; **153**: 523–25.

9. ABU J I, HABIBA M A, BAKER R, HALLIGAN A W F, NAFTALIN N J, HSU R, *et al*. Quantitative and qualitative assessment of women's experience of a one-stop menstrual clinic in comparison with traditional gynaecology clinics. *BJOG* 2001; **108**: 993–9.

2 Normal pelvic anatomy

LIL VALENTIN AND STURLA EIK-NES

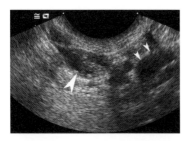

FIGURE 2.1 a

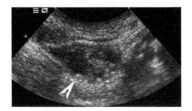

FIGURE 2.1 b

To see more details, activate the zoom function: **a)** ovary before zoom (one large arrow), the two smaller arrows show the iliac vessels; **b)** ovary after zoom

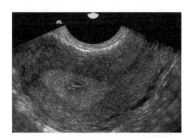

FIGURE 2.2 a

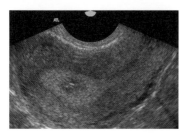

FIGURE 2.2 b

You will have maximal lateral resolution where the focus is **a)** the focus (arrow to the right) gives maximum lateral resolution very close to the transducer head **b)** placing the focus (arrow to the right) at the level of the endometrium gives maximum lateral resolution at the level of the endometrium

Optimisation and systemisation

A gynaecological ultrasound examination can be performed transabdominally, transvaginally or, in exceptional cases, transrectally (using a transvaginal probe). Irrespective of the route of examination it is always important to optimise the image and to perform a systematic examination.

Optimising the image

The image depth, magnification, focus, gain and frequency usually need to be changed during every examination. At the beginning of the examination or when you are searching for a particular organ or structure use low magnification (high depth). When you have found what you want to see, magnify the image to fill the ultrasound screen with that object. This can be achieved by decreasing the depth, diminishing the scan angle or by activating the zoom function (Figure 2.1). Place the focus on the area of interest to achieve the best lateral resolution (Figure 2.2). Adjust the gain to make your image darker or lighter (Figure 2.3). Always choose the highest ultrasound frequency possible. However, if the object of interest is situated far away from the ultrasound transducer you may need to reduce the frequency to optimise the image. This is because the depth of penetration is inversely related to the ultrasound frequency. However, a disadvantage of low frequency is a reduction in image (axial) resolution (Figure 2.4).

There are many other functions in an ultrasound system that can be used to change the appearance of the ultrasound image (such as pre-processing or edge enhancement, post-processing, log compression or dynamic range, persistence) but, unlike those discussed above, these functions do not need to be adjusted for every patient.

In some cases, it is important to work with a high frame rate; for example, if you want to detect or study a moving structure such as an embryonic heart. To increase the frame rate, use low magnification and a single ultrasound focus. Moving structures are also seen more easily if you decrease persistence (the persistence function 'averages' several images into one, so when you decrease persistence there is no 'averaging').

Unfortunately, different companies use diverse terms to describe the same ultrasound functions. Ask a representative of your ultrasound company to explain the functions of the system you are using.

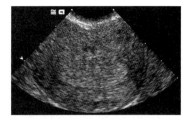

FIGURE 2.3 a

Image orientation

Irrespective of whether you perform a transabdominal, transvaginal or transrectal scan, there is general agreement that, in transverse section, the patient's right side should be shown on the left side of the ultrasound screen. When you perform a transabdominal scan, superficial structures should be shown in the upper part and deeper structures in the lower part of the image. In a longitudinal view, the cranial structures should be shown on the left side of the screen and caudal on the right side. Unfortunately, there is no consensus on the image orientation during transvaginal scans. Some prefer to show the image with the transducer head ('footprint', 'apex of the pie') in the upper part of the image and others prefer to show it with the transducer head in the lower part of the image. For longitudinal sections through the pelvis, some show the bladder on the left side of the screen and others show it on the right side. To avoid confusion, it is useful to standardise image orientation. To obtain transvaginal images that are similarly orientated to those of transabdominal images, the logical orientation would be one where the scan head is shown in the lower part of the image and the bladder is shown on the right side of the ultrasound screen (Figure 2.5). This orientation makes transvaginal images clearly distinguishable from transabdominal views and facilitates correlation between the two approaches to ultrasound scanning.

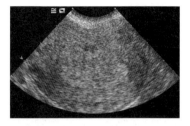

FIGURE 2.3 b

Adjust the gain to make your image
a) darker or **b)** lighter

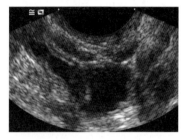

FIGURE 2.4 a

A systematic scanning technique

There are two reasons to adopt a systematic scanning technique. First, it will ensure that a complete pelvic examination is performed. For example: immediately after starting the scan you notice a large ovarian cyst. You focus on the cyst, only to realise, once the patient has left, that you did not examine either her uterus or the other ovary. Second, if you always scan all the organs in the pelvis in a systematic way as described below, you will build up a reference of what is normal, which will increase your confidence in detecting pelvic pathology.

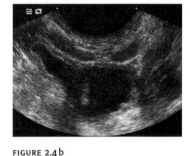

FIGURE 2.4 b

The same image obtained with a) low (5 MHz) and b) high (8 MHz) frequency. For maximum axial resolution always choose the highest ultrasound frequency possible

Transvaginal examination

It is mandatory that transvaginal scans are performed with a completely empty bladder. Scanning a woman with an incompletely empty bladder

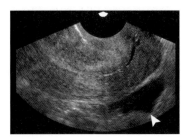

FIGURE 2.6 a

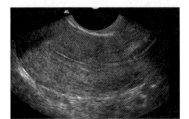

FIGURE 2.6 b

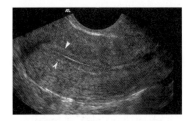

FIGURE 2.6 c

The first step of a transvaginal ultrasound examination is to show: **a)** a sagittal section through the cervix with the cervical canal on the ultrasound screen. The arrow points to a normal amount of fluid in the fossa Douglasi. Then, follow the cervical canal upwards towards the fundus uteri so that **b)** the cervical canal can be seen to join the endometrium **c)** Measurement of endometrial thickness. Measure from the endometrial-myometrial border on one side to that on the other on that longitudinal section through the uterus where the endometrium appears to be at its thickest

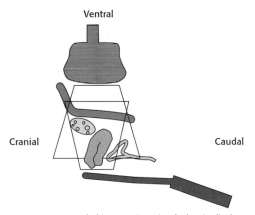

FIGURE 2.5 Recommended image orientation for longitudinal scans through the pelvis. When scanning transabdominally, the transducer head ('footprint', 'apex of the pie') is shown on the top of the screen; when scanning transvaginally, it is shown at the bottom of the screen. In both cases, the cranial end of the patient is shown to the left on the screen and the caudal end (bladder) is shown to the right on the screen. For transabdominal imaging this image orientation is internationally agreed, for transvaginal scanning we recommend it. On transverse scans, however they are obtained, the patient's right side is always shown on the left side of the screen and vice versa

increases examination time and decreases image quality.

All probes should be thoroughly cleaned after each patient examination. All examinations should be performed with the operator properly gloved during the procedure. The probe should be covered with a protective sheath before insertion. Following each examination the sheath should be disposed of and the probe wiped clean and appropriately disinfected. The type of antimicrobial solution and method of disinfection depends on manufacturer and infectious disease recommendations.[1] There must be enough coupling gel between the transducer head and the cover (so that there is no air between the transducer head and the cover) and the covered probe should be lubricated. The patient should be informed how the examination will be carried out and she should be warned before the probe is inserted. Some patients may want to watch the screen during the examination (if technically feasible) while others might prefer not to. Ask the patient about her preference.

The ultrasound probe is slowly introduced into the vagina in such a way that a longitudinal section of the uterus will appear on the screen. Watch the screen while introducing the probe. When the cervix comes into view, the examination starts.

Move the probe so that a longitudinal section through the cervical canal is shown on the screen. Follow the cervical canal upwards towards the fundus uteri so the cervical canal can be seen to join the endometrium (Figure 2.6). Look through the corpus uteri from one side to the other until the whole uterine body has been scanned in a longitudinal section. Turn the transducer through 90 degrees so that a transverse section through the corpus uteri comes into view (Figure 2.7). Now scan the uterus from the fundus to the portio of the cervix and back again.

To find the ovaries, start from a transverse section through the uterine body. Identify the 'corner' of the uterus where the tube starts (Figure 2.7) and follow the tube to the iliac vessels on the pelvic wall. A transverse view through the ovary will now come into view (Figure 2.8a). Scan the ovary on a transverse section from 'bottom' to 'top', then turn the transducer through 90 degrees so that a longitudinal section of the ovary is shown on the screen (Figure 2.8b). Scan the ovary from one side to the other. Scan the area below and above the ovary on a transverse scan through the pelvis and scan the area laterally and medially of the ovary on a sagittal scan through the pelvis. Are there any masses adjacent to the ovary?

Go back to a transverse section of the uterus and perform exactly the same manoeuvre to find and examine the contralateral ovary. Scan the pouch of Douglas. Is there any fluid? Suspicion of peritoneal implants? Masses (Figure 2.6a)? Scan the urinary bladder. Are the walls of the bladder normal (Figure 2.9)?

Measuring endometrial thickness is an essential part of the examination in women with history of postmenopausal bleeding. Measure endometrial thickness on a longitudinal scan through the uterus where the endometrium seems to be at its thickest. Measure from the endometrial-myometrial border on one side to that on the other (Figure 2.6c). The value of measuring the uterine and ovarian size is unclear. However, should you wish to assess the uterine size, the length should be measured from the external cervical os to the top of the uterine fundus. Measure the anterior–posterior diameter of the uterus where it appears to be at its widest. The width of the uterus is measured on a transverse section through the uterine body where it appears to be at its widest. The width of the ovary is measured on a transverse section through the ovary where it appears to be at its widest. The length and anterior–posterior diameter of the ovary are measured where they appear to be at their largest on a longitudinal scan through the ovary. Reference values for uterine and ovarian size can be found in the literature.[2,3]

Transrectal examination

A transrectal scan can be suggested to the patient as an alternative to a transvaginal scan if a transvaginal scan is impossible and if a transabdominal scan yields insufficient information. The examination technique of a transrectal scan is the same as that of a transvaginal scan.

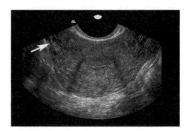

FIGURE 2.7 Transvaginal scan showing a transverse section through the uterus. The width of the uterus is measured on a transverse section through the uterine body where it appears to be at its widest. The arrow shows the 'corner' of the uterus where the tube starts. If one is scanning transvaginally this is the starting point when searching for the ovary

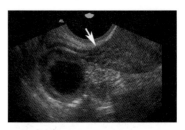

FIGURE 2.8 a

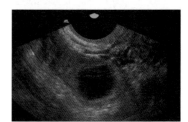

FIGURE 2.8 b

a) Transvaginal scan showing a transverse section through the ovary. The width of the ovary is measured on a transverse section through the ovary where it appears to be at its widest. Scan the ovary from bottom to top. The arrow shows the 'corner' of the uterus where the tube starts. If one is scanning transvaginally this is the starting point when searching for the ovary; **b)** Longitudinal view of the same ovary as in 2.8a. Scan the ovary from one side to the other. The length and anterior-posterior diameter of the ovary are measured where they appear to be at their largest on a longitudinal scan through the ovary

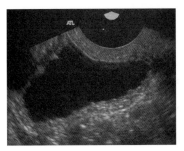

FIGURE 2.9 Normal urinary bladder. The mucosa of the bladder is seen clearly

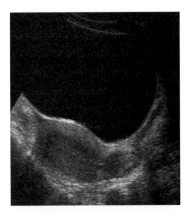

FIGURE 2.10 a

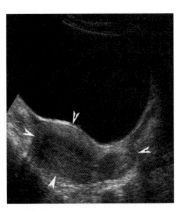

FIGURE 2.10 b

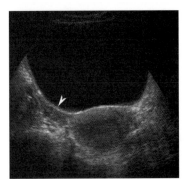

FIGURE 2.10 c

Abdominal ultrasound images of the uterus: **a)** longitudinal section through the uterus. Fundus uteri is shown to the left of the screen. The caudal end (cervix) is shown to the right of the screen; **b)** the full length of the uterus is measured from the outer cervical os to the fundus (arrows). The anterior-posterior diameter of the uterus is measured on a longitudinal sonogram where it appears to be at its widest (arrows), and the endometrial thickness is measured on a longitudinal sonogram where it seems to be at its thickest; **c)** Transverse view of the uterus. The right ovary can also be seen on the image (arrow). Measure the width of the uterus where it appears to be at its widest

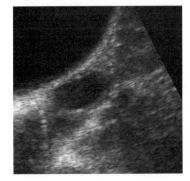

FIGURE 2.11 a

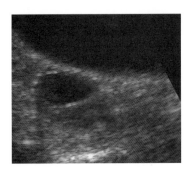

FIGURE 2.11 b

Abdominal ultrasound images of an ovary: **a)** longitudinal section through the ovary; **b)** transverse section through the same ovary

Transabdominal examination

Transabdominal ultrasound examinations must be performed with a full urinary bladder in women in whom a transvaginal scan is contraindicated or unacceptable. A full bladder will displace gas filled bowel and allow the ultrasound beams to travel thorough fluid (urine) until they reach the uterus and ovaries. When a transabdominal scan is performed in conjunction with a vaginal scan the full bladder technique is not required.

You should start the examination by obtaining a longitudinal view of the uterus. Try to see the cervical canal adjoining the endometrium. Scan the uterus from one side to the other and measure the endometrial thickness as previously described. Turn the transducer through 90 degrees to obtain a transverse view of the uterus. Scan the uterus in the transverse plane from the fundus to the portio of the cervix and back again to the fundus (Figure 2.10).

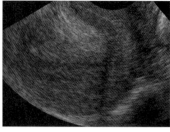

FIGURE 2.12 a

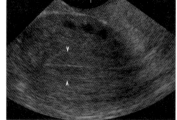

FIGURE 2.12 b

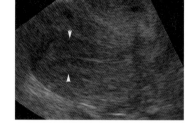

FIGURE 2.12 c

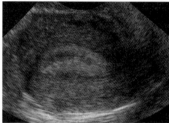

FIGURE 2.12 d

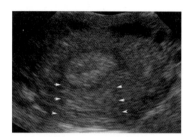

FIGURE 2.12 e

Longitudinal sections through the uterus obtained by transvaginal sonography during the same menstrual cycle: **a)** cycle day 3: the uterus is at its smallest and the endometrium is thin; in this case the endometrium is difficult to discern; **b)** 3 days before ovulation: the uterus has increased in size, the endometrium has become thicker and manifests a 'triple-layer' appearance; the arrows show the border between the endometrium and myometrium; **c)** 1 day before ovulation: the 'triple layer' is still seen but less clearly than before; the arrows show the border between the endometrium and myometrium **d)** 6 days after ovulation; the endometrium is homogenously hyperechoic and the triple layer appearance has disappeared; **e)** transverse section through the uterus 6 days after ovulation (echo enhancement is delineated by arrows) echo enhancement is often seen behind a secretory endometrium

To find the ovaries, start from a longitudinal section through the uterus. With a longitudinal view of the uterus on the screen, angle – do not slide – the transducer towards the iliac vessels on the pelvic wall where you will find the ovary. Scan through the whole ovary from one side to the other in the longitudinal scan plane. Then go back to the uterus, angle the transducer towards the contralateral pelvic wall until the contralateral ovary comes into view and scan the contralateral ovary in the same manner as described above.

Go back to a transverse section through the uterus, slide the transducer up and down – you might also need to angle it and rotate it – until you find a transverse section through one of the ovaries. Scan through the whole ovary in the transverse plane. Then do the same for the contralateral ovary (Figure 2.11). The measurements of the uterine and ovarian size and performed in a similar way as described in the subsection on the technique of transvaginal scan.

Normal ultrasound morphology of the uterus and ovaries

Women of fertile age

Uterine ultrasound morphology changes during the menstrual cycle (Figure 2.12).[4] At the beginning of the menstrual cycle, the uterus is at its smallest and the endometrium is thin. During the follicular phase, the uterus increases in size and the endometrium becomes thicker and

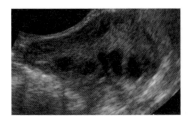

FIGURE 2.13 a

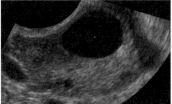

FIGURE 2.13 b

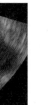

FIGURE 2.13 c

Longitudinal sections through the dominant ovary obtained by transvaginal sonography during the same menstrual cycle: **a)** cycle day 3: both ovaries contain several small follicles <10 mm. In this phase of the cycle it is not possible to determine which ovary is going to become the dominant one, i.e., the one carrying the follicle destined to ovulate. The non-dominant ovary retains this appearance throughout the menstrual cycle;[3] **b)** dominant ovary 3 days before ovulation. The dominant follicle has a diameter of 17 mm; **c)** dominant ovary 1 day before ovulation. The dominant follicle has a diameter of 20 mm; **d)** corpus luteum 6 days after ovulation. Note the echoes inside the corpus luteum. They reflect that bleeding has occurred into the corpus luteum; **e)** power Doppler image of the corpus luteum. The corpus luteum is well vascularised.[4] The large arrow points to the 'feeding vessel' of the corpus luteum, the small arrows delineate the corpus luteum itself. Vessels surround the corpus luteum. This is reflected in the colour Doppler image as a ring of colour surrounding the corpus luteum[4]

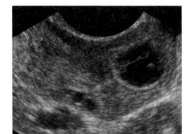

FIGURE 2.13 d

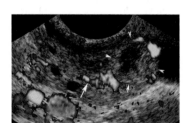

FIGURE 2.13 e

manifests a 'triple-layer' appearance. After ovulation, the 'triple-layer' appearance of the endometrium disappears and the endometrium becomes homogenously hyperechoic. Echo enhancement is often seen behind a secretory endometrium.

Ovarian ultrasound morphology changes during the menstrual cycle (Figure 2.13).[2,5] At the beginning of the menstrual cycle, both ovaries contain 3–11 follicles (usually 6–7) 10 mm or less in diameter. The non-dominant ovary retains this appearance throughout the menstrual cycle.[5] In the early follicular phase it is not possible to determine which ovary is going to become dominant; that is, the ovary carrying the follicle destined to ovulate. The dominant ovary can usually be identified 9–6 days (mean 7 days) before the luteinising hormone (LH) surge; that is between cycle days 5 and 12 (mean cycle day 8) as the ovary carrying a follicle larger than any of the other follicles and with a diameter of greater than 10 mm. The dominant follicle displays a linear growth rate of 1.4–2.2 mm/day (mean 1.7 days). At the time of the luteinising hormone (LH) surge, the leading follicle has a diameter of 18–22 mm.[5] After ovulation, the follicle becomes a corpus luteum. The corpus luteum is usually smaller than the dominant follicle. Its wall is thicker and with high-resolution ultrasound systems it may be possible to see the crenated appearance of the wall. Bleeding into the corpus luteum explains the presence of echoes in the corpus luteum at ultrasound examination.[2] The corpus luteum is well vascularised so it appears to be well-vascularised on colour Doppler ultrasound examination.[6]

Postmenopausal women

The uterus and ovaries are smaller in postmenopausal women than in women of fertile age.[2,3] The endometrium has uniform ultrasound morphology because there are no cyclical hormonal changes. It is thin (usually no more than 5 mm thick) and hyperechoic.[2,3] The ovaries contain no follicles but one or more inclusion cysts no larger than 10 mm are often seen in healthy postmenopausal women.[7] Ultrasound images of normal postmenopausal uteri and ovaries are shown in Figures 2.14 and 2.15.

The urinary bladder

The urinary bladder should be empty at transvaginal ultrasound examination. Nonetheless, it usually contains a small amount of urine, which makes it possible to examine the walls of the urinary bladder (Figure 2.9).

The pouch of Douglas

In women of fertile age fluid is almost always seen in the pouch of Douglas, at least in the late follicular phase and in the secretory phase of the menstrual cycle (Figure 2.6a). In the early luteal phase, the pouch of Douglas normally contains 15–25 ml fluid.[2] It is not possible to give an exact cut-off point in millimetres for what is a normal amount of pelvic fluid in a woman of fertile age but fluid outside the pouch of Douglas (for example, in the space between the uterus and the bladder) must be regarded as abnormal or at least extremely unusual.

An ultrasound finding of even a small amount of fluid in the pouch of Douglas in a postmenopausal woman is unusual and a follow-up is advisable to monitor its size.

Conclusion

A successful performance of a gynaecological ultrasound examination is possible only if the examiner knows how to optimise the image (magnification, gain, focus, frequency), applies a systematic examination technique and is familiar with the normal appearances of pelvic organs.

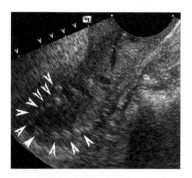

FIGURE 2.14 a

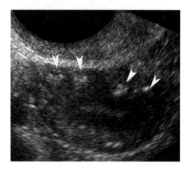

FIGURE 2.14 b

Transvaginal ultrasound images of normal postmenopausal uteri: **a)** longitudinal section through a small postmenopausal uterus. It is difficult to see the endometrium. Note the presence of calcifications (arrows) symmetrically surrounding the uterus. These are supposed to be calcifications in vessel walls and are common findings in postmenopausal women; **b)** transverse section through another postmenopausal uterus with peripheral calcifications (arrows). The endometrium is thin and hyperechoic (but the thickness of the endometrium should not be measured on a transverse section through the uterus but on a longitudinal section through the uterus)

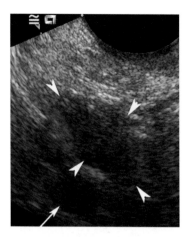

FIGURE 2.15 a

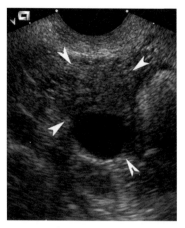

FIGURE 2.15 b

Transvaginal ultrasound images of normal ovaries in postmenopausal women: **a)** small ovary with no visible cystic spaces; the small arrows delineate the outline of the ovary, the longer arrow points to the iliac vessel on the pelvic wall; **b)** small ovary with one small 'cystic space', probably an inclusion cyst; the small arrows delineate the outline of the ovary

Acknowledgements

The studies from the author's institution were supported by grants from the Malmö General Hospital Cancer Foundation, funds administered by the Malmö Health Care Administration, the Faculty of Medicine of Lund University, the Anna-Lisa och Sven-Erik Lundgren Foundation for Medical Research, the Ingabritt and Arne Lundberg Research Foundation and the Swedish Medical Research Council (grants no. B96-17X-11605-01A, K98-17X-11605-03A, K2001-72X-11605-06A).

REFERENCES

1. American Institute of Ultrasound in Medicine. Guidelines for Cleaning and Preparing Endocavitary Ultrasound Transducers Between Patients. Approved June 4, 2003 [www.aium.org/publications/statements/_statementSelected.asp?statement=27].

2. MERZ E, MIRIC-TESANIC D, BAHLMAN F, WEBER G, WELLEK S. Sonographic size of uterus and ovaries in pre and postmenopausal women. *Ultrasound Obstet Gynecol* 1996; **7**: 38–42.

3. SLADKEVICIUS P, VALENTIN L, MARSÁL K. Transvaginal grey-scale and Doppler ultrasound examinations of the uterus and ovaries in healthy postmenopausal women. *Ultrasound Obstet Gynecol* 1995; **6**: 81–90.

4. RITCHIE W G. Sonographic evaluation of normal and induced ovulation. *Radiology* 1986; **161**: 1–10.

5. PACHE T, HOP W C, WLADIMIROFF J W, FAUSER B C J M, DE JONG F H. Growth patterns of non dominant ovarian follicles during the normal menstrual cycle. *Fertil Steril* 1990; **54**: 638–42.

6. SLADKEVICIUS P, VALENTIN L, MARSÁL K. Blood flow velocity in the uterine and ovarian arteries during the normal menstrual cycle. *Ultrasound Obstet Gynecol* 1993; **3**: 199–208.

7. VALENTIN L, SKOOG L, EPSTEIN E. The frequency and type of adnexal lesions in an autopsy material comprising postmenopausal women. An ultrasound study with histological correlation. *Ultrasound Obstet Gynecol* 2003; **22**: 284–9.

3   The uterus

REHAN SALIM AND DAVOR JURKOVIC

Introduction

The central location, relatively large size and easily identifiable shape of the uterus make it the central landmark of the female pelvis. The uterus is divided into four anatomical parts. The fundus is the uppermost part and extends into the interstitial portion of the fallopian tubes laterally. The corpus is the main body of the uterus and the isthmus is the lowermost portion, which extends into the cervix. The lower uterine segment in the pregnant uterus forms at the isthmus, which is at the level of the reflection of the urinary bladder in the nonpregnant uterus. Scars from previous caesarean sections are demonstrable at this level as deficiencies in the continuum of the endometrium that extend into the myometrium.

The cervix is fixed to the upper vagina by the uterosacral ligaments. However, the upper body of the uterus is relatively mobile and may project anteriorly towards the urinary bladder (anteverted) or posteriorly towards the rectum (retroverted). Anteflexion and retroflexion of the uterus describe the angle of the uterine body relative to the axis of the body of the cervix, either projecting forwards or backwards. The position of the uterus and flexion of the cervix are significant, as they provide useful information for clinicians performing procedures such as endometrial sampling and insertion of intrauterine contraceptive devices.

On transabdominal scanning, an anteverted uterus is usually easily demonstrated but a retroverted uterus may be difficult to see, as it projects away from the transducer and lies behind the cervix (Figure 3.1). Transvaginal ultrasound imaging provides more accurate and informative views of the uterus (Figure 3.2). Occasionally, the uterus lies parallel to the ultrasound beam, in the same axis as the vagina and cervix, and is termed as axial. This position can pose diagnostic difficulties, particularly in the assessment of the uterine cavity. Although the uterus usually lies in the midline, slight lateral deviation is often found and should be considered a normal anatomical variation. However, extreme lateroflexion may be caused by an adnexal mass or pelvic adhesions.

The wall of the uterus is made of three layers: the serosa, the myometrium and the endometrium. The serosal surface of the uterus is its peritoneal covering and is usually seen on ultrasound as a bright

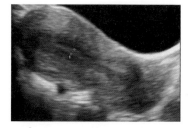

FIGURE 3.1 Longitudinal view of an anteverted uterus obtained on a transabdominal scan

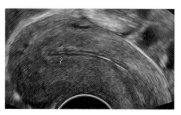

FIGURE 3.2 Longitudinal view of a retroverted uterus on transvaginal scan. The uterine fundus is lying posteriorly opposite the urinary bladder

hyperechoic outline around the uterus. The myometrium is composed of smooth muscle fibres and blood vessels. The muscular component in a normal uterus displays characteristic homogeneous low-level echogenicity. Within this hypoechoic area are small circular anechoic spaces that represent the arcuate and radial vessels in cross-section.

The inner layer of the uterus, the endometrium, is the hormone responsive tissue that varies in appearance depending on the circulating hormonal milieu. The area of myometrium closest to the endometrium is known as the junctional zone, which usually appears less echogenic than the main body of uterine myometrium (Figure 3.3).

The use of ultrasound in the examination of the uterus has evolved over time. Initially, ultrasound was mostly used to raise a suspicion of a possible uterine abnormality, while more invasive techniques, such as laparoscopy or hysteroscopy, were used to establish the final diagnosis of uterine lesion. Improvements in ultrasound technology and, in particular, the use of high frequency transvaginal probes, have helped to transform the role of ultrasound from a general screening tool to a definitive diagnostic test for most pathological conditions affecting the uterus.

Congenital uterine anomalies

Congenital morphological anomalies of the uterus, which arise during organogenesis, have been a source of much debate concerning their clinical significance. Traditionally, they have been associated with poor reproductive outcomes, specifically recurrent early pregnancy loss and preterm labour. However, clear evidence regarding the prevalence of congenital anomalies and the benefits of treatment has always been lacking. The major factor underlying this lack has been the need for invasive diagnostic methods, such as hysterosalpingography or hysteroscopy and laparoscopy, to make a diagnosis. These invasive tests are not applicable to all women so comprehensive screening is difficult. Additionally, anomalies are often encountered incidentally in women who attend for pelvic imaging for indications unrelated to reproductive performance and it has been unclear how these anomalies should be managed in asymptomatic women.

The advent of three-dimensional ultrasound in gynaecological practice has significantly enhanced our ability to detect uterine abnormalities. This technology collates a set of ultrasound data, which can then be manipulated and viewed at any arbitrary angle and plane. In the context of uterine assessment, it allows the operator to view the coronal plane of the uterus, which is often unobtainable on the conventional B-mode two-dimensional transvaginal ultrasound examination,

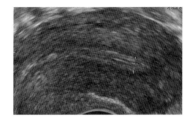

FIGURE 3.3 Longitudinal section of the uterus showing the endometrium, with a clear midline echo, junctional zone and the hypoechoic myometrium

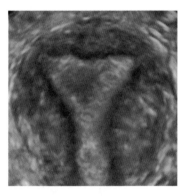

FIGURE 3.4 Coronal view of the uterus obtained on three-dimensional scan. The outer uterine contour is convex and the upper aspect of the uterine cavity is straight. These are typical features of a normal uterus

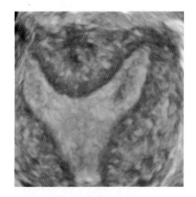

FIGURE 3.5 An arcuate uterus demonstrated on three-dimensional scan is characterised by a normal outer uterine contour and a concave shape of the fundal aspect of the uterine cavity

Uterine morphology	Fundal contour	External contour
Normal	Straight or convex	Uniformly convex or with indentation < 10 mm
Arcuate	Fundal indentation with central point of indentation at obtuse angle (>90°)	Uniformly convex or with indentation < 10 mm
Subseptate	Presence of septum, which does not extend to cervix, with central point of septum at an acute angle (<90°)	Uniformly convex or with indentation < 10 mm
Bicornuate	Two well formed uterine cornua; fundal contour convex in each	Fundal indentation > 10 mm dividing the two cornua
Unicornuate	Single well-formed uterine cavity with a single interstitial portion of fallopian tube and concave fundal contour	Fundal indentation > 10 mm dividing the two cornua if rudimentary horn present

TABLE 3.1 Three-dimensional ultrasound classification of congenital uterine anomalies

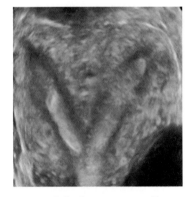

FIGURE 3.6 A subseptate uterus with a normal outer uterine contour and a deep septation extending into the lower half of the uterine cavity

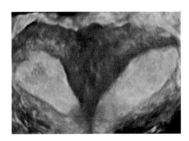

FIGURE 3.7 A bicornuate uterus with two well formed uterine cornua

as it is lying perpendicularly to the ultrasound beam. The importance of this plane is that it allows for the differentiation between the most common duplication anomalies including the arcuate, subseptate and bicornuate uterus. This is important, as each of these anomalies carries different reproductive implications and they have very different management strategies – an attempt to resect a septum in a bicornuate uterus could lead to perforation of the fundus (Figure 3.4–3.8).

Two early studies examined the diagnostic accuracy of two- and three-dimensional ultrasonography for the diagnosis of congenital uterine anomalies, using hysterosalpingography as the gold standard.[1,2] Both showed a good agreement between three-dimensional ultrasound and hysterosalpingography in classifying the uterus as normal or abnormal. This result was superior to that of two-dimensional ultrasound, which also identified all cases of abnormal uterus but also gave a number of false positive findings.

The reproducibility of three-dimensional ultrasound diagnosis of uterine anomalies has also been tested using a modified American Fertility Society Classification of Congenital Uterine Anomalies (Table 3.1).[3] Good intra- and inter-observer agreement has been reported, with only occasional differences between the operators, mainly in cases of arcuate and subseptate uteri (Table 3.2).[4] Three-dimensional ultrasound is, at present, the only imaging technique that has been systematically assessed for the reproducibility of the diagnosis of congenital uterine anomalies.

Using three-dimensional ultrasound, a large-scale screening study of women at low risk for the presence of congenital uterine anomalies was performed by Jurkovic et al. (1997).[5] The reported prevalence of major anomalies was 2.3%, which was similar to the results of previous studies which used more invasive methods to diagnose uterine

Operator A	Operator B				Total
	Normal	*Arcuate*	*Subseptate*	*Unicornuate*	
Normal	27	0	0	0	**27**
Arcuate	0	33	0	0	**33**
Subseptate	0	1	19	0	**20**
Unicornuate	0	0	0	3	**3**
Total	27	34	19	3	**83**

TABLE 3.2 Interobserver diagnosis of congenital uterine anomalies

defects.[6] Subsequently, the reproductive impact of anomalies in the low-risk group was reported by Woelfer *et al.* (2001)[7] who used three-dimensional ultrasonography to screen 1089 women presenting for pelvic imaging for indications unrelated to their past reproductive performance. The study showed that, even in women with an incidental finding of uterine anomaly, the risk of first-trimester miscarriage was significantly increased in those diagnosed with a subseptate uterus compared with women with normal uteri. There was also a slightly higher risk of second-trimester miscarriage and preterm delivery in women with arcuate uteri. A further study, which used the same diagnostic criteria and methods to compare congenital uterine anomalies in low-risk women and those with history of recurrent miscarriage, showed a four times higher prevalence of anomalies in those who suffered repeated pregnancy losses.[8] In addition, the study also showed that uterine anomalies in women with recurrent pregnancy loss tend to be more severe compared with the anomalies that were diagnosed incidentally on screening.

These studies provide strong objective evidence to support the widely held view that congenital uterine anomalies have a significant detrimental effect of on women's reproductive performance. However, it is still not clear what benefits, if any, that surgical correction of uterine anomalies may have on women's future reproductive performance. The ability to perform a detailed, non-invasive assessment of uterine anomalies, including the measurements of uterine cavity dimensions before and after surgery may help to improve selection of patients and to provide an objective measure of the success of anatomical reconstruction of the uterine cavity.

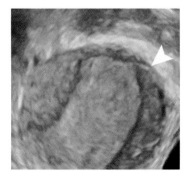

FIGURE 3.8 A unicornuate uterus, which is detected by the presence of a single interstitial tube (arrow)

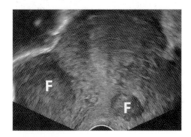

FIGURE 3.9 Uterine fibroids (F), which typically present as well-defined hypoechoic lesions within the myometrium

Uterine fibroids

Uterine fibroids are the most common uterine abnormality encountered in women of reproductive age, being present in at least 40% of women over the age of 40 years. Clinically, women often present with menstrual problems, classically menorrhagia and dysmenorrhoea, but fibroids may also cause pressure symptoms on surrounding organs, such as the bladder, leading to urinary frequency. Uterine fibroids can also be found during investigations for infertility, where they may be associated with a reduced chance of successful assisted reproduction treatment.

The ultrasound appearance of fibroids is variable but, most commonly, they appear as well defined, echo dense, single or multiple myometrial tumours (Figure 3.9). Histologically, fibroids are composed of densely packed whorls of smooth muscle and connective tissue, which causes reflection of the ultrasound beam, seen as acoustic shadowing. Occasionally, fibroids may undergo degeneration or they may contain areas of calcifications, which can alter their ultrasound appearances quite significantly (Figures 3.10, 3.11). These changes often occur in pregnancy when the trophic action of increased circulating estrogens stimulates fibroids to grow rapidly. This rapid enlargement of a fibroid may result in outgrowth of its blood supply leading to infarction and degeneration.

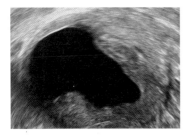

FIGURE 3.10 A uterine fibroid which has undergone cystic degeneration

Clinically, degeneration of fibroids can be the cause of significant pain in pregnancy. The degenerated fibroid is located at the site of maximal tenderness and it usually has a cystic centre, which may be filled with hypoechoic fluid and septa of the remnants of the necrotic myometrium. These appearances can be alarming and may be mistaken for more significant pathology, such a sarcoma or an ovarian mass. The differentiation is generally easy, as an ovarian mass is separate from the uterus and sarcoma is exceedingly rare in premenopausal women. Similar ultrasound appearances sometimes occur in uterine fibroids following embolisation. This iatrogenic method of causing vascular occlusion and degeneration usually results in cystic necrosis similar to that found in pregnancy. However, over time, fibroids that have undergone embolisation may become calcified and appear hyperechoic on ultrasound scan.[9]

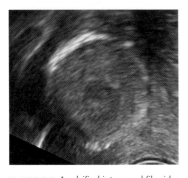

FIGURE 3.11 A calcified intramural fibroid, common in postmenopausal women

Although uterine fibroids are easily diagnosed on ultrasonography, it is their location, rather than their presence, which is often the most significant factor in determining their clinical significance and management options (Figure 3.12). Intramural fibroids are predominantly located within the myometrium and they rarely cause significant clinical problems unless they are large (greater than 5 cm) when they may

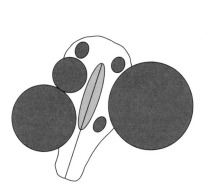
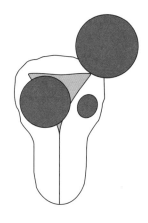

FIGURE 3.12 Two examples of fibroid mapping on ultrasound scan: left – intramural and subserous fibroids; right – submucous, intramural and subserous fibroids

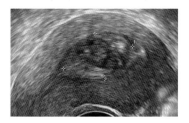

FIGURE 3.13 A longitudinal view of the uterus showing a submucous fibroid protruding deep into the uterine cavity

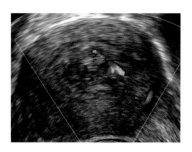

FIGURE 3.14 On Doppler examination it is possible to visualise blood vessels on the surface of the fibroid

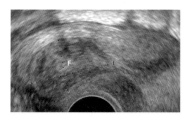

FIGURE 3.15 A submucous fibroid expelled into the cervical canal

cause pressure effect on surrounding organs, specifically the urinary bladder, causing pain or urinary frequency. Subserous fibroids project from the uterine serosa and they, too, are only problematic when large and indenting surrounding organs. Occasionally, subserous fibroids may be entirely extrauterine and connected to the uterus by a small pedicle. These are classified as pedunculated fibroids, which may sometimes undergo torsion and present with an acute abdomen. Occasionally, they may be mistaken for an ovarian tumour but this is overcome by using B-mode to identify an ipsilateral normal ovary and Doppler to demonstrate the stalk connecting the fibroid to the uterus.

Identifying and describing the location of all fibroids on ultrasound examination is of importance, as it enables the clinician to make a more complete assessment regarding the contribution of uterine fibroids to the clinical symptomatology. It also helps to plan further management, selection of the appropriate procedure and the chances of success of removal and subsequent resolution of symptoms. Thus, a small intramural fibroid on the posterior wall of the uterus is unlikely to be the cause of any significant menstrual irregularities. However, the knowledge that the uterine cavity is morphologically normal would enable the woman who is suffering from heavy dysfunctional uterine bleeding

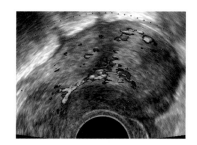

FIGURE 3.16 On Doppler examination, a vascular pedicle can be demonstrated, which shows the origin of the fibroid at the upper posterior aspect of the uterine cavity

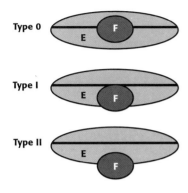

FIGURE 3.17 A schematic demonstration of the classification of the submucous uterine fibroids according the European Society of Hysteroscopy; E=endometrium, F=fibroid

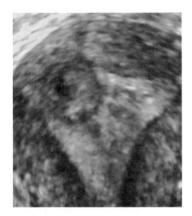

FIGURE 3.18 A three-dimensional rendered scan showing a submucous fibroid distorting the right upper aspect of the uterine cavity

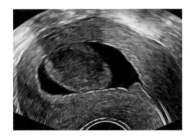

FIGURE 3.19 A type 0 anterior submucous fibroid as demonstrated on saline infusion sonohysterography

to consider either endometrial ablation or an intrauterine progestogen releasing device to control the symptoms.

Clinically, the most important uterine fibroids are submucous fibroids, which account for only 5% of all uterine fibroids. These are the cause of the most classical symptoms associated with uterine fibroids: dysmenorrhoea and menorrhagia. Submucous fibroids protrude into the uterine cavity to varying degrees, with some causing only a minor indent while others lie entirely within the endometrial cavity forming fibroid polyps (Figures 3.13–3.16). It is important to attempt to provide an estimate of the degree of protrusion of a fibroid into the uterine cavity, as fibroids that are predominantly within the cavity may be amenable to hysteroscopic resection. A classification system for this is already in use by hysteroscopic surgeons, who define submucous fibroids as either:

▷ type 0 (polyps), which are pedunculated and entirely within the cavity
▷ type 1, which are sessile and have less than 50% of the total fibroid within the myometrium
▷ type 2, which have 50% or more of the total fibroid within the myometrium (Figure 3.17).[10]

Type 2 fibroids may be unsuitable for hysteroscopic resection or may require a two-stage procedure. In either case, this classification system is aimed at improved patient selection for hysteroscopic resection and this is conventionally done by a diagnostic hysteroscopy. However, whether hysteroscopy should be the imaging modality to select those fibroids that are amenable to hysteroscopic resection remains uncertain. Vercellini et al. (1997)[11] reported that only 69% of submucous fibroids deemed amenable to hysteroscopic resection were actually successfully removed at operative hysteroscopy. This suggests that preoperative assessment by hysteroscopy may not be accurate in predicting the success of fibroid resection.

Ultrasound has the advantages of being a widely available outpatient imaging modality, with the ability to measure and assess the depth of fibroid involvement into the myometrium more accurately than any other imaging technique. However, conventional B-mode transvaginal ultrasound is not accurate enough for the detection of intracavitary pathology or for the measurement of extension of fibroids into the uterine cavity.[11] A refinement, saline infusion sonohysterography, provides a clearer view of the uterine cavity by providing an acoustic contrast within the uterine cavity. This enables more accurate detection of focal pathology in the uterine cavity, including submucous fibroids, with results comparable to diagnostic hysteroscopy (Figures 3.18, 3.19).[12]

Hysteroscopy type	3-D SIS			Total
	Type 0	*Type 1*	*Type 2*	
(fibroid polyp) 0	11	1	0	**12**
1	0	34	3	**37**
2	0	9	9	**12**
Total	11	12	12	**61**

TABLE 3.3 Comparison between three-dimensional saline infusion sonohysterography (3D SIS) and diagnostic hysteroscopy for classification of submucous fibroids

Three-dimensional ultrasound may further facilitate the assessment of the relationship of submucous fibroids and the uterine cavity (Figure 3.20). Preliminary data indicate that three-dimensional ultrasound is a reproducible method for the assessment of uterine fibroids, which may provide a more effective alternative to diagnostic hysteroscopy for preoperative assessment of submucous fibroids (Table 3.3).[13]

Submucous fibroids may be a cause of infertility in some women as conception rates are improved following fibroid removal. Eldar-Geva *et al.* (1998)[14] reported a 33.8% miscarriage rate in women with submucous fibroids compared with 16.8% in controls. Bernard *et al.* (2000)[15] reported that removal of even solitary submucous fibroids improves livebirth rates. Although these results are encouraging, there are no prospective randomised controlled studies to assess the true impact of these interventions.

The significance of intramural fibroids in women complaining of infertility remains uncertain. However, a study by Hart *et al.* (2001)[16] investigated the impact of small (less than 5 cm) intramural fibroids on conception rates in 112 women using conventional B ultrasound. They reported that the presence of small intramural fibroids reduced the chances of conception by 50%. These findings are of some concern and it remains to be seen whether they will be confirmed in future studies.

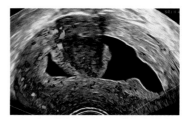

FIGURE 3.20 Colour Doppler examination shows circumferential blood supply typical of a fibroid. Doppler also facilitates better delineation of the endometrium overlying the fibroid

Uterine sarcoma

Uterine sarcoma is a rare tumour of the uterine myometrium that is usually diagnosed after hysterectomy. The clinical presentation is usually of a rapidly enlarging uterus in a postmenopausal woman. Although pain is generally not a feature, the rapid growth of the tumour may cause it to outgrow its blood supply, leading to necrosis and subsequent pain. The condition is rare and thought to complicate around 0.03% of benign fibroids, although this figure is highly speculative. The natural history of sarcoma uteri remains unknown and there is no clear evidence to link benign uterine fibroids with subsequent malignant transformation into sarcoma.

Preoperative detection has been problematic, as the rarity of the tumour has not enabled collation of morphological data from significant number of women. The ultrasound features are nonspecific and the most useful finding is the presence of wide areas of tumour necrosis (Figure 3.21) Only limited data regarding ultrasound features of sarcomata are available. On Doppler examination, sarcomas may display increased vascularity (Figure 3.22). Hata *et al.* (1997)[17] compared blood flow indices between five uterine sarcomata and 41 uterine fibroids. They reported that using a cut-off of 41 cm/second for peak systolic velocity, on colour Doppler, the detection rate for sarcoma was 80% with a false-positive rate of 2.4% with no significant difference in resistance index between the two groups. Szabo *et al.* (1997)[18] reported on the comparison of 12 women with sarcomas and 117 women with benign fibroids. In contrast to the former study, in this group there was a reduction in the resistance index with an increase in blood velocity within sarcomas. This study also reported that subjective assessment of vascularity demonstrated irregular blood vessel patterns within uterine sarcoma. The differences between the two studies highlight the difficulties in a correct preoperative ultrasound diagnosis of uterine sarcoma.

Adenomyosis

Adenomyosis is a common condition that is associated with a range of symptoms including pelvic pain, dysmenorrhoea and menorrhagia. As these symptoms are also commonly encountered in other gynaecological conditions, the reported accuracy of clinical diagnosis of adenomyosis ranges from 2.6% to 26.0%.[19] Adenomyosis may be found in up to 20% of hysterectomy specimens but it is asymptomatic in around 30% of these cases. It is more common in older multiparous women and those who have had previous uterine surgery, especially curettage and caesarean section. Advances in endometrial ablation have reduced the need for hysterectomy in many women but, if adenomyosis is present, the risk of subsequent hysterectomy is increased. Preoperative screening for adenomyosis may play a role in better triaging women who are likely to benefit from endometrial ablation.

On clinical examination, there may be diffuse uterine enlargement, although the posterior uterine wall may be disproportionately larger. This is usually more pronounced in the premenstrual phase. Diagnosis with ultrasound is difficult, as there are no characteristic features. Early studies used transabdominal ultrasound and described the myometrium as having a 'focal honeycomb' appearance with irregular

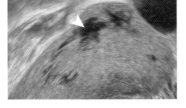

FIGURE 3.21 Uterine sarcoma originating from the posterior aspect of the uterus. The tumour was relatively echogenic and contained large areas of necrosis, which is highly suspicious of sarcomatous changes (arrow)

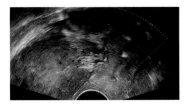

FIGURE 3.22 On Doppler examination, the sarcoma showed moderate to high blood supply

5–7mm cystic spaces (Figure 3.23). These findings confirmed adenomyosis in four of nine subjects.[20] Subsequently, Bohlman et al. (1987)[21]
diagnosed adenomyosis on the basis of hypoechogenicity of the myometrium, posterior uterine wall thickening and anterior displacement
of the endometrial cavity (Figures 3.24, 3.25). However, these findings
were confirmed at histology in only 50% of cases. Siedler et al. (1987)[22]
also used similar criteria and reported a sensitivity of only 63% but a
specificity of 97% with a positive predictive value of 71%.

Transvaginal ultrasound, with its improved resolution, enables evaluation of more subtle features that may be suggestive of adenomyosis.
Several features have been reported that would be suggestive of adenomyosis, including uterine enlargement not explained by leiomyomas,
asymmetrical thickening of the anterior or posterior uterine walls, lack of
contour or abnormality effect, heterogeneous and poorly circumscribed
areas in the myometrium, increased echotexture of the myometrium
and anechoic cysts or lacunae within the myometrium.[23] In isolation,
however, these features are neither sensitive nor specific.[24]

Diagnostic difficulties may arise in differentiating adenomyosis
from fibroids, which may also be coexistent pathology in up to 60%
of women. Several features have been proposed that would be more
suggestive of adenomyosis including:

▷ poorly defined hypoechogenic area
▷ lack of edge shadowing
▷ echogenic nodules and linear striations radiating out from the
   myometrium and into the endometrium
▷ normal distribution of uterine vessels on colour Doppler
   examination.[25]

Conclusion

Ultrasound examination, in conjunction with clinical history and assessment, provides a conclusive and accurate diagnosis of most congenital and acquired uterine abnormalities. This helps to correlate clinical
symptoms with pathological changes and decide whether the detected
abnormalities are a likely cause of the woman's complaint or whether
they are simply incidental findings of limited clinical relevance. The other

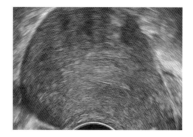

FIGURE 3.23 Longitudinal section
through the retroverted uterus showing
a thickened anterior uterine wall with
parallel shadowing on ultrasound scan,
a typical feature of diffuse adenomyosis

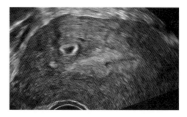

FIGURE 3.24 Oblique section of the
uterus showing four cystic lesions typical
of focal adenomyosis

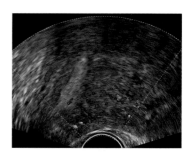

FIGURE 3.25 Doppler assessment of
uterus with extensive adenomyosis
showing abnormal distribution of radial
arteries

important advantage of non-invasive diagnosis is the ability to improve selection of women for various conservative and surgical management options available to them. In women who opt for surgery, ultrasound examination may be used to assess the likelihood of successful surgery and the risk of complications. Following surgery, ultrasound can help to assess objectively the success of operation and detect early recurrence of condition such as fibroids or intrauterine adhesions.

REFERENCES

1. JURKOVIC D, GEIPEL A, GRUBOECK K, JAUNIAUX E, NATUCCI M, CAMPBELL S. Three-dimensional ultrasound for the assessment of uterine anatomy and detection of congenital anomalies: a comparison with hysterosalpingography and two-dimensional sonography. *Ultrasound Obstet Gynecol* 1995; **5**: 233–7.

2. RAGA F, BONILLA-MUSOLES F, BLANES J, OSBORNE N G. Congenital Müllerian anomalies; diagnostic accuracy of three-dimensional ultrasound. *Fertil Steril* 1996; **65**: 523–8.

3. BUTTRAM V C, GIBBONS W E. Müllerian anomalies: a proposed classification (an analysis of 144 cases). *Fertil Steril* 1979; **32**: 40–6.

4. SALIM R, WOELFER B, BACKOS M, REGAN L, JURKOVIC D. Reproducibility of three-dimensional ultrasound diagnosis of congenital uterine anomalies. *Ultrasound Obstet Gynecol* 2003; **21**: 578–82.

5. JURKOVIC D, GRUBOECK K, TAILOR A, NICOLAIDES K H. Ultrasound screening for congenital uterine anomalies. *Br J Obstet Gynaecol* 1997; **104**: 1320–1.

6. SIMON C, MARTINEZ L, PRADO F. Müllerian defects in women with normal reproductive outcome. *Fertil Steril* 1991; **56**: 1192–3.

7. WOELFER B, SALIM R, BANERJEE S, ELSON J, REGAN L, JURKOVIC D. Reproductive outcomes in women with congenital uterine anomalies detected by three-dimensional ultrasound screening. *Obstet Gynecol* 2001; **98**: 1099–103.

8. SALIM R, REGAN L, WOELFER B, BACKOS M, JURKOVIC D. A comparative study of the morphology of congenital uterine anomalies in women with and without a history of recurrent first trimester miscarriage. *Hum Reprod* 2003; **1**: 162–6.

9. MUELLER G C, GEMMETE J J, CARLOS R C. Diagnostic imaging and vascular embolization for uterine leiomyomas. *Semin Reprod Med* 2004; **22**: 131–42.

10. WAMSTEKER K, EMANUEL M H, DE KRUIF J H. Transcervical hysteroscopic resection of submucous fibroids for abnormal uterine bleeding: results regarding the degree of intramural extension. *Obstet Gynecol* 1993; **82**: 736–40.

11. VERCELLINI P, CORTESI I, OLDANI S, MOSCHETTA M, DE GIORGI O, CROSIGNANI P. The role of transvaginal ultrasonography and outpatient diagnostic hysteroscopy in the evaluation of patients with menorrhagia. *Hum Reprod* 1997; **12**: 1768–71.

12. FARQUHAR C, EKEROMA A, FURNESS S, ARROLL B. A systematic review of transvaginal ultrasonography, sonohysterography and hysteroscopy for the investigation of abnormal uterine bleeding in premenopausal women. *Acta Obstet Gynecol Scand* 2003; **82**: 493–504.

13. SALIM R, LEE C, DAVIES A, JOLAOSO B, OFUASIA E, JURKOVIC D. A comparative study of three-dimensional saline infusion sonohysterography and diagnostic hysteroscopy for the classification of submucous fibroids. *Hum Reprod* 2005; **20**: 253–7.

14. ELDAR-GEVA T, MEAGHER S, HEALY D L, MacLACHLAN V, BREHENY S, WOOD C. Effect of intramural, subserosal, and submucosal uterine fibroids on the outcome of assisted reproductive technology treatment. *Fertil Steril* 1998; **70**: 687–91.

15. BERNARD G, DARAI E, PONCELET C, BENIFLA J L, MADELENAT P. Fertility after hysteroscopic myomectomy: effect of intramural myomas associated. *Eur J Obstet Gynecol Reprod Biol* 2000; **88**: 85–90.

16. HART R, KHALAF Y, YEONG C T, SEED P, TAYLOR A, BRAUDE P. A prospective controlled study of the effect of intramural uterine fibroids on the outcome of assisted conception. *Hum Reprod* 2001; **16**: 2411–17.

17. HATA K, HATA T, MARUYAMA R, HIRAI M. Uterine sarcoma: can it be differentiated from uterine leiomyoma with Doppler ultrasonography? A preliminary report. *Ultrasound Obstet Gynecol* 1997; **9**: 101–4.

18. SZABO I, SZANTHO A, PAPP Z. Uterine sarcoma: diagnosis with multiparameter sonographic analysis. *Ultrasound Obstet Gynecol* 1997; **10**: 220–5.

19. REINHOLD C, ATRI M, MEHIO A, ZAKARIA R, ALDIS A E, BRET P M. Diffuse uterine adenomyosis: morphologic criteria and diagnostic accuracy of endovaginal sonography. *Radiology* 1995; **197**: 609–14.

20. WALSH J W, TAYLOR KJ, ROSENFIELD A T. Gray scale ultrasonography in the diagnosis of endometriosis and adenomyosis. *Am J Roentgenol* 1979; **132**: 87–90.

21. BOHLMAN M E, ENSOR R E, SANDERS R C. Sonographic findings in adenomyosis of the uterus. *Am J Roentgenol* 1987; **148**: 765–6.

22. SIEDLER D, LAING F C, JEFFREY R B JR, WING V W. Uterine adenomyosis. a difficult sonographic diagnosis. *J Ultrasound Med* 1987; **6**: 345–9.

23. HIRAI M, SHIBATA K, SAGAI H, SEKIYA S, GOLDBERG B B. Transvaginal pulsed and color Doppler sonography for the evaluation of adenomyosis. *J Ultrasound Med* 1995; **14**: 529–32.

24. BROSENS J J, BARKER F G. The role of myometrial needle biopsies in the diagnosis of adenomyosis. *Fertil Steril* 1995; **63**: 1347–9.

25. DEVLIEGER R, D'HOOGHE T, TIMMERMAN D. Uterine adenomyosis in the infertility clinic *Hum Reprod Update* 2003; **9**: 139–47.

Postmenopausal bleeding: presentation and investigation

CHRISTOPHER LEE AND DAVOR JURKOVIC

Introduction

Postmenopausal bleeding is the most common presentation of malignant disorders of the endometrium. Its prevalence in the general population is estimated to be 40.9% (95% CI 21.8–77.1%) immediately after the first 12 months of amenorrhoea following menopause, falling to 4.2% (95% CI 1.7–10.2%) more than 3 years after menopause.[1] The reported prevalence of malignancy in women presenting with bleeding after menopause varies between 5% and 15%.[2–4] It is therefore mandatory that all women presenting with postmenopausal bleeding undergo further investigation. Investigation is directed towards differentiating benign from malignant causes of bleeding, in particular maximising the sensitivity for detection of malignancy, while avoiding unnecessary invasive testing and hospital admissions. Women experiencing irregular bleeding on hormone replacement therapy (HRT) also warrant further investigation, although the time interval between presentation and initiation of investigation is less critical as the risk of malignancy is significantly lower in this group (relative risk 1.3%).[5]

The initial assessment of women presenting with postmenopausal bleeding includes a thorough history and examination. Particular attention should be paid to risk factors including advanced age, obesity, infertility, low parity, family history and history of tamoxifen usage.[6,7]

This chapter reviews current evidence on various investigative modalities and management planning for women presenting to the gynaecology clinic with postmenopausal bleeding and discusses some of the issues to be considered when planning a cost-effective, clinic-based service for these women.

Investigations

Endometrial biopsy

Dilatation and curettage (D&C) was for many years the investigation of choice in women presenting with postmenopausal bleeding. However, blind endometrial biopsy in the form of D&C is an inadequate technique for either the diagnosis or treatment of intrauterine lesions.[8-11] It is now considered obsolete for the investigation of postmenopausal bleeding.

More recently, several devices have been developed to enable endometrial sampling in the outpatient clinic setting. The Pipelle de Cornier® (Unimar, Wilton, CT) is a widely used system. This is a narrow plastic catheter, which is passed through the cervical canal into the uterine cavity. There is an internal piston to generate negative pressure within the lumen of the catheter and a sharp aperture at the distal end to facilitate endometrial sampling. Stovall et al.[12] assessed the accuracy of the Pipelle system in the detection of endometrial cancer. The study included women with histological confirmation of endometrial cancer following D&C. Histological findings of the Pipelle biopsy were compared with those from the hysterectomy specimen. The reported sensitivity of the Pipelle system to detect endometrial cancer was 97.5%.[12] However, these findings should be interpreted with caution. Women included in this study had an established diagnosis of endometrial carcinoma; the study was therefore susceptible to operator bias. Furthermore, only women whose endometrial carcinoma was diagnosed on D&C were included. Given the diagnostic inadequacy of dilatation and curettage,[8-11] it is likely that the women included had relatively advanced disease. It follows that the study therefore almost certainly overestimated the sensitivity of the Pipelle device for the detection of endometrial cancers.

In another study of similar design,[13] the sensitivity of Pipelle to detect endometrial cancer was lower with 11 of 65 (17%) patients having false negative results. Of these, five (8%) had tumours confined to an endometrial polyp and three (5%) had disease localised to less than 5% of the surface area of the endometrium. The Pipelle missed none of the tumours in which more than 50% of the endometrium was involved (30 of 65 patients or 46%). Although the Pipelle is useful for detecting global processes in the endometrium, tumours localised to a polyp or small area of the endometrium may go undetected.[13] Pal et al.[14] found that blind endometrial biopsy in the office setting missed small lesions in up to 50% of cases. It can be concluded from these studies that blind endometrial sampling in the absence of any form of endometrial imaging has no place in the modern gynaecology clinic.

Transvaginal ultrasound

Transvaginal ultrasound (TVS) is an accurate, non-invasive diagnostic modality that enables examination of the uterine cavity and endometrium in the outpatient setting. With the uterus visualised in a longitudinal plane, the thickness of the endometrial echo can be measured.

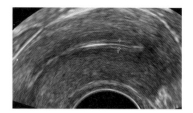

FIGURE 4.1 Longitudinal scan through the uterus illustrating the technique of endometrial thickness measurement. Callipers are placed on the outer borders of the endometrium with the midline echo lying perpendicular to the axis of the cavity

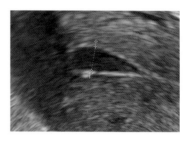

FIGURE 4.2 Endometrial thickness measurement in a postmenopausal woman with an accumulation of fluid within the uterine cavity caused by cervical stenosis. The total anterior and posterior diameter of the cavity is measured and then thickness of the fluid is subtracted to calculate the endometrial thickness

Measurement of the endometrial thickness is the discriminatory parameter used in classifying women into those at low risk of endometrial pathology and those requiring further investigation. The endometrium is measured across the thickest part from anterior to posterior, perpendicular to the axis of the cavity (Figure 4.1). The hypoechoic layer of surrounding myometrium should not be included in the measurement. By convention, the endometrial thickness includes both anterior and posterior layers of the endometrium. This is because the endometrial–myometrial interface is often more easy to visualise than the interface between the anterior and posterior endometrial layers. The examination should only be considered complete if the whole endometrium has been visualised. If there is fluid present within the uterine cavity, the thickness of the fluid layer should be subtracted from the total cavity diameter (Figures 4.2, 4.3).[15] Anechoic fluid within the cavity is a common finding in postmenopausal women and, in conjunction with a thin regular endometrial echo, may be considered a normal finding. This does not require further investigation.[16]

In cases in which the endometrial thickness cannot be measured, the scan should be considered non-diagnostic and a second-line investigative modality employed, such as hysteroscopy or saline-infusion sonohysterography.[16]

Epstein and Valentin tested the reproducibility of endometrial thickness measurement by TVS.[16] Inter-observer agreement in classifying endometrial thickness as ≤4.4 mm or ≥4.5 mm was good (kappa 0.81) and reproducibility was deemed clinically acceptable. It was also concluded that, in clinical practice, it is sufficient to take just one measurement of endometrial thickness.[17]

Endometrial thickness is used in women presenting with postmenopausal bleeding to discriminate between those women who are unlikely to have endometrial pathology (≤4 mm) from those who are at high risk (≥5 mm) and require further investigation.[18–21] A meta-analysis looking at almost 6000 women with postmenopausal bleeding found that using a cut-off of 5 mm for endometrial thickness, the risk of disease following a 'normal' test result (i.e. ≤4 mm) was reduced ten-fold to 1% compared with the pre-test risk of 10% (the background risk of endometrial cancer in women presenting with postmenopausal bleeding). This finding was applicable whether or not the woman was using HRT.[21] This corresponded to an overall sensitivity to detect endometrial cancer of 96% (95% CI 94–98) at the 5 mm cut-off level and an overall sensitivity to detect any endometrial disease (including cancer, hyperplasia and polyps) of 92% (95% CI 90–93). Specificity was lower in those women taking HRT at all endometrial thickness cut-off levels. At the 5-mm threshold, among women with normal histological

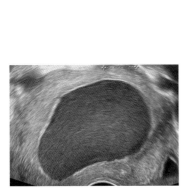

FIGURE 4.3 Pathological haematometra in a postmenopausal woman. The uterine cavity is distended with a large amount of thick echogenic fluid, which is suspicious of endometrial pathology

findings, 8% (95% CI 6–10%) of women using no HRT had an abnormal test result, whereas 23% (95% CI 21–25%) of women with a histologically normal endometrium who were using HRT had an abnormally thickened endometrium on TVS.[21]

In a multicentre study, Karlsson et al.[18] measured endometrial thickness using TVS before curettage in 1168 women presenting with postmenopausal bleeding. They did not find a single malignancy when the endometrial thickness measured less than 5 mm. They concluded that, in women with an endometrium of ≤4 mm, it is justified to refrain from curettage.[18]

Thus, in women presenting with postmenopausal bleeding, an endometrial thickness of ≤4 mm is sufficient to reassure the woman that a sinister cause for the bleeding is extremely unlikely. She may be discharged with no further investigations or follow-up. However, should the woman experience recurrent episodes of postmenopausal bleeding, reassessment is indicated, using TVS. The implications of further bleeding following a reassuring TVS were investigated.[22] The study showed that further bleeding and endometrial growth are common during a 12-month follow-up period in women with postmenopausal bleeding and an endometrial thickness of less than 5 mm. There was no difference in rates of further bleeding whether or not D&C was carried out. If the endometrial thickness is found to be ≥5 mm at follow-up TVS, a histological diagnosis should be obtained by endometrial biopsy but not necessarily for further bleeding without endometrial growth.[22]

In addition to endometrial thickness, it is important to assess the morphology of the endometrium using TVS. Endometrial polyps are a common finding in postmenopausal women and when they occur in association with postmenopausal bleeding they should be removed for histopathological diagnosis (Figures 4.4–4.8). Endometrial polyps are discrete focal thickenings of the endometrium, which are hyperechoic compared with the surrounding endometrium and myometrium on TVS. In pre- or perimenopausal women, visualisation of polyps may be enhanced if the scan is performed in the follicular phase of the cycle, when the endometrium will be relatively less echogenic, resulting in a greater contrast between polyp and endometrium. The interface between polyp and endometrium may be visualised directly on TVS. This observation may be facilitated by gentle pressure applied with the tip of the ultrasound probe while visualising both polyp and endometrium. This causes the polyp to 'slide' against the endometrium, a phenomenon that can be clearly seen on scan.

Various studies have examined the usefulness of colour Doppler imaging in the assessment of the endometrium. Timmerman et al.[23] first described the pedicle artery sign, which uses colour flow Doppler

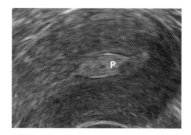

FIGURE 4.4 An endometrial polyp visualised as a well-defined hyperechoic lesion surrounded by normal hypoechoic endometrium; a clear interruption of the midline echo facilitates the diagnosis of a polyp

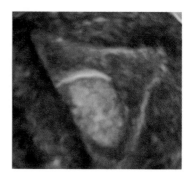

FIGURE 4.5 Visualisation of an endometrial polyp on three-dimensional scan gives clear information about the size of the polyp in relation to the uterine cavity and its exact location

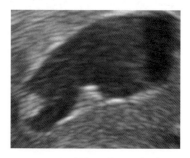

FIGURE 4.6 Multiple endometrial polyps in a postmenopausal woman with haematometra

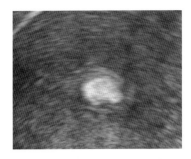

FIGURE 4.7 A polyp, which appeared unusually hyperechoic on ultrasound scan; the diagnosis of a benign polyp was confirmed on histological examination

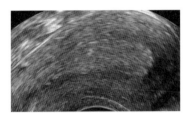

FIGURE 4.8 A diffusely thickened endometrium, which is suspicious of endometrial hyperplasia rather than a polyp

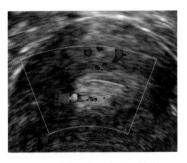

FIGURE 4.9 Colour Doppler used in the diagnosis of endometrial polyp; a feeding vessel is clearly seen arising from the right lateral aspect of the cavity, entering the polyp

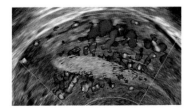

FIGURE 4.10 The uterine vascular network seen on colour Doppler examination

examination to visualise the pedicle artery supplying the endometrial polyp (Figure 4.9). The test had a positive predictive value of 81.3% and negative predictive value of 93.8% for endometrial polyps. When the test was applied to the prediction of any focal intracavitary pathology, the positive predictive value was increased to 94.2%.[23] They concluded that this test may replace more established second-stage tests such as saline infusion sonohysterography and outpatient hysteroscopy in women with an endometrial polyp.[23] Jakab et al.[24] compared diagnostic sensitivity of TVS alone with TVS plus power Doppler to assess presence of a pedicle artery in the detection of endometrial polyps. In their study, 20/41 (49%) polyps were correctly identified on non-enhanced greyscale TVS. With the use of power Doppler, the pedicle artery was correctly identified in 39/41 (95%) cases.[24] Alcazar at al.[25] also found a high sensitivity of 95% and specificity of 80% using colour Doppler to identify the pedicle artery in the diagnosis of endometrial polyps.

The usefulness of Doppler imaging to accurately differentiate benign from malignant endometrial pathology remains less clear (Figure 4.10). Wilailak et al.,[26] in their study examining the endometrium of 81 women presenting with postmenopausal bleeding, found that transvaginal Doppler did not enable the operator to differentiate normal from abnormal endometrium. Endometrial thickness was the only significant differentiating parameter.[26] Vuento et al.,[27] in their study including 1074 postmenopausal women, also found no improvement in the detection of premalignant and malignant endometrial lesions when using Doppler imaging, compared with non-enhanced ultrasound. Chan et al.[28] concluded from their study that colour Doppler did not confer additional information over that of TVS alone in the assessment of women with postmenopausal bleeding. Conversely, several studies reported Doppler imaging to be a valuable diagnostic technique for endometrial cancer.[29–33] Epstein et al.[34] attempted to objectify Doppler data using a 'vascularity index' calculated as vascularised area/endometrial area. This, together with endometrial thickness and HRT, was used to calculate an 'objective probability of endometrial malignancy'. From this study, they concluded that power Doppler can contribute to a correct diagnosis of endometrial malignancy, especially if the endometrial thickness measures 5–15 mm.[34]

There are inconsistencies between the findings of these studies and the usefulness of Doppler in diagnosing endometrial cancer remains unresolved. However, it is likely that the role of Doppler imaging in diagnosis of endometrial cancer is in providing additional information to an overall picture established by multiple techniques, rather than as a useful test in isolation.

SALINE INFUSION SONOHYSTEROGRAPHY

In 1981, a new technique of enhanced endometrial examination was described. This was termed 'echohysteroscopy'. Now commonly known as saline infusion sonohysterography (SIS) or hydrosonography, this ultrasound technique involves instillation of sterile saline through the cervix into the uterine cavity during TVS examination. SIS is simple to perform in the outpatient setting and allows enhanced visualisation of the endometrium at the fluid-endometrial interface. This provides increased sensitivity compared with conventional TVS for detection of uterine cavity abnormalities including endometrial polyps, submucous fibroids and endometrial carcinoma (Figures 4.11–4.13).[36–41] The technique is less painful than outpatient hysteroscopy and is better tolerated by patients. It is also less expensive, requiring minimal additional equipment, and can be performed as part of the transvaginal ultrasound examination.[42–44]

The accuracy of SIS has been evaluated in several studies. Epstein *et al.*[45] compared TVS, SIS and hysteroscopy for the investigation of women with postmenopausal bleeding and an endometrial thickness greater than 5 mm. They found almost perfect agreement (96%) between SIS and hysteroscopy in the diagnosis of focally growing lesions. This was supported by the findings of Krampl *et al.*,[37] who evaluated the diagnostic accuracy of TVS, SIS and hysteroscopy in women presenting with abnormal uterine bleeding. They found SIS to be significantly better than TVS in detecting focal intrauterine pathology. Direct visualisation of the endometrium at hysteroscopy did not improve the rates of detection or exclusion of focal intrauterine pathology, compared with SIS.[37]

SIS is therefore indicated in women in whom non-enhanced TVS reveals a thickened endometrium but it is inconclusive as to whether the thickening is focal or diffuse. The risk of infection as a result of SIS is small and has been reported to be less than 1%.[46] Antibiotic prophylaxis may therefore be limited to women deemed to be at particular risk, such as those with a history of pelvic infection, unexplained pelvic tenderness or immune suppression. Discomfort during the procedure is common and appears to be more common in nulliparous compared to multiparous women. Failure of SIS may occasionally occur because of discomfort or cervical stenosis. This is an indication for hysteroscopy performed under anaesthesia.

Outpatient hysteroscopy

Outpatient hysteroscopy facilitates direct inspection of the uterine cavity in the clinic setting. Kremer *et al.*[47] found no difference in patient

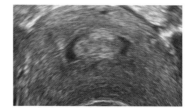

FIGURE 4.11 An endometrial polyp clearly visualised on ultrasound scan following instillation of saline inside the uterine cavity

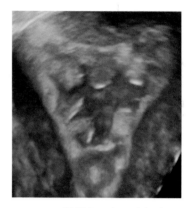

FIGURE 4.12 Multiple endometrial polyps demonstrated on three-dimensional saline infusion sonohysterography

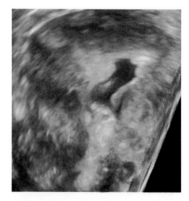

FIGURE 4.13 Uterine adhesions can create confusing appearances on two-dimensional scan. On three-dimensional saline infusion sonohysterography, the irregularity in the cavity is clearly demonstrated

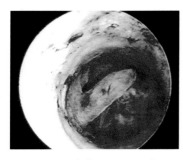

FIGURE 4.14 Typical appearances of benign endometrial polyp on outpatient hysteroscopy

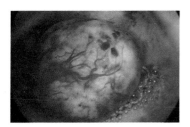

FIGURE 4.15 A submucous fibroid polyp seen on hysteroscopy

acceptability of outpatient hysteroscopy when compared with daycase hysteroscopy under general anaesthesia. In addition, in their study population, recovery time was significantly shorter in women who underwent outpatient hysteroscopy.[47]

This technique has been employed both as a first- and second-line test in the investigation of abnormal uterine bleeding. However, we propose that diagnostic hysteroscopy is best used as a second-line investigative tool, in view of the invasive nature of the procedure compared with TVS. Indications are similar to those for SIS; it may be used in patients for whom TVS demonstrates a thickened endometrium of ≥5mm[21] and the nature of the thickening is not clearly established on scan. Several studies have demonstrated a good level of diagnostic accuracy and a high degree of feasibility of diagnostic hysteroscopy carried out as an outpatient procedure (Figures 4.14, 4.15).[47-51] Distension of the uterus is necessary for visual inspection of the uterine cavity.[52] This is achieved either by the instillation of fluid, such as saline, or insufflation with CO_2 gas.[53] Although CO_2 gas is generally well tolerated, uterine distension with saline has been shown to be more comfortable, more cost-effective and to provide superior views in the presence of uterine bleeding.[53]

Outer sheaths are available with an operating channel through which it is possible to perform minor surgical procedures such as polypectomies and directed biopsies.[52,54,55] This is important as hysteroscopic visualisation of the endometrium alone is not sufficiently accurate for the diagnosis of endometrial cancer. Lo and Yuen[56] found a low sensitivity (58.8%) and positive predictive value (20.8%) in the detection of endometrial cancer. They therefore felt it necessary to perform biopsy during hysteroscopy in all cases.[56] De Wit et al.[57] also reported a low diagnostic accuracy of hysteroscopy in the detection of endometrial carcinoma. In their study, only two of seven proven cases of endometrial carcinoma (29%) were suspected of having cancer at the diagnostic hysteroscopy. One case of endometrial carcinoma was missed following hysteroscopy and endometrial biopsy (although the authors do not specify whether this was a guided biopsy).[57]

There are also reports of endometrial carcinoma detected incidentally at hysteroscopic endometrial resection, following a reportedly normal endometrium at diagnostic hysteroscopy.[58,59] A further consideration is whether diagnostic hysteroscopy may cause dissemination of malignant cells from the uterine cavity into the peritoneal cavity via the fallopian tubes. Several studies have reported positive cytology for endometrial cells in peritoneal washings after hysteroscopy.[60-63] Currently, the risk of peritoneal metastases as a result of hysteroscopy remains unclear.

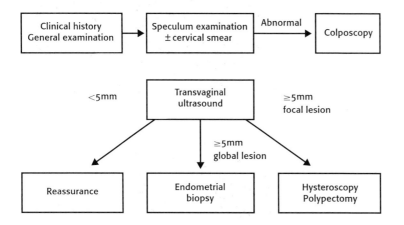

FIGURE 4.16 Summary of ultrasound-based triage of women with history of postmenopausal bleeding

The rapid access clinic

Rapid access clinics have been established throughout the UK to facilitate early diagnosis and treatment of gynaecological cancers. The main objective is to minimise the interval between presentation and initiation of appropriate treatment in women with gynaecological cancers. In the UK, the current maximum waiting time for patients to attend for the initial assessment is 2 weeks. Therefore, it is important that the clinics are organised in a way that ensures optimal use of limited resources. The service should be designed to complete the diagnostic process on an outpatient basis, using methods that facilitate accurate differentiation between benign gynaecological conditions and cancer. A flowchart outlining a management strategy for women presenting with postmenopausal bleeding is illustrated (Figure 4.16). A full clinical history and examination should precede investigations.

Some 0.8–1.8% of women with postmenopausal bleeding will have cervical carcinoma.[18, 64] The speculum examination with cervical smear test if indicated are therefore essential components of the investigation of women presenting with postmenopausal bleeding. This is even more important following a normal endometrial thickness measurement on TVS, as the risk of cervical pathology will consequently be increased.

According to current evidence, TVS is the method of choice for the initial assessment of women presenting with postmenopausal bleeding. Using an endometrial thickness of ≤4mm as the discriminatory parameter, 40–50% of women presenting with postmenopausal bleeding can be reassured that their risk of endometrial cancer is low, without undergoing further, more invasive, testing.[18] This approach ensures that the resources are used effectively, with the aim of minimising unnecessary interventions in women with no uterine pathology. However, this approach is less suitable for women with a history of vaginal bleeding

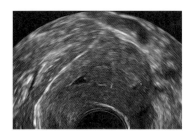

FIGURE 4.17 Advanced endometrial cancer presents as an irregular mass distending the uterine cavity

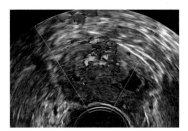

FIGURE 4.18 On colour Doppler examination the tumour appears highly vascular

on tamoxifen treatment, as almost 90% of them will have increased endometrial thickness on ultrasound scan. Many of these women will have tamoxifen-induced polyps which should be removed for histological analysis. Thus, hysteroscopy may be a more appropriate first-line investigation for this group of women.[65]

In women demonstrated on TVS to have a uniformly thickened endometrium (Figures 4.17, 4.18), the secondary test may be either outpatient endometrial sampling, with a device such as the Pipelle, or hysteroscopy. Van den Bosch et al.[66] advocated the combined use of TVS with outpatient endometrial sampling. They found a sensitivity of 100% in the detection of endometrial carcinoma by Pipelle endometrial sampling after TVS. They suggested that endometrial sampling is indicated in women with an endometrial thickness of greater than 4 mm. For women with focal endometrial lesions, however, hysteroscopy is indicated (Figure 4.2). This may be performed in the outpatient setting, as a daycase procedure or, if necessary, the woman may be admitted for an inpatient operation. The choice of the method will depend on several factors including the size of the lesion, degree of vaginal and cervical atrophy and availability of facilities locally.

In women in whom TVS is inconclusive regarding the nature of the endometrial thickening, the choice of secondary investigation is either SIS or hysteroscopy. With saline infusion into the uterine cavity, the sensitivity of transvaginal ultrasound to detect subtle focal pathology within the uterine cavity can be enhanced to a level similar to hysteroscopy.[42,43,45,67,68] This allows triage into those requiring an operative procedure and directed biopsy and those for whom an endometrial biopsy in the outpatient clinic is likely to provide information accurate enough to inform management decisions.

SIS has been found to be more acceptable to patients[69] and less costly with lower complication rates than hysteroscopy. De Kroon et al.[70] commented that diagnostic hysteroscopy can be restricted to women in whom SIS is inconclusive or fails. Again, the choice between these methods will depend on the level of ultrasound expertise available locally.

Hysteroscopy may be used as the primary test when ultrasound is not available. However, this approach is more expensive and carries the risk of surgical and anaesthetic complications. Women who are most likely to suffer complications are those with bleeding as a result of atrophic changes of the genital organs. This population of women are less likely to harbour endometrial disease.

After the triage process and secondary investigations, those women with a histological diagnosis of endometrial cancer should be referred directly to the regional cancer centres for further expert management.

Conclusion

Advances in ultrasound and hysteroscopy have facilitated the rapid diagnosis of endometrial cancer in the outpatient setting. The ability to discriminate between women with a normal endometrium and those with pathological lesions, while avoiding the need for operative intervention, has significantly improved the quality of care provided to women presenting with postmenopausal bleeding. The facility to establish the diagnosis of cancer by non-invasive investigative modalities is particularly important in postmenopausal women, many of whom are elderly and have additional medical problems, which increases the risk of both surgical and anaesthetic complications. However, it remains to be seen whether shortened waiting times for clinic appointments and more effective diagnostic workup will result in improved long-term cure outcomes in women with endometrial cancer.

REFERENCES

1. Astrup K, Olivarius Nde F. Frequency of spontaneously occurring postmenopausal bleeding in the general population. *Acta Obstet Gynecol Scand* 2004; **83**:203–7.

2. Lidor A, Ismajovich B, Confino E, David MP. Histopathological findings in 226 women with post-menopausal uterine bleeding. *Acta Obstet Gynecol Scand* 1986; **65**:41–3.

3. Danero S, Ricci MG, La Rosa R, Massafra C, Franchi F, Pitino C, et al. Critical review of dilatation and curettage in the diagnosis of malignant pathology of the endometrium. *Eur J Gynaecol Oncol* 1986; **7**:162–5.

4. O'Connell LP, Fries MH, Zeringue E, Brehm W. Triage of abnormal postmenopausal bleeding: a comparison of endometrial biopsy and transvaginal sonohysterography versus fractional curettage with hysteroscopy. *Am J Obstet Gynecol* 1998; **178**:956–61.

5. Beral V, Banks E, Reeves G, Appleby P. Use of HRT and the subsequent risk of cancer. *J Epidemiol Biostat* 1999; **4**:191–215.

6. Bristow R. Endometrial cancer. *Curr Opin Oncol* 1999; **11**:388–93.

7. Farquhar CM, Lethaby A, Sowter M, Verry J, Baranyai J. An evaluation of risk factors for endometrial hyperplasia in premenopausal women with abnormal menstrual bleeding. *Am J Obstet Gynecol* 1999; **181**:525–9.

8. Bettochi S, Ceci O, Vicino M, Marello F, Impedovo L, Selvaggi L. Diagnostic inadequacy of dilatation and curettage. *Fertil Steril* 2001; **75**:803–5.

9. Emanuel MH, Wamsteker K, Lammes FB. Is dilatation and curettage obsolete for diagnosing intrauterine disorders in premenopausal patients with persistent abnormal uterine bleeding? *Acta Obstet Gynecol Scand* 1997; **76**:65–8.

10. Stock RJ, Kanbour A. Prehysterectomy curettage. *Obstet Gynecol* 1975; **45**:537–41.

11. Lerner HM. Lack of efficacy of prehysterectomy curettage as a diagnostic procedure. *Am J Obstet Gynecol* 1984; **148**:1055–6.

12. Stovall TG, Photopulus GJ, Poston WM, Ling FW, Sandles LG. Pipelle endometrial sampling in patients with known endometrial carcinoma. *Obstet Gynecol* 1991; **77**:954–6.

13. Guido RS, Kanbour-Shakir A, Rulin MC, Christopherson WA. Pipelle endometrial sampling. Sensitivity in the detection of endometrial cancer. *J Reprod Med* 1995; **40**:553–5.

14. Pal L, Lapensee L, Toth TL, Isaacson KB. Comparison of office hysteroscopy, transvaginal ultrasonography and endometrial biopsy in evaluation of abnormal uterine bleeding. *J Soc Laparoendosc Surg* 1997; **1**:125–30.

15. Fleischer AC, Kalemeris GC, Entman SS. Sonographic depiction of the endometrium during normal cycles. *Ultrasound Med Biol* 1986; **12**:271–7.

16. Epstein E, Valentin L. Managing women with post-menopausal bleeding. *Best Prac Res Clin Obstet Gynaecol* 2004; **18**:125–43.

17. VALENTIN L. Intraobserver and interobserver reproducibility of ultrasound measurements of endometrial thickness in postmenopausal women. *Ultrasound Obstet Gynecol* 2002;**20**:486–91.

18. KARLSSON B, GRANBERG S, WIKLAND M, YLOSTALO P, TORVID K, MARSAL K, et al. Transvaginal ultrasonography of the endometrium in women with postmenopausal bleeding: a Nordic multicenter study. *Am J Obstet Gynecol* 1995;**172**:1488–94.

19. GUPTA J K, CHIEN PF, VOIT D, CLARK TJ, KHAN K S. Ultrasonographic endometrial thickness for diagnosing endometrial pathology in women with postmenopausal bleeding: a meta-analysis. *Acta Obstet Gynecol Scand* 2002;**81**:799–816.

20. GOLDSTEIN R B, BREE R L, BENSON C B, BENACERRAF B R, BLOSS J D, CARLOS R, et al. Evaluation of the woman with postmenopausal bleeding: Society of Radiologists in Ultrasound-Sponsored Consensus Conference statement. *J Ultrasound Med* 2001;**20**:1025–36.

21. SMITH-BINDMAN R, KERLIKOWSKE K, FELDSTEIN V A, SUBAK L, SCHEIDLER J, SEGAL M, et al. Endovaginal ultrasound to exclude endometrial cancer and other endometrial abnormalities. *JAMA* 1998;**280**:1510–17.

22. EPSTEIN E, VALENTIN L. Rebleeding and endometrial growth in women with postmenopausal bleeding and endometrial thickness <5 mm managed by dilatation and curettage or ultrasound follow-up: a randomized controlled study. *Ultrasound Obstet Gynecol* 2001;**18**:499–504.

23. TIMMERMAN D, VERGUTS J, KONSTANTINOVIC M L, MOERMAN P, VAN SCHOUBROECK D, DEPREST J, et al. The pedicle artery sign based on sonography with color Doppler imaging can replace second-stage tests in women with abnormal vaginal bleeding. *Ultrasound Obstet Gynecol* 2003;**22**:166–71.

24. JAKAB A, OVARI L, JUHASZ B, BIRINYI L, BACSKO G, TOTH Z. Detection of feeding artery improves the ultrasound diagnosis of endometrial polyps in asymptomatic patients. *Eur J Obstet Gynecol Reprod Biol* 2005;**119**:103–7.

25. ALCAZAR J L, GALAN M J, MINGUEZ J A, GARCIA-MANERO M. Transvaginal color Doppler sonography versus sonohysterography in the diagnosis of endometrial polyps. *J Ultrasound Med* 2004;**23**:743–8.

26. WILAILAK S, JIRAPINYO M, THEPPISAI U. Transvaginal Doppler sonography: is there a role for this modality in the evaluation of women with postmenopausal bleeding? *Maturitas* 2005;**50**:111–16.

27. VUENTO M H, PIRHONEN J P, MAKINEN J I, TYRKKO J E, LAIPPALA P J, GRONOOS M, et al. Screening for endometrial cancer in asymptomatic postmenopausal women with conventional and colour Doppler sonography. *Br J Obstet Gynaecol* 1999;**106**:1229–30.

28. CHAN FY, CHAU MT, PUN TC, LAM C, NGAN HY, LEONG L, et al. Limitations of transvaginal sonography and color Doppler imaging in the differentiation of endometrial carcinoma from benign lesions. *J Ultrasound Med* 1994;**13**:623–8.

29. SAWICKI V, SPIEWANKIEWICZ B, STELMACHOW J, CENDROWSKI K. Color Doppler assessment of blood flow in endometrial cancer. *Eur J Gynaecol Oncol* 2005;**26**:279–84.

30. SZPUREK D, SAJDAK S, MOSZYNSKI R, ROSZAK A. Estimation of neovascularisation in hyperplasia and carcinoma of endometrium using a 'power' angio-Doppler technique. *Eur J Gynaecol Oncol* 2000;**21**:405–7.

31. BALLESTER M J, GIRONES R, TORRES J V, GUILLEN P, OSBORNE NG, BONILLA-MUSOLES F. Diagnosis of endometrial carcinoma: predictive value of transvaginal color Doppler. *J Gynecol Surg* 1994;**10**:173–83.

32. KURJAK A, SHALAN H, SOSIC A, BENIC S, ZUDENIGO D, KUPESIC S, et al. Endometrial carcinoma in postmenopausal women: evaluation by transvaginal color Doppler ultrasonography. *Am J Obstet Gynecol* 1993;**169**:1597–603.

33. DRAGOJEVIC S, MITROVIC A, DIKIC S, CANOVIC F. The role of transvaginal colour Doppler sonography in the evaluation of abnormal uterine bleeding. *Arch Gynecol Obstet* 2005;**271**:332–5.

34. EPSTEIN E, SKOOG L, ISBERG PE, DE SMET F, DE MOOR B, OLOFSSON PA, et al. An algorithm including results of gray-scale and power Doppler ultrasound to predict endometrial malignancy in women with postmenopausal bleeding. *Ultrasound Obstet Gynecol* 2002;**20**:370–6.

35. NANNINI R, CHELO E, BRANCONI F, TANTINI C, SCARSELLI G F. Dynamic echohysteroscopy: a new diagnostic technique in the study of female infertility. *Acta Eur Fertil* 1981;**12**:165–71.

36. BRONZ L, SUTER T, RUSCA T. The value of transvaginal sonography with and without saline instillation in the diagnosis of uterine pathology in pre and postmenopausal women with abnormal bleeding or suspect sonographic findings. *Ultrasound Obstet Gynecol* 1997;**9**:53–8.

37. KRAMPL E, BOURNE T, HURLEN-SOLBAKKEN H, ISTRE O. Transvaginal ultrasonography sonohysterography and operative hysteroscopy for the evaluation of abnormal uterine bleeding. *Acta Obstet Gynecol Scand* 2001;**80**:616–22.

38. LINDHEIM S R, ADSUAR N, KUSHNER D M, PRITTS E A, OLIVE D L. Sonohysterography: a valuable tool in evaluating the female pelvis. *Obstet Gynecol Surv* 2003;**58**:770–84.

39. DUEHOLM M, FORMAN A, JENSEN M L, LAURSEN H, KRACHT P. Transvaginal sonography combined with saline contrast sonohysterography in evaluating the uterine cavity in premenopausal patients with abnormal uterine bleeding. *Ultrasound Obstet Gynecol* 2001;**18**:54–61.

40. Nanda S, Chadha N, Sen J, Sangwan K. Transvaginal sonography and saline infusion sonohysterography in the evaluation of abnormal uterine bleeding. *Aust N Z J Obstet Gynaecol* 2002;**42**:530–4.

41. Valenzano M, Costantini S, Cucuccio S, Dugnani M C, Paoletti R, Ragni N. Use of hysterosonography in women with abnormal postmenopausal bleeding. *Eur J Gynaecol Oncol* 1999;**20**:217–22.

42. Widrich T, Bradley L D, Mitchinson A R, Collins R L. Comparison of saline infusion sonography with office hysteroscopy for the evaluation of the endometrium. *Am J Obstet Gynecol* 1996;**174**:1327–34.

43. Bernard J P, Lécuru F, Darles C, Robin F, de Bievre P, Taurelle R. Saline contrast sonohysterography as first-line investigation for women with uterine bleeding. *Ultrasound Obstet Gynecol* 1997;**10**:121–5.

44. Rogerson L, Bates J, Weston M, Duffy S. A comparison of outpatient hysteroscopy with saline infusion hysterosonography. *BJOG* 2002;**109**:800–4.

45. Epstein E, Ramirez A, Skoog L, Valentin L. Transvaginal sonography, saline contrast sonohysterography and hysteroscopy for the investigation of women with postmenopausal bleeding and endometrium >5 mm. *Ultrasound Obstet Gynecol* 2001;**18**:157–62.

46. Bonnamy L, Marret H, Perrotin F, Body G, Berger C, Lansac J. Sonohysterography: a prospective survey of results and complications in 81 patients. *Eur J Obstet Gynecol Reprod Biol* 2002;**102**:42–7.

47. Kremer C, Duffy S, Moroney M. Patient satisfaction with outpatient hysteroscopy versus day case hysteroscopy: randomised controlled trial. *BMJ* 2000;**320**:279–82.

48. Downes E, al-Azzawi F. The predictive value of outpatient hysteroscopy in a menopause clinic. *Br J Obstet Gynaecol* 1993;**100**:1148–9.

49. Nagele F, O'Connor H, Davies A, Badawy A, Mohamed H, Magos A. Two thousand five hundred outpatient diagnostic hysteroscopies. *Obstet Gynecol* 1996;**88**:87–92.

50. Cicinelli E, Didonna T, Ambrosi G, Schonauer LM, Fiore G, Matteo M G. Topical anaesthesia for diagnostic hysteroscopy and endometrial biopsy in postmenopausal women: a randomised placebo-controlled double-blind study. *Br J Obstet Gynaecol* 1997;**104**:316–19.

51. Tahir M M, Bigrigg M A, Browning J J, Brookes ST, Smith P A. A randomized controlled trial comparing transvaginal ultrasound, outpatient hysteroscopy and endometrial biopsy with inpatient hysteroscopy and curettage. *Br J Obstet Gynaecol* 1999;**106**:1259–64.

52. Wieser F, Tempfer C, Kurz C, Nagele F. Hysteroscopy in 2001: a comprehensive review. *Acta Obstet Gynecol Scand* 2001;**80**:773–83.

53. Nagele F, Bournas N, O'Connor H, Broadbent M, Richardson R, Magos A L. A comparison of carbon dioxide and normal saline for uterine distension in outpatient hysteroscopy. *Fertil Steril* 1996;**65**:305–9.

54. Campo R, Van Belle Y, Rombauts L, Brosens I, Gordts S. Office mini-hysteroscopy. *Hum Reprod Update* 1999;**5**:73–81.

55. Gimpelson R J. Office hysteroscopy. *Clin Obstet Gynecol* 1992;**35**:270–81.

56. Lo K W K, Yuen P M. The role of outpatient diagnostic hysteroscopy in identifying anatomic pathology and histopathology in the endometrial cavity. *J Am Assoc Gynecol Laparosc* 2000;**7**:381–5.

57. de Wit A C, Vleugels M P, de Kruif J H. Diagnostic hysteroscopy: a valuable diagnostic tool in the diagnosis of structural intra-cavital pathology and endometrial hyperplasia or carcinoma? Six years of experience with non-clinical diagnostic hysteroscopy. *Eur J Obstet Gynecol Reprod Biol* 2003;**110**:79–82.

58. Dwyer N A, Stirrat G M. Early endometrial carcinoma: an incidental finding after endometrial resection. *Br J Obstet Gynaecol* 1991;**98**:733–4.

59. Colafranceschi M, Bettochi S, Mencaglia L, van Herendael B J. Missed hysteroscopic detection of uterine carcinoma before endometrial resection: report of three cases. *Gynecol Oncol* 1996;**62**:298–300.

60. Ranta H, Aine R, Oksanen H, Heinonen P K. Dissemination of endometrial cells during carbon dioxide hysteroscopy and chromotubation among infertile patients. *Fertil Steril* 1990;**53**:751–3.

61. Egarter C, Krestan C, Kurz C. Abdominal dissemination of malignant cells with hysteroscopy. *Gynecol Oncol* 1996;**63**:143–4.

62. Leveque J, Goyat F, Dugast J, Loeillet L, Grall JY, Le Bars S. Value of peritoneal cytology after hysteroscopy in surgical stage I adenocarcinoma of the endometrium. *Oncol Rep* 1998;**5**:713–15.

63. Nagele F, Wieser F, Deery A, Hart R, Magos A. Endometrial cell dissemination at diagnostic hysteroscopy: a prospective randomized cross-over comparison of normal saline and carbon dioxide uterine distension. *Hum Reprod* 1999;**14**:2739–42.

64. Gredmark T, Kvint S, Havel G, Mattson LA. Histopathological findings in women with postmenopausal bleeding. *Br J Obstet Gynaecol* 1995;**102**:133–6.

65. Assikis V J, Neven P, Jordan V C, Vergote I. A realistic clinical perspective of tamoxifen and endometrial carcinogenesis. *Eur J Cancer* 1996;**32A**:1464–76.

66. Van den Bosch T, Vandendael A, Van Schoubroeck D, Wranz P A B, Lombard C J. Combining vaginal ultrasonography and office endometrial sampling in the diagnosis of endometrial disease in postmenopausal women. *Obstet Gynecol* 1995;**85**:349–52.

67. WILLIAMS C D, MARSHBURN P B. A prospective study of transvaginal hydrosonography in the evaluation of abnormal uterine bleeding. *Am J Obstet Gynecol* 1998; **179**: 292–8.

68. KAMEL H S, DARWISH A M, MOHAMED S A. Comparison of transvaginal ultrasonography and vaginal sonohysterography in the detection of endometrial polyps. *Acta Obstet Gynecol Scand* 2000; **79**: 60–4.

69. TIMMERMAN D, DEPREST J, BOURNE T, VAN DEN BERGHE I, COLLINS W P, VERGOTE I. A randomized trial on the use of ultrasonography or office hysteroscopy for endometrial assessment in postmenopausal patients with breast cancer who were treated with tamoxifen. *Am J Obstet Gynecol* 1998; **179**: 62–70.

70. DE KROON C D, JANSEN F W, LOUWÉ L A, DIEBEN S W M, VAN HOUWELINGEN H C, TRIMBOS J B. Technology assessment of saline contrast hysterosonography. *Am J Obstet Gynecol* 2003; **188**: 945–9.

5

HRT, contraceptives and other drugs affecting the endometrium

LOUISE MELSON AND TIMOTHY HILLARD

Introduction

The endometrium undergoes cellular and structural changes that are essential for its function. These changes are cyclical and are controlled by the production of estrogen and progesterone by the ovaries. The ultrasonographic appearances of the endometrium therefore vary, depending on the phase of the menstrual cycle. The endometrium is thin in the first few days of the menstrual cycle, after menstruation, usually less than 4 mm double-layer thickness (Figure 5.1). Throughout the follicular phase, the endometrium proliferates in response to estrogen (Figure 5.2). It then becomes secretory in response to progesterone produced from the corpus luteum (Figure 5.3). In the normal cycle, endometrial thickness ranges from 6 mm to 12 mm in the late follicular phase.[1] The endometrial thickness reaches a peak 5 days after the luteinising hormone (LH) surge with an average of 14 mm.[2]

Drugs with estrogenic or progestogenic modes of action also lead to alterations in the ultrasonographic appearances of the endometrium. This chapter will help the sonographer to interpret appearances of the endometrium in women who are on these drugs.

Hormone replacement therapy

Some 15–20% of menopausal women will take hormone replacement therapy (HRT) at some time in their lives. The majority will take it for a relatively short time for the relief of troublesome menopausal symptoms in the perimenopausal and early postmenopausal period. Women with a uterus who are taking estrogen replacement therapy should receive additional progesterone, to reduce the incidence of endometrial hyperplasia[3] and cancer.[4] Irregular or unscheduled bleeding is a common adverse effect of taking HRT, which requires appropriate management. Up to 50% women stop HRT within 6–12 months of commencing it, abnormal bleeding being one of the main causes of dissatisfaction with treatment. In one series, unexpected bleeding episodes were reported in 38% women on sequential and 41% women on period-free HRT over a 2-year period.[5] Clearly, this is an important problem that requires appropriate investigation and use of resources.

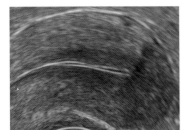

FIGURE 5.1 Longitudinal section through the uterus showing thin, normal, postmenstrual endometrium

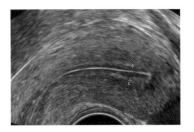

FIGURE 5.2 Endometrium in the late follicular phase is thickened and appears hypoechoic compared with the surrounding myometrium

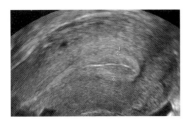

FIGURE 5.3 Hyperechoic, thick endometrium is a normal finding in the luteal phase of the cycle

Ultrasound assessment has an important role in the management of these women with abnormal bleeding.

Prescribing HRT

There has been controversy over HRT usage and the reporting of two large studies attracted much media attention. The Women's Health Initiative (WHI)[6,7] was a large randomised controlled trial in the USA in women with an average age of 63 years using estrogen and progesterone in combination or estrogen alone. The Million Women Study[8] was an observational study of women in the UK with a mean age 55 years using a wide range of preparations of HRT.

Although there has been considerable controversy surrounding these studies (the Million Women Study in particular has been heavily criticised[9,10]), they now form the basis of current prescribing habits. The known benefits of HRT from these and previous studies include symptom relief, the prevention of osteoporotic fractures and, in the WHI study, a reduction in colon cancer. There was no reduction in cardiovascular disease and no improvement in quality of life for asymptomatic women.[4] Combined HRT was associated with an increased risk of breast cancer (RR 1.3–2.0); the risk was dependent on duration of treatment with all types of combined therapy.[4,6] Estrogen alone was not associated with an increased risk of breast cancer with over 7 years of usage in the WHI trial.[5] HRT was associated with a small increase risk of thrombosis, ischaemic heart disease and stroke.

The Committee on Safety of Medicines (CSM)[11] has advised that HRT is beneficial for the treatment of menopausal symptoms, as it is highly effective in the relief of vasomotor symptoms and hormone-related mood changes. The lowest effective dose should be used for the shortest duration. They recommend that all women on HRT should have the benefits and risks of treatment reassessed at regular intervals. They do not recommend HRT as a first-line treatment solely for the prevention of osteoporosis, as they concluded the potential benefits are outweighed by the overall risks of HRT. However, it can be used in women who are unable to tolerate other osteoporosis prevention treatments or clearly those still suffering menopausal symptoms. Importantly, the CSM and other regulatory bodies have emphasised that women who have had a premature menopause should take HRT for symptom relief and prevention of osteoporosis at least until the age of 50 years and then have their treatment reviewed. The main indications for HRT are:

▷ premature menopause
▷ relief of menopausal symptoms

▷ treatment of urogenital atrophy

▷ prevention of osteoporosis (see text).

Types of HRT

There are many HRT preparations available commercially that incorporate a number of different combinations and different routes of administration. Estrogen is the principal component of HRT and is usually given on a continuous basis with progestogen being added cyclically on a monthly basis (sequential), cyclically on a 3-monthly basis (tricyclic or long cycle) or continuously (period-free or no bleed) (Figure 5.4).

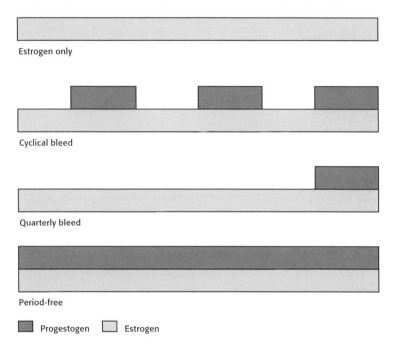

Estrogen only

Cyclical bleed

Quarterly bleed

Period-free

■ Progestogen   □ Estrogen

FIGURE 5.4 Schematic representation of types of HRT available

Women who are experiencing menopausal symptoms and who are still having regular or irregular cycles are likely to still have some endogenous ovarian activity and should be commenced on a sequential therapy. Women who have had amenorrhoea for more than 12 months or women over 54 years on sequential treatment can be safely started on continuous combined therapy on the assumption that endogenous ovarian activity has ceased. Women who cannot tolerate progestogens can consider quarterly-bleed HRT to minimise the time exposed to the progestogenic component (Figure 5.5).

Choosing the wrong type of HRT is likely to increase the chances of abnormal bleeding. Unlike the contraceptive estrogens, HRT is prescribed at physiological doses and does not suppress endogenous ovarian activity. Thus, breakthrough bleeding is more likely to occur on

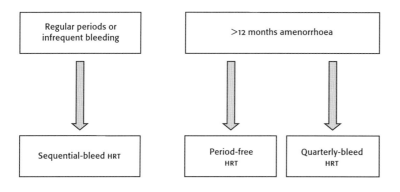

FIGURE 5.5 Selection of appropriate type of HRT based on menstrual history

period-free HRT if the woman is not truly postmenopausal. Breakthrough bleeding can occur in the estrogen-only phase of quarterly-bleed HRT. The levonorgestrel intrauterine system (Mirena®, Schering Health) is an alternative option for providing progestogen for endometrial protection. Mirena has obtained a license for use with estrogen as HRT and also provides contraceptive cover for the perimenopausal woman.

Abnormal bleeding on HRT

Abnormal bleeding on HRT is a common clinical problem. In the WHI study,[6] 40% of women reported abnormal bleeding, which was comparable to Ettinger's figures quoted earlier.[5] In Ettinger's series, 12.3% of the sequential group and 20.1% in the period-free group required an endometrial biopsy, although the bleeding episodes declined with more than 2 years usage in the no-bleed HRT group. On sequential HRT, 85% of women will experience a withdrawal bleed but up to 15% may have no bleeding.[10] The withdrawal bleed should occur towards the end of the progestogen phase and not be unduly heavy or painful. A change in the timing of the withdrawal bleed, the development of heavy or painful withdrawal bleeding, or intermenstrual bleeding, should all be considered abnormal. Compliance, particularly with the progestogen component, should be checked and a pelvic examination performed. Broad-spectrum antibiotics may interfere with hormone absorption leading to breakthrough bleeding.

On period-free HRT progestogen is taken continuously to oppose the proliferative effects of estrogen on the endometrium. Bleeding episodes initially are quite common and may take months to settle[12] (Figure 5.6). However, most women will achieve amenorrhoea by 6 months and bleeding in the first 3–6 months is considered normal, provided that it is not heavy or painful. Women should be advised of this, to aid compliance with treatment during the first 6 months. Persistent bleeding after 6 months or bleeding after a period of amenorrhoea should always be investigated.

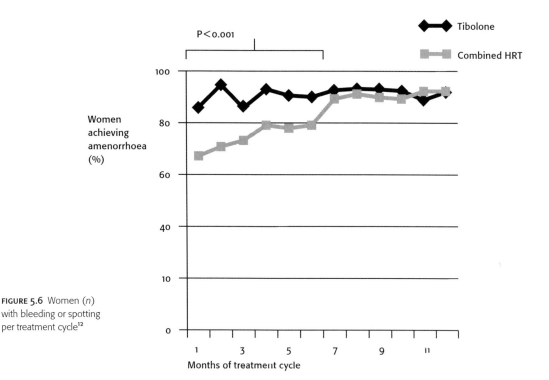

FIGURE 5.6 Women (*n*) with bleeding or spotting per treatment cycle[12]

- **Poor compliance**
- **Antibiotics**
- **Continuing endogenous ovarian activity**
- **Gastrointestinal upset**
- **Lower genital tract pathology**
- **Cervical lesion**
- **Endometrial hyperplasia**
- **Endometrial polyps**
- **Endometrial carcinoma**
- **Bleeding diatheses**
- **Concurrent medication, e.g. warfarin**

BOX 5.1 Causes of abnormal bleeding on HRT

Benign pathology, such as endometrial polyps and sub-mucous fibroids, is common and may occur in up to 40% of women with a history of abnormal uterine bleeding on HRT (Box 5.1).[13] The risk of endometrial hyperplasia on sequential HRT is around 2.7–5.0%[3,14] and is probably higher on tricyclic HRT. The incidence of endometrial hyperplasia is rare with combined estrogen and progestogen HRT, less than 1%.[3] Unopposed estrogen therapy is known to increase the risk of endometrial cancer.[3] Studies have shown an increase in the risk of endometrial cancer with long-term use (more than 5 years) of sequential HRT and a reduction in endometrial cancer with continuous no-bleed HRT.[15] The risks of endometrial cancer with cyclical or continuous HRT are shown in Table 5.1. Women continuing HRT for the medium to long term should therefore be advised to switch to no-bleed HRT once they have been on 5 years of sequential therapy or are past the menopause. Tibolone is not thought to have any adverse effects on endometrial cancer although the 2003 Million Women Study publication does suggest there may be a small increase.[8] However, these data are observational and randomised trials are in progress assessing this issue.

Endometrial assessment is recommended in women on cyclical HRT who experience change in pattern of bleeding such as intermenstrual, persistent or heavy bleeding. In women on period-free HRT the endometrium should be checked in cases of continued bleeding after

HRT	Cyclic, OR (95% CI)	Continuous, OR (95% CI)	Estrogen alone, OR (95% CI)
Never	1.0	1.0	1.0
Ever	2.0 (1.4–2.7)	0.7 (0.4–1.0)	
< 5 years	1.5 (1.0–2.2)	0.8 (0.5–1.3)	
> 5 years	2.9 (1.8–4.6)	0.2 (0.1–0.8)	6.2 (3.1–12.6)

6 months of use or bleeding after a period of amenorrhoea. Investigations are also advised in women with painful bleeding and in cases of unopposed estrogen use.

TABLE 5.1 The risk of endometrial cancer with duration and type of hormone replacement therapy (HRT)[13]

Initial assessment should involve a pelvic examination and a smear if indicated. Further investigation will depend on local hospital protocols and should involve a transvaginal ultrasound scan (TVS), an endometrial biopsy and/or a hysteroscopy. Hysteroscopy is an invasive test, which provides detailed endometrial assessment with the possibility of performing targeted biopsies. It can detect small polyps or submucous fibroids that can be missed by endometrial biopsy procedures, dilatation and curettage or ultrasound investigations. TVS is used to assess the endometrial thickness, endometrial morphology and the presence of other pelvic pathology such as ovarian cysts. TVS is preferable to transabdominal pelvic ultrasound because of the better quality of images. The endometrium is measured as a double layer. The accuracy of detection of polyps, submucous fibroids and pathology can be increased by saline infusion sonography (SIS) (Figures 5.7, 5.8). These techniques are all discussed in more detail elsewhere in this book.

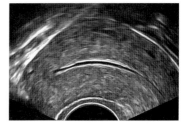

FIGURE 5.7 Longitudinal section of the uterine cavity following saline instillation shows a thin normal endometrium

Effects of HRT on the endometrium

In postmenopausal bleeding there is a cut off of 4 mm for double-layer endometrial thickness on TVS (see Chapter 4) but for women on HRT there is no agreed cut-off point. The effects of different types of HRT on endometrial thickness are shown in Table 5.2.

Sequential HRT, by its very nature, is likely to have a variable effect on the endometrium, mimicking as it does the monthly cycle. The endometrial thickness has been shown to have a maximal thickness at midcycle (days 13–23)[16] and be thinnest around day 7. The endometrial thickness in women on sequential HRT measured soon after withdrawal bleeding is not significantly different from women on combined HRT regimens.[17] This is therefore the optimal time to investigate.

The largest series on HRT effects on the endometrium is from the meta-analysis by Smith-Bindam et al.[18] but, even here, only 471 of the 5892 women were on HRT. This seminal study showed that TVS has

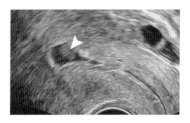

FIGURE 5.8 A small fundal endometrial polyp (arrow) is clearly visualised following saline instillation into the uterine cavity

Study	E only	E+P cyclical	E+P continuous	Tibolone
Levine 1995[37]	6.6	8.3	6.2	
Van den Bosch 2002[38]		5.7	4.3	4.6
Omodei 2002[17]		3.6	3.2	
Affinito 2001[16]		4.2		
Van den Bosch 2003[39]		5.5	3.5	4.1
Omodei 2004[40]		3.7	3.5	

E = estrogen   P = progestogen

TABLE 5.2 Mean endometrial thickness with different types of hormone replacement therapy

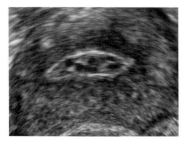

FIGURE 5.9 Cystic, hyperplastic endometrium in a woman with a history of irregular bleeding on hormone replacement therapy

a high sensitivity for detecting abnormalities of the endometrium on women with and without HRT, although both sensitivity and specificity were compromised by HRT. Using a cut-off of 5 mm, TVS had a sensitivity of 96% (95% CI 94–98%) and specificity of 92% (95% CI 90–93%) for postmenopausal women not on HRT and a sensitivity of 92% (95% CI 90–94%) and specificity 77% (95% CI 75–79%) for women on HRT. Increasing the threshold for endometrial thickness reflects a compromise between sensitivity and specificity. Thus, while a cut-off for HRT of 5 mm may detect the majority of malignancies, a much larger number of investigations would have to be performed to detect one cancer.

The PEPI study[3] compared the mean endometrial thickness with the endometrial biopsy findings in asymptomatic women on HRT. The study showed a high negative predictive value (99%) when the threshold for endometrial thickness was 5 mm, indicating that there is little additional information to be obtained from a biopsy after ultrasound has shown an endometrial thickness of <5 mm. These women can be therefore be reassured and discharged, avoiding the need for further invasive investigations. Granberg et al.[19] compared transvaginal ultrasound findings with histological findings in women with postmenopausal bleeding on HRT. The results showed endometrial pathology more likely in women with an endometrial thickness greater than 8 mm. The incidence increased with increasing endometrial thickness but endometrial cancer occurred more often in the non-HRT group (Figure 5.9).

Thus, when interpreting TVS results for women on HRT, the different effects of various types of HRT on the endometrium should be considered. Period-free HRT should induce endometrial atrophy so a 4-mm or 5-mm cut-off as for postmenopausal bleeding should be sufficient. Women on sequential therapy require investigation at endometrial thickness of more than 8 mm but between 4.0 mm and 7.9 mm there is no consensus. The need for further investigation should be based on clinical judgement but one option would be to rescan at the beginning of the next cycle when the endometrium should be at its thin-

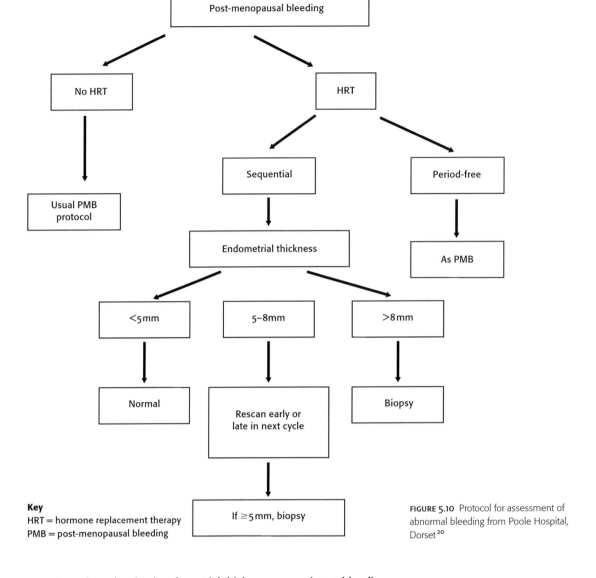

Key
HRT = hormone replacement therapy
PMB = post-menopausal bleeding

FIGURE 5.10 Protocol for assessment of abnormal bleeding from Poole Hospital, Dorset [20]

nest. A persistently raised endometrial thickness or persistent bleeding should initiate further investigation. A suggested protocol used at St Mary's Maternity Unit, Poole Hospital, is shown in Figure 5.10.[20] Recurrent bleeding despite normal endometrial thickness on HRT requires investigation.[21]

Other drugs affecting the endometrium

Tamoxifen

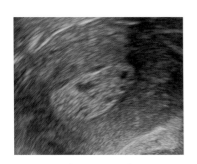

FIGURE 5.11 A large, cystic polyp occupying most of the uterine cavity in a woman taking tamoxifen

Tamoxifen is currently indicated for the treatment and prevention of breast cancer. The Early Breast Cancer Collaborative Group[22] showed that tamoxifen treatment reduced mortality from breast cancer by almost 25% and recurrence by 50%. Tamoxifen has an anti-estrogenic action on breast tissue but has an estrogen agonist-like action on the endometrium and bone. Treatment with tamoxifen is associated with an increased risk of endometrial carcinoma (RR 2.0, 95% CI 1.2–3.2 over 2–5 years of use; and RR 6.9, 95% CI 2.4–19.4 over more than 5 years of use.[23] The cancers that develop are more likely to be late stage at presentation and a more aggressive histological type, with poorer 5-year survival rates. The development of polyps is also more common.[24]

Abnormal bleeding with current or past tamoxifen use must be investigated. Transvaginal ultrasound examination of the endometrium often shows irregular thickening of the endometrium with cystic spaces and glandulocystic polyps (Figure 5.11). The endometrium may appear thickened in up to 75% women without pathological significance.[25] There is no established correlation between endometrial histology and ultrasonic findings. Many of the sonographic changes may be subendometrial and saline sonography will help to differentiate these cases from endometrial pathology such as polyps.[26] Hysteroscopy and directed biopsy is advised if polyps are suspected.

Currently, screening asymptomatic women with breast cancer on tamoxifen for endometrial abnormalities is not advocated as it is unlikely to be cost-effective and may do more harm with increased interventions and associated complications.[27] However, screening healthy women who are taking tamoxifen for prevention of breast cancer on a long-term basis should be considered. Neven et al.[28] have suggested a baseline TVS assessment and yearly TVS after 3 years of tamoxifen treatment.

Raloxifene

Raloxifene is a selective estrogen receptor modulator (SERM). It is indicated for the prevention and treatment of postmenopausal osteoporosis. Unlike tamoxifen, it does not stimulate the endometrium in healthy postmenopausal women. The effect of raloxifene on the endometrium has been studied in the Euralox 1 trial.[29] No increase in endometrial thickness was found in postmenopausal women on raloxifene compared with baseline measurements and use of continuous combined HRT.

Contraceptives

Hormonal contraceptives and intrauterine contraceptive devices (IUCD) have multiple effects leading to their contraceptive action. The effect on the endometrium can either be a by-product of this action or the main contraceptive effect as with the levonorgestrel intrauterine system.

Combined oral contraceptives

Combined oral contraceptives exert their main contraceptive effect by inhibiting ovulation. The administration of estrogen and progestogen together causes inhibition of follicular development, ovulation and therefore corpus luteum formation. The inhibitory action is at the level of the hypothalamus, blocking normal production of gonadotrophin-releasing hormone (GnRH), thereby reducing pituitary production of follicle-stimulating hormone (FSH) and luteinising hormone (LH).[30] There is also a smaller action at the pituitary level. The predominant anti-ovulatory effect is from the progestogenic component. The estrogenic component potentiates the effects of progestin and stabilises the endometrium, preventing irregular shedding.[30] This gives better cycle control and less breakthrough bleeding. The endometrium does not undergo the normal phases of proliferation and secretory changes and is thinner on ultrasound examination compared with normal cycles.[31]

Progestogen-only contraceptives

Progestogen-only contraceptives prevent pregnancy through a combination of mechanisms. The main action is disturbance of hypothalamic–pituitary function suppressing ovulation, particularly the midcycle LH surge. Low doses do not have an anti-ovulatory effect but act by the alteration of the cervical mucus, which becomes hostile to sperm.[32] The volume of mucus is reduced and it is thicker, with altered cell content and structure. These changes result in little or no sperm penetration. The effects on the endometrium of progestogen-only contraception varies between atrophy, suppressed proliferation and sometimes normal activity.[33] On histology, the endometrial glands are reduced in number and diameter. These changes result in the appearance of a thin endometrium on ultrasonography.[34] The effect of injectable depot medroxyprogesterone acetate (DMPA) on the endometrium is particularly marked.

The levonorgestrel intrauterine system has minimal effect on the ovarian–pituitary axis, with up to 85% women ovulating.[35] The main effect is local suppression of the endometrium, which prevents implan-

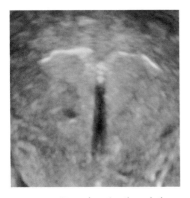

FIGURE 5.12 Coronal section through the uterus showing a Mirena® intrauterine system located in the centre of the uterine cavity

tation. On ultrasound examination, it has been shown to significantly reduce the endometrial thickness after 4 months of use (Figure 5.12).[36]

Conclusions

Bleeding problems on sequential and continuous combined HRT are common, especially in the first 6 months, and may reduce compliance with treatment. There are many causes of abnormal bleeding: the most common pathologies are submucous fibroids and polyps. Although unscheduled bleeding on HRT requires investigation, the underlying malignancy risk is low. Ultrasound has an important role in investigation in the management of abnormal bleeding on HRT.

All drugs with estrogenic or progestogenic actions lead to alterations of the ultrasound appearance of the endometrium. Because of this, and the high frequency with which they are used in the population, it is important for the sonographer to take a drug history and to incorporate this information into the interpretation of the ultrasound image.

REFERENCES

1. FORREST TS, ELYADERANI M K, MUILENBURG M I, BEWTRA C, KABLE WT, SULLIVAN P. Cyclic endometrial changes: US assessment with histologic correlation. *Radiology* 1988;**167**:233–7.

2. RANDALL J M, FISK N M, McTAVISH A, TEMPLETON A. Transvaginal ultrasonic assessment of endometrial growth in spontaneous and hyperstimulated menstrual cycles. *BJOG* 1989;**96**:954–9.

3. Writing group for the PEPI trial. Effects of oestrogen and progestins on the biochemistry and morphology of the postmenopausal endometrium. *JAMA* 1996;**275**:370–5.

4. PERSSON I, ADAMI H O, BERGKVIST L, LINDGREN A, PETTERSSON B, HOOVER R, *et al*. Risk of endometrial cancer after treatment with oestrogen alone or in combination with progestogens: results of a prospective study. *BMJ* 1989;**298**:147–51.

5. ETTINGER B, LI D K, KLEIN R. Unexpected vaginal bleeding and associated gynaecological care in postmenopausal women using hormone replacement therapy: comparison of cyclical versus continuous combined schedules. *Fertil Steril* 1998;**69**:865–9.

6. Writing Group for the Women's Health Initiative Investigators. Risks and benefits of estrogen plus progestin in healthy postmenopausal women. *JAMA* 2002;**288**:321–33.

7. Writing Group for the Women's Health Initiative Investigators. Effects of conjugated equine estrogen in postmenopausal women with hysterectomy. *JAMA* 2004;**291**:1701–12.

8. Million Women Study Collaborators. Breast cancer and hormone replacement therapy in the Million Women Study. *Lancet* 2003;**362**:419–27.

9. SHAPIRO S. The Million Women Study: potential biases do not allow uncritical acceptance of the data. *Climacteric* 2004;**7**:415–16.

10. WHITEHEAD M, FARMER R. The Million Women Study: a critique. *Endocrine* 2004;**24**:187–93.

11. Committee on Safety of Medicines. Further advice on safety of hormone replacement therapy (HRT). Press release, 3 December 2003; reference no. 2003/0492 [www.dh.gov.uk/PublicationsAndStatistics/PressReleases/].

12. HAMMAR M, CHRISTAU S, NATHORST-BOOS J, RUD T, GARRE K. A double-blind randomised trial comparing the effects of tibolone and continuous combined hormone replacement therapy in postmenopausal women with menopausal symptoms. *BJOG* 1998;**105**:904–11.

13. NAGELE F, O'CONNOR H, BASKETT T F, DAVIES A, MOHAMMED H, MAGOS A L. Hysteroscopy in women with abnormal uterine bleeding on hormone replacement therapy: a comparison with postmenopausal bleeding. *Fertil Steril* 1996;**65**:1145–50.

14. STURDEE D W, ULRICH L G, BARLOW D H, BARLOW D H, WELLS M, CAMPBELL M J, *et al*. The endometrial response to sequential and continuous combined oestrogen-progestogen replacement therapy. *BJOG* 2000;**107**:1392–400.

15. WEIDERPASS E, ADAMI HO, BARON J A, MAGNUSSON C, BERGSTROM R, LINDGREN A, et al. Risk of endometrial cancer following with and without progestins. J Natl Cancer Inst 1999;**91**:1131–7.

16. AFFINITO P, PALOMBA S, SAMMARTINO A, BONIFACIO M, NAPPI C. Ultrasonographic endometrial monitoring during continuous-sequential hormonal replacement therapy regimen in postmenopausal women. Maturitas 2001;**39**:239–44.

17. OMODEI U, FERRAZZIA E, RUGGERI C, PALAI N, DORDONI D, PERUGINOA G. Endometrial thickness and histological abnormalities in women on hormonal replacement therapy: a transvaginal ultrasound/hysteroscopy study. Ultrasound Obstet Gynaecol 2000;**15**:317–20.

18. SMITH-BINDAM R, KERLIKOWSKE K, FELDSTEIN V, SUBAK L, SCHEIDER J, SEGAL M, et al. Endovaginal ultrasound to exclude endometrial cancer and other endometrial abnormalities. JAMA 1998;**280**:1510–17.

19. GRANBERG S, YLOSTALO P, WIKLAND M, KARLSSON B. Endometrial sonographic and histological findings in women with and without hormonal replacement therapy suffering from postmenopausal bleeding. Maturitas 1997;**27**:35–40.

20. MELSON L, HILLARD T C. The management of abnormal bleeding on HRT: a proposed protocol and early audit of results. Br J Menopause Soc 2002;**4 Suppl 2**:23.

21. GULL B, KARLSSON B, MILSOM I, GRANBERG S. Can ultrasound replace dilation and curettage? A longitudinal evaluation of postmenopausal bleeding and transvaginal sonographic measurement of the endometrium as predictors of endometrial cancer. Am J Obstet Gynecol 2003;**188**:401–8.

22. Early Breast Cancer Collaborative Group. Tamoxifen for early breast cancer: an overview of the randomised trials. Lancet 1998;**351**:1451–67.

23. BERGMAN L, BEELEN M L, GALLEE M P, HOLLEMA H, BENRAADT J, VAN LEEUWEN F, and the Comprehensive Cancer Centres' ALERT Group. Risk and prognosis of endometrial cancer after tamoxifen for breast cancer. Lancet 2000;**356**:881–7.

24. TIMMERMAN D, DEPREST J, BOURNE T, VAN DEN BERGHE I, COLLINS W, VERGOTE I. A randomised trial on the use of ultrasonography or office hysteroscopy for endometrial assessment in postmenopausal patients with breast cancer who were treated with tamoxifen. Am J Obstet Gynecol 1998;**179**:62–70.

25. PERROT N, GUYNOT B, ANTOINE M. The effects of tamoxifen on the endometrium. Ultrasound Obstet Gynecol 1994;**4**:83–4.

26. GOLDSTEIN S R. Unusual ultrasonographic appearance of the uterus in patients receiving tamoxifen. Am J Obstet Gynecol 1994;**170**:447–51.

27. VOSSE M, RENARD F, COIBION M, NEVEN P, NOGARET J M, HERTENS D. Endometrial disorders in 406 breast cancer patients on tamoxifen: the case for less intensive monitoring. Eur J Obstet Gynecol 2002;**101**:58–63.

28. NEVEN P, VERNAEVE H. Guidelines for monitoring patients taking tamoxifen. Drug Saf 2000;**22**:1–11.

29. NEVEN P, LUNDE T, BENEDETTI-PANICI P, TIITINEN A, MARINESCU B, DEVILLIERS T, et al. A multicentre randomised trial to compare uterine safety of raloxifene with a continuous combined hormone replacement therapy containing oestradiol and norethisterone acetate. BJOG 2003;**110**:157–67.

30. LOBO R A, STANCZYK F Z. New physiology of hormonal contraceptives. Am J Obstet Gynecol 1994;**170**:1499–507.

31. LUDICKE F, JOHANNISSON E, HELMERHORST FM, CAMPANA A, FOIDART J. HEITHECKER R. Effect of a combined oral contraceptive containing 3 mg of drospirenone and 30 micrograms of ethinyl estradiol on the human endometrium. Fertil Steril 2001;**76**:102–7.

32. MACKAY EV, KHOO S K, ADAM R R. Contraception with a six-monthly injection of progestogen. Part 2. Effects on cervical mucus secretion and endocrine function. Aust N Z J Obstet Gynaecol 1971;**1**:156–63.

33. MOGHISSI K S, MARKS C. Effects of microdose progestogens on endogenous gonadotrophic and steroid hormones, cervical mucus properties, vaginal cytology and endometrium. Fertil Steril 1971;**22**:424–34.

34. KAEWRUDEE S, TANEEPANICHSKUL S. Norplant users with irregular bleeding. Ultrasonographic assessment and evaluation of serum concentrations of estradiol and progesterone. J Reprod Med 2000;**45**:983–6.

35. LAHTEENMAKI P, RAURAMO I, BACKMAN T. The levonorgestrel intra uterine system in contraception. Steroids 2000;**65**:693–7.

36. ZALEL Y, GAMZU R, SHULMAN A, ACHIRON R, SCHIFF G, LIDOR A. The progestative effect of the levonorgestrel-releasing intrauterine system: when does it manifest? Contraception 2003;**67**:473–6.

37. LEVINE D, GOSINK B B, JOHNSON L A. Change in endometrial thickness in postmenopausal women undergoing hormone replacement therapy. Radiology 1995;**197**:603–8.

38. VAN DEN BOSCH T, DONDERS G G, RIPHAGEN I, DEBOIS P, AMEYE L, DE BRABANTER J, et al. Ultrasonographic features of the endometrium and the ovaries in women on etonogestrel implant. Ultrasound Obstet Gynecol 2002;**20**:377–80.

39. VAN DEN BOSCH T, VAN SCHOUBROECK D, AMEYE L, DE BRABANTER J, VAN HUFFEL S, TIMMERMAN D. Ultrasound assessment of endometrial thickness and endometrial polyps in women on hormonal replacement therapy. Am J Obstet Gynecol 2003;**188**:1249–53.

40. OMODEI U, FERRAZZI E, RAMAZZOTTO F, BECORPI A, GRIMALDI E, SCARSELLI G, et al. Endometrial evaluation with transvaginal ultrasound during hormone therapy: a prospective multicenter study. Fertil Steril 2004;**81**:1632–7.

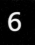

Diagnosis and management of adnexal masses

LIL VALENTIN

Introduction

Transvaginal ultrasound examination is an excellent tool for solving clinical problems in women with symptoms suggesting the presence of an adnexal mass. A gynaecologist experienced in ultrasound diagnosis using good-quality equipment is usually able to establish with confidence the nature of a pelvic tumour from its ultrasound image.[1–13] This helps to individualise and optimise the management of a woman with a palpable pelvic mass.

Ultrasound morphology for discrimination between benign and malignant adnexal masses

Subjective evaluation of the greyscale ultrasound image (that is, pattern recognition) for discrimination between benign and malignant tumours can be learned by performing gynaecological ultrasound examinations on a regular basis. However, the diagnostic accuracy of subjective assessment of tumour morphology increases with increasing experience.[3] An experienced ultrasound examiner can confidently discriminate between benign and malignant pelvic tumours in the adnexal region using pattern recognition. The reported sensitivity of pattern recognition varies between 88% and 100% and the reported specificity between 62% and 96%.[2,14–20] Pattern recognition has been shown to be superior to all other ultrasound methods (such as simple classification systems, scoring systems or mathematical models for calculating the risk of malignancy) for discrimination between benign and malignant extrauterine pelvic masses.[2,19] Adding Doppler ultrasound examination to subjective evaluation of the greyscale ultrasound image does not seem to yield much improvement in diagnostic precision,[2,14,15,18] but it may increase the confidence with which a correct diagnosis of benignity or malignancy is made.[2,14] A useful Doppler variable is the colour score (that is, the subjective evaluation of the colour content of the scan).[21,22] The higher the colour content of the tumour scan the greater the risk of malignancy.[21]

My personal experience is that the absence of solid components and absence of irregularities in an adnexal mass at ultrasound examination suggests benignity, whereas any irregularity – be it in the outline, the cyst wall or in the echogenicity of a tumour – suggests malignancy (Figure 6.1). Some cysts with an extremely large number of locules may be malignant even in the absence of irregularities or unequivocal solid components (Figure 6.2). In cystic tumours with solid components, the larger and more irregular the solid components are, the greater the risk of malignancy. In solid tumours, the more irregular the outline and echogenicity of the tumour, the greater the risk of malignancy. Using these simple rules, my detection rate (sensitivity) of malignant tumours including borderline tumours was 88% (21/24) with a specificity of 96% (143/149) in one series of patients undergoing preoperative ultrasound examination.[2] In a later series, the sensitivity and specificity were 83% (30/36) and 91% (91/100), respectively.[19] In these two series, all but two of the nine malignancies that were misdiagnosed as more likely to be benign than malignant were borderline tumours, the other two being a tubal cancer and a dysgerminoma.

Papillary projections – (solid projections into a cyst cavity from the cyst wall of more than 3 mm in height)[22] – are a strong sign of malignancy.[23–28] Papillary projections are particularly common in borderline tumours.[29] However, papillary projections are also quite common in ovarian adenofibromas (5/7; 70%), and may be seen in serous cystadenomas (4/11; 37%) and mucinous cystadenomas (3/14; 21%).[19] Papillary projections in benign tumours explain many false-positive ultrasound diagnoses of malignancy. The difficulty of correctly classifying tumours with papillary projections is illustrated in Figure 6.3.

Using ultrasound to characterise an adnexal mass

Some tumours – for example, endometriomas, dermoid cysts, hydro-pyo- and haematosalpinx, peritoneal pseudocysts, paraovarian cysts, haemorrhagic corpus luteum cysts, myomas, abscesses and ovarian fibromas, thecomas and Brenner tumours – may present with typical appearances at greyscale imaging.[4, 9, 10, 30–41] Therefore, an experienced ultrasound examiner can often make a correct specific diagnosis based on the greyscale ultrasound findings.[1, 14, 15, 37] Doppler assessment of intra-tumoral blood flow contributes little to the correct specific diagnosis of an adnexal mass.[1]

The ability to make a correct specific diagnosis in a series of pelvic tumours is highly dependent upon the types of tumour in the tumour series studied. My own series [1, 2, 19] contain a mixture of different types of tumour that in all likelihood is fairly representative of the types of pelvic tumour currently considered appropriate to treat with surgery.

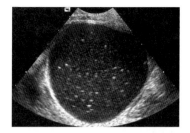

FIGURE 6.1a

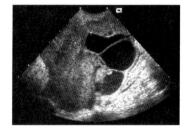

FIGURE 6.1b

a) Benign tumour characterised by the absence of solid components and absence of irregularities; **b)** malignant tumour characterised by irregular solid components

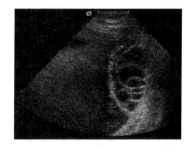

FIGURE 6.2 Malignant tumour (borderline) without solid components and without irregularities

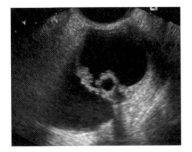

FIGURE 6.3 a

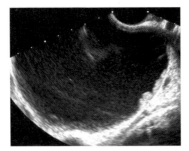

FIGURE 6.3 b

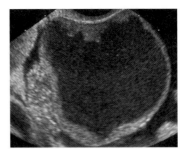

FIGURE 6.3 c

Papillary projections in: **a)** benign cyst; **b)** borderline tumour; **c)** primary invasive ovarian cancer. Note the overlapping ultrasound characteristics between benign and borderline tumours with papillary projections

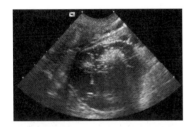

FIGURE 6.4 a

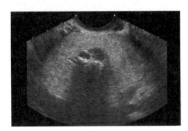

FIGURE 6.4 b

Dermoid cyst with typical: **a)** 'white ball' and long echogenic lines and bright prominent spots representing hair in fluid; **b)** shadowing

Ultrasound characteristics of dermoid cysts

Most dermoid cysts are easily recognised at greyscale imaging by their content of fat and hair.[35,39] The most characteristic ultrasound features of a dermoid cyst are the presence of:

▷ 'white ball' (corresponding to hair and sebum) filling part of or the whole tumour

▷ long, echogenic (white) lines and prominent echogenic dots in cyst fluid (corresponding to hair floating freely in fluid)

▷ shadowing.[35,39,42]

Shadowing often makes it difficult to measure accurately the size of dermoid cysts. Some may be impossible to detect, even when they are clearly palpable, because their echogenicity is similar to surrounding bowel. Confusion of dermoid cysts with endometrioma, mucinous cystadenoma, struma ovarii, serous cystadenoma, cystadenofibroma and Brenner tumour have been reported.[1,5,9,11,13,34,35] Typical ultrasound images of dermoid cysts are shown in Figure 6.4.

Ultrasound characteristics of endometriomas

Endometriomas are known to manifest typical 'ground glass' appearance at greyscale imaging.[9,30,34,43] One or more small 'solid foci' may be seen to protrude from the cyst wall into the cyst lumen, which probably represent blood clots or fibrin.[43] At greyscale imaging, endometriomas may be confused with dermoid cysts, abscesses, ovarian adenofibromas, ovarian fibromas, unspecified benign ovarian cysts, mucinous and serous cystadenomas and haemorrhagic cysts.[1,5,9,11–13,43] Typical ultrasound images of endometriomas are shown in Figure 6.5.

Ultrasound characteristics of haemorrhagic corpus luteum cysts

A haemorrhagic corpus luteum cyst typically contains web-like material.[30,43] Blood clots within the cyst sometimes appear bizarre and they may be misinterpreted as solid component within the cyst.[30,43] This explains why there is a risk of misclassifying a corpus luteum cyst as a malignant tumour. Colour Doppler ultrasound examination may help to discriminate between a clot which contains no detectable blood flow and a solid component with detectable colour Doppler signals. When in doubt, a follow-up examination 6–8 weeks later helps to establish the correct diagnosis. However, in my experience, some haemorrhagic cysts may take up to 4 months to regress. Typical ultrasound images of haemorrhagic corpus luteum cysts are shown in Figure 6.6.

Ultrasound characteristics of hydro-pyo-haematosalpinx

In most cases, a fluid-filled diseased tube is easily distinguishable from other types of cystic adnexal masses at greyscale ultrasound examination. The most characteristic ultrasound features are 'sausage' shape lesions and the presence of 'incomplete septa', (septa that are not seen to reach the opposite wall of the cystic structure). Mucosal folds protruding into the lumen of a swollen tube create a 'cog-wheel' appearance. However, if the tube is not swollen, the mucosal folds form a 'beads-on-a-string' appearance.[4,44] An inexperienced ultrasound examiner may confuse swollen mucosal folds in a tube with papillary projections and incorrectly suggest a diagnosis of malignancy. Typical ultrasound images of diseased tubes are shown in Figure 6.7.

Ultrasound characteristics of paraovarian cysts

Paraovarian cysts may arise from embryonic ducts and are usually located between the tube and the ovary.[30] They may be of mesothelial, mesonephric or paramesonephric origin.[45,46] On ultrasound examination some paraovarian cysts are seen to be clearly separated from a normal ovary. However, if no ovary is seen separately from the cyst, it may be impossible to distinguish an ovarian cyst from a paraovarian cyst.[30] The cyst fluid may be anechoic or echogenic.[30] Papillary projections and septa are fairly common.[47] Malignancy may develop in a paraovarian cyst, borderline tumours probably being more common than invasive cancers. Malignancy is more common in paraovarian cysts greater than 5 cm with papillary projections than in other types of paraovarian cysts.[30,47,48,49] A typical ultrasound image of a paraovarian cyst is shown in Figure 6.8.

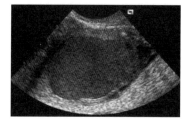

FIGURE 6.5 a

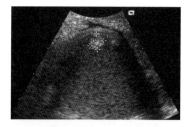

FIGURE 6.5 b

Endometrioma with typical: **a)** homogenously echogenic cyst fluid representing chocolate sauce-like old blood; **b)** 'wall nodularity' (callipers)

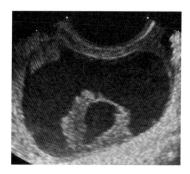

FIGURE 6.6 a

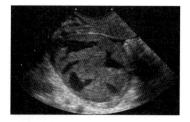

FIGURE 6.6 b

Haemorrhagic corpus luteum with bizarre blood clots **a)** and **b)**

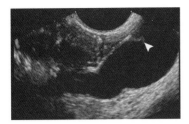

FIGURE 6.7a

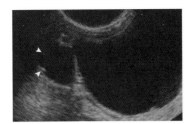

FIGURE 6.7b

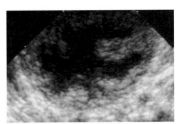

FIGURE 6.7c

Diseased tube with typical: **a)** sausage shape and small mucosal folds (arrow); **b)** beads on a string (arrows); **c)** cogwheel appearance: this appearance is explained by swollen mucosal folds protruding in to the fluid filled lumen of an inflamed tube

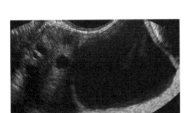

FIGURE 6.8 Paraovarian cyst close to but separated from a normal ovary

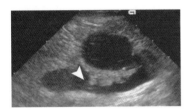

FIGURE 6.9 Peritoneal pseudocyst; note the fimbriae of the tube (arrow) protruding into the triangular cystic space (the peritoneal pseudocyst)

Ultrasound characteristics of peritoneal pseudocysts

Peritoneal pseudocysts are fluid collections among adhesions occurring after an inflammatory process in the peritoneal cavity or after an operation. The typical ultrasound morphology of a peritoneal pseudocyst is that of a cystic mass following the contours of the pelvis – even though pseudocysts may also be oval or round – and with a deformed ovary suspended among adhesions centrally or peripherally in the cyst. The cyst fluid may be anechoic or echoic and the cyst may contain both septa and papillary projections.[30,50–54] A typical ultrasound image of a peritoneal pseudocyst is shown in Figure 6.9.

Ultrasound characteristics of ovarian fibromas, fibrothecomas, thecofibromas, thecomas, Brenner and other benign solid ovarian tumours

Fibromas and fibrothecomas usually yield an echo pattern indistinguishable from that of pedunculated myomas (that is, they are solid, round or oval tumours with a smooth outline and a regular 'stripy' echogenicity). Different types of solid benign ovarian tumour, such as fibroma, thecoma, fibrothecoma and Brenner tumour, may manifest similar echogenicity at greyscale sonography.[30,33,40,41] Guerriero *et al.*[9] reported confusion of ovarian endometrioma and fibroma at greyscale sonography and such confusion also occurred in one of my own series.[1] Typical ultrasound images of benign solid pelvic lesions are shown in Figure 6.10.

Ultrasound characteristics of tubo-ovarian abscess

The ultrasound morphology of a tubo-ovarian abscess may be that of a unilocular cystic structure or that of complex multicystic structure with thick walls and thick septae, filled with homogenously echogenic material ('ground glass' appearance). Given the complex and varied echogenicity of tubo-ovarian abscesses, it is not surprising that they may be confused with a variety of other conditions, such as endometriomas or malignancies.[1,4,55,56] It is not always possible to distinguish a tubo-ovarian abscess from a pelvic abscess of other origin, such as a periappendiceal or diverticular abscess.[4] Knowledge of the patient's history and clinical findings is a prerequisite for making a correct diagnosis. Detailed description of the ultrasound morphology of different types of pelvic inflammatory disease are available elsewhere.[44,57,58]

Ultrasound characteristics of ovarian serous cystadenoma, mucinous cystadenoma and adenofibroma

In my experience, the greyscale ultrasound images of serous cyst(aden)oma, mucinous cyst(aden)oma and adenofibroma manifest overlapping characteristics. Overlapping characteristics have also been found by others.[33] However, Fleischer et al.,[7] Buy et al.[37] and Guerriero et al.[8] found it possible to diagnose serous and mucinous cyst(aden)omas with greyscale sonography. Buy et al.[37] considered the characteristic features of a serous cystadenoma to be 'a unilocular or bilocular cystic mass with homogenous water echogenicity, thin regular wall, thin regular septum (when present) and no vegetations', and those of a mucinous cystadenoma to be 'a multilocular cyst containing fluid of different echogenicities, with regular wall and septa and no vegetations'. Using these criteria, they diagnosed serous cystadenomas with a sensitivity of 70% and a specificity of 98% and mucinous cystadenomas with a sensitivity of 50% and a specificity of 96%. Fleisher et al.[7] and Guerriero et al.[8] found the sensitivity of greyscale imaging for diagnosing serous cystadenoma to be 75% and 78%, respectively, and the specificity to be 75% and 96%, respectively. The sensitivity and specificity of greyscale imaging for diagnosing mucinous cystadenomas were reported by Fleischer et al.[7] to be 95% and 99%, respectively.

Incidentally detected pelvic tumours

Many adnexal masses that would almost certainly have remained undetected before the ultrasound era are now found incidentally at transvaginal ultrasound examination of women without symptoms of an adnexal tumour. The natural history of incidentally detected pelvic masses with benign ultrasound morphology is not known. We do not know how often such tumours will cause problems in the future (such as torsion, pain, infertility), if there is a risk of some of them becoming malignant or the magnitude of any such a risk.

In one study by Caspi et al.,[59] 86 asymptomatic women (72 premenopausal and 14 postmenopausal) with an adnexal mass with sono-

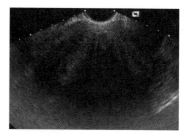

FIGURE 6.10 a

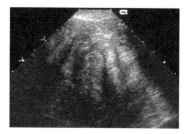

FIGURE 6.10 b

Benign, solid ovarian tumour may be confused with a pedunculated uterine myoma if no connection is seen between the pedunculated myoma and the uterus: **a)** ovarian fibroma; **b)** uterine leiomyoma. At ultrasound examination, an ovarian fibroma may appear denser than a uterine leiomyoma (as in this case) but it may also have an ultrasound appearance that is indistinguishable from that of a uterine leiomyoma

graphic morphology compatible with a dermoid cyst not larger than 6 cm were managed expectantly and followed up for a mean of 3 years. Torsion or other complications did not occur. Twenty-eight women who desired pregnancy became pregnant and had one or more uncomplicated pregnancies during follow-up. Growth rate of the dermoid cysts was low.

Hundreds of postmenopausal women with adnexal cysts – most of the cysts being simple cysts ≤5 cm in diameter – have been managed expectantly for up to 9 years without any adverse effects being noted.[60–68] There are also other data supporting that it is probably safe to manage this type of cyst expectantly.[69,70]

It is by no means obvious that adnexal masses with benign ultrasound morphology incidentally detected at ultrasound examination should be surgically removed. Surgery is associated with risks. The intraoperative and postoperative complication rate associated with adnexal surgery is reported to vary between 0.3% and 8%.[71–76] The mortality associated with adnexal surgery is difficult to estimate but mortality associated with gynaecological laparoscopic procedures may be 1/25 000.[77] Long-term complications after gynaecological surgery include adhesion formation,[78] which, in turn, may cause infertility or bowel obstruction.[78–80] I have found no published information on the incidence of small bowel obstruction after adnexal surgery but one may expect one death because of postoperative small bowel obstruction per 625 hysterectomies (my own calculations made on the basis of information from Al-Took *et al.*[78] and Fevang *et al.*[81]). To determine whether surgical removal of adnexal masses with benign ultrasound morphology incidentally detected at ultrasound examination in asymptomatic women is beneficial, it would be necessary to conduct a randomised controlled trial comparing surgery with expectant management. However, it would probably be difficult to conduct such a trial. Experts in gynaecological ultrasound would have to perform all ultrasound examinations, because confusion of benign and malignant tumours resulting in inclusion of malignancies in the trial would be unacceptable. Moreover, the primary endpoint of such a trial is not obvious, follow-up time would need to be very long, the trial would need to be very large and individual preferences of women might make it difficult to recruit patients.

My personal opinion is that one should not examine asymptomatic women with ultrasound – or with gynaecological palpation – because there is no evidence that detection of pelvic masses that do not cause symptoms is beneficial. This is true even of malignant masses. We have to await the results of randomised trials evaluating ultrasound screening for ovarian cancer before we will know if detection of ovarian cancer at an asymptomatic stage improves the prognosis.[82]

Acknowledgements

The studies from the author's institution were supported by grants from the Malmö General Hospital Cancer Foundation, funds administered by the Malmö Health Care Administration, the Faculty of Medicine of Lund University, the Anna-Lisa och Sven-Erik Lundgren Foundation for Medical Research, the Ingabritt and Arne Lundberg Research Foundation, two governmental grants (Landstingsfinansierad regional forskning, Region Skåne and ALF-medel) and the Swedish Medical Research Council (grant nos. B96-17X-11605-01A, K98-17X-11605-03A, K2001-72X-11605-06A AND K2002-72X-11605-07B).

REFERENCES

1. VALENTIN L. Pattern recognition of pelvic masses by gray-scale ultrasound imaging: the contribution of Doppler ultrasound. *Ultrasound Obstet Gynecol* 1999; **15**:338–47.

2. VALENTIN L. Prospective cross-validation of Doppler ultrasound examination and gray-scale ultrasound imaging for discrimination of benign and malignant pelvic masses. *Ultrasound Obstet Gynecol* 1999; **14**:273–83.

3. TIMMERMAN D, SCHWARZLER P, COLLINS W P, CLAERHOUT F, COENEN M, AMANT F, *et al.* Subjective assessment of adnexal masses with the use of ultrasonography: an analysis of interobserver variability and experience. *Ultrasound Obstet Gynecol* 1999; **13**:11–16.

4. PATTEN R M. The Fallopian tube and pelvic inflammatory disease. In: Nyberg D A, Hill L M, Böhm-Velez M, Mendelson E B, editors. *Transvaginal Ultrasound.* St Louis: Mosby Year Book; 1992. p. 209–21.

5. KURJAK A, KUPESIC S. Scoring system for prediction of ovarian endometriosis based on transvaginal color Doppler sonography. *Fertil Steril* 1994; **62**:81–8.

6. BENACERRAF B R, FINKLER N J, WOJCIECHOWSKI C, KNAPP R C. Sonographic accuracy in the diagnosis of ovarian masses. *J Reprod Med* 1990; **35**:491–5.

7. FLEISHER A C, JAMES A E, MILLIS J B, JULIAN C. Differential diagnosis of pelvic masses by grey scale sonography. *Am J Radiol* 1978; **131**:469–76.

8. GUERRIERO S, MALLARINI G, AJOSSA S, RISALVATO A, SATTA R, MAIS V, *et al.* Transvaginal ultrasound and computed tomography combined with clinical parameters and CA-125 determinations in the differential diagnosis of persistent ovarian cysts in premenopausal women. *Ultrasound Obstet Gynecol* 1997; **9**:339–43.

9. GUERRIERO S, MAIS V, AJOSSA S, PAOLETTI A M, ANGIOLUCCI M, LABATE F, *et al.* The role of endovaginal ultrasound in differentiating endometriomas from other ovarian cysts. *Clin Exp Obstet Gynecol* 1995; **22**:20–2.

10. KIM J S, WOO S K, SUH S J, MORETTIN L B. Sonographic diagnosis of paraovarian cysts: value of detecting a separate ipsilateral ovary. *Am J Radiol* 1995; **164**:1441–4.

11. MAIS V, GUERRIERO S, AJOSSA S, ANGIOLUCCI M, PAOLETTI A M, MELIS G B. Transvaginal sonography in the diagnosis of cystic teratoma. *Obstet Gynecol* 1995; **85**:48–52.

12. GUERRIERO S, MAIS V, AJOSSA S, PAOLETTI A M, ANGIOLUCCI M, MELIS G B. Transvaginal ultrasonography combined with Ca-125 plasma levels in the diagnosis of endometrioma. *Fertil Steril* 1996; **65**:293–8.

13. MAIS V, GUERRIERO S, AJOSSA S, ANGIOLUCCI M, PAOLETTI A M, MELIS G B. The efficiency of transvaginal ultrasonography in the diagnosis of endometrioma. *Fertil Steril* 1993; **60**:776–80.

14. JAIN K A. Prospective evaluation of adnexal masses with endovaginal grey-scale and duplex and color Doppler US: correlation with pathologic findings. *Radiology* 1994; **191**:63–7.

15. BUY J N, GHOSSAIN M A, HUGOL D, HASSEN K, SCIOT C, TRUC J B, *et al.* Characterization of adnexal masses: combination of color Doppler and conventional sonography compared with spectral Doppler analysis alone and conventional sonography alone. *Am J Roentgenol* 1996; **166**:385–93.

16. LEVINE D, FELDSTEIN V A, BABCOOK C J, FILLY R A. Sonography of ovarian masses: poor sensitivity of resistive index for identifying malignant lesions. *Am J Roentgenol* 1994; **162**:1355–9.

17. SALEM S, WHITE LM, LAI J. Doppler sonography of adnexal masses: the predictive value of the pulsatility index in benign and malignant disease. *Am J Roentgenol* 1994; **163**: 1147–50.

18. STEIN S M, LAIFER-NARIN S, JOHNSON M B, ROMAN LD, MUDERSPACH LI, TYSZKA J M, et al. Differentiation of benign and malignant adnexal masses: relative value of grey-scale, color Doppler, and spectral Doppler sonography. *Am J Roentgenol* 1995; **164**: 381–6.

19. VALENTIN L, HAGEN B, TINGULSTAD S, EIK-NES S. Comparison of 'pattern recognition' and logistic regression models for discrimination between benign and malignant pelvic masses. A prospective cross-validation. *Ultrasound Obstet Gynecol* 2001; **18**: 357–65.

20. GUERRIERO S, AJOSSA S, RISALVATO A, LAI M P, MAIS V, ANGIOLUCCI M, MELIS G B. Diagnosis of adnexal malignancies by using color Doppler energy imaging as a secondary test in persistent masses. *Ultrasound Obstet Gynecol* 1998; **11**: 277–82.

21. VALENTIN L. Gray scale sonography, subjective evaluation of the color Doppler image and measurement of blood flow velocity for distinguishing benign and malignant tumors of suspected adnexal origin. *Eur J Obstet Gynecol Reprod Biol* 1997; **72**: 63–72.

22. TIMMERMAN D, VALENTIN L, BOURNE TH, COLLINS W P, VERRELST H, VERGOTE I. Terms, definitions and measurements to describe the sonographic features of adnexal tumors: a consensus opinion from the International Ovarian Tumor Analysis (IOTA) group. *Ultrasound Obstet Gynecol* 2000; **16**: 500–5.

23. GRANBERG S, WIKLAND M, JANSSON I. Macroscopic characterization of ovarian tumors and the relation to the histological diagnosis: criteria to be used for ultrasound evaluation. *Gynecol Oncol* 1989; **35**: 139–44.

24. GRANBERG S, NORSTROM A, WIKLAND M. Tumors in the lower pelvis as imaged by vaginal sonography. *Gynecol Oncol* 1990; **37**: 224–9.

25. TAILOR A, JURKOVIC D, BOURNE TH, COLLINS W P, CAMPBELL S. Sonographic prediction of malignancy in adnexal masses using multivariate logistic regression analysis. *Ultrasound Obstet Gynecol* 1997; **10**: 41–7.

26. TIMMERMAN D, BOURNE TH, TAILOR A, COLLINS W P, VERRELST H, VANDENBERGHE K, et al. A comparison of methods for preoperative discrimination between malignant and benign adnexal masses: the development of a new logistic regression model. *Am J Obstet Gynecol* 1999; **181**: 57–65.

27. MARRET H, ECOCHARD R, GIRAUDEAU B, GOLFIER F, RAUDRANT D, LANSAC J. Color Doppler energy prediction of malignancy in adnexal masses using logistic regression models. *Ultrasound Obstet Gynecol* 2002; **20**: 597–604.

28. ALCAZAR J L, MERCE LT, LAPARTE C, JURADO M, LOPEZ-GARCIA G. A new scoring system to differentiate benign from malignant adnexal masses. *Am J Obstet Gynecol* 2003; **188**: 685–92.

29. EXACOUSTOS C, ROMANINI ME, RINALDO D, AMOROSO C, SZABOLCS B, ZUPI E, et al. Preoperative sonographic features of borderline ovarian tumors. *Ultrasound Obstet Gynecol* 2005; **25**: 50–9.

30. GRANT E G. Benign conditions of the ovary. In: Nyberg D A, Hill LM, Böhm-Velez M, Mendelson EB, editors. *Transvaginal Ultrasound*. St Louis, MO: Mosby Year Book; 1992. p. 187–208.

31. FLEISCHER A C, KEPPLE D M. Benign conditions of the uterus, cervix, and endometrium. In: Nyberg D A, Hill LM, Böhm-Velez M, Mendelson EB, editors. *Transvaginal Ultrasound*. St Louis, MO: Mosby Year Book; 1992. p. 21–41.

32. BAZOT M, GHOSSAIN M A, BUY J N, DELIGNE L, HUGOL D, TRUC J B, et al. Fibrothecomas of the ovary: CT and US findings. *J Comput Assist Tomogr* 1993; **17**: 754–9.

33. CARTER J R, CARSON LF, TWIGGS LB. Gynecologic oncology. In: Nyberg D A, Hill LM, Böhm-Velez M, Mendelson EB, editors. *Transvaginal Ultrasound*. St Louis, MO: Mosby Year Book; 1992. p. 241–65.

34. KUPFER M C, SCHWIMER S R, LEBOVIC J. Transvaginal sonographic appearance of endometriomata: spectrum of findings. *J Ultrasound Med* 1992; **11**: 129–33.

35. CASPI B, APPELMAN Z, RABINERSON D, ELCHALAL U, ZALEL Y, KATZ Z. Pathognomonic echo patterns of benign cystic teratomas of the ovary: classification, incidence and accuracy rate of sonographic diagnosis. *Ultrasound Obstet Gynecol* 1996; **7**: 275–9.

36. SOHAEY R, GARDNER TL, WOODWARD PJ, PETERSON C M. Sonographic diagnosis of peritoneal inclusion cysts. *J Ultrasound Med* 1995; **14**: 913–17.

37. BUY J N, GHOSSAIN M A, SCIOT C, BAZOT M, GUINET C, PREVOT S, et al. Epithelial tumours of the ovary: CT findings and correlation with US. *Radiology* 1991; **178**: 811–18.

38. JAIN K A, FRIEDMAN D L, PETTINGER T W, ALAGAPPAN R, JEFFREY R B Jr, SOMMER F G. Adnexal masses: comparison of specificity of endovaginal US and pelvic MR imaging. *Radiology* 1993; **186**: 697–704.

39. COHEN L, SABBAGHA R. Echo patterns of benign cystic teratomas by transvaginal ultrasound. *Ultrasound Obstet Gynecol* 1993; **3**: 120–3.

40. ATHEY P A, MALONE R S. Sonography of ovarian fibromas/thecomas. *J Ultrasound Med* 1987; **6**: 431–6.

41. ATHEY P A, SIEGEL M F. Sonographic features of Brenner tumour of the ovary. *J Ultrasound Med* 1987; **6**: 367–72.

42. BRONSHTEIN M, YOFFE N, BRANDES J M, BLUMENFELD Z. Hair as a sonographic marker of ovarian teratomas: improved identification using transvaginal sonography and simulation model. *J Clin Ultrasound* 1991; **19**: 351–5.

43. PATEL M D, FELDSTEIN V A, CHEN D C, LIPSON S D, FILLY R A. Endometriomas: diagnostic performance of US. *Radiology* 1999; **210**: 739–45.

44. TIMOR-TRITSCH I E, LERNER J P, MONTEAGUDO A, MURPHY K E, HELLER D S. Transvaginal sonographic markers of tubal inflammatory disease. *Ultrasound Obstet Gynecol* 1998; **12**: 56–66.

45. GENADRY R, PARMLEY T, WOODRUFF J D. The origin and clinical behavior of the paraovarian tumor. *Am J Obstet Gynecol* 1977; **129**: 873–80.

46. GARDNER G H, GREENE R R, PECKHAM B M. Normal and cystic structures of the broad ligament. *Am J Obstet Gynecol* 1948; **55**: 917–39.

47. KORBIN C D, BROWN D L, WELCH W R. Paraovarian cystadenomas and cystadenofibromas: sonographic characteristics in 14 cases. *Radiology* 1998; **208**: 459–62.

48. STEIN A L, KOONINGS P P, SCHLAERTH J B, GRIMES D A, D'ABLAING G 3rd. Relative frequency of malignant paraovarian tumors: should paraovarian tumors be aspirated? *Obstet Gynecol* 1990; **75**: 1029–31.

49. CLARK J E, WOOD H, JAFFURS W J, FABRO S. Endometrioid-type cystadenocarcinoma arising in the mesosalpinx. *Obstet Gynecol* 1979; **54**: 656–8.

50. HOFFER F A, KOZAKEWICH H, COLODNY A, GOLDSTEIN D P. Peritoneal inclusion cysts: ovarian fluid in peritoneal adhesions. *Radiology* 1988; **169**: 189–91.

51. McFADDEN D E, CLEMENT P B. Peritoneal inclusion cysts with mural mesothelial proliferation. A clinicopathological analysis of six cases. *Am J Surg Pathol* 1986; **10**: 844–54.

52. KIM J S, LEE H J, WOO S K, LEE T S. Peritoneal inclusion cysts and their relationship to the ovaries: evaluation with Sonography. *Radiology* 1997; **204**: 481–4.

53. JAIN K A. Imaging of peritoneal inclusion cysts. *AJR Am J Roentgenol* 2000; **174**: 1559–63.

54. SAVELLI L, DE IACO P, GHI T, BOVICELLI L, ROSATI F, CACCIATORE B. Transvaginal sonographic appearance of peritoneal pseudocysts. *Ultrasound Obstet Gynecol* 2004; **23**: 284–8.

55. HATA K, HATA T, AOKI S, TAKAMIYA O, KITAO M. Ultrasonographic evaluation of pelvic inflammatory disease. *Nippon Sanka Fujinka Gakkai Zasshi* 1989; **41**: 895–8.

56. VARRAS M, POLYZOS D, PEROULI E, NOTI P, PANTAZIS I, AKRIVIS C. Tubo-ovarian abscesses: spectrum of sonographic findings with surgical and pathological correlations. *Clin Exp Obstet Gynecol* 2003; **30**: 117–21.

57. MOLANDER P, SJOBERG J, PAAVONEN J, CACCIATORE B. Transvaginal power Doppler findings in laparoscopically proven acute pelvic inflammatory disease. *Ultrasound Obstet Gynecol* 2001; **17**: 233–8.

58. TAIPALE P, TARJANNE H, YLOSTALO P. Transvaginal sonography in suspected pelvic inflammatory disease. *Ultrasound Obstet Gynecol* 1995; **6**: 430–4.

59. CASPI B, APPELMAN Z, RABINERSON D, ZALEL Y, TULANDI T, SHOHAM Z. The growth pattern of ovarian dermoid cysts: a prospective study in premenopausal and postmenopausal women. *Fertil Steril* 1997; **68**: 501–5.

60. LEVINE D, GOSINK B B, WOLF S I, FELDESMAN M R, PRETORIUS D H. Simple adnexal cyst: the natural history in postmenopausal women. *Radiology* 1992; **184**: 653–9.

61. KROON E, ANDOLF E. Diagnosis and follow-up of simple ovarian cysts detected by ultrasound in postmenopausal women. *Obstet Gynecol* 1995; **85**: 211–4.

62. ANDOLF E, JORGENSEN C. Simple adnexal cysts diagnosed by ultrasound in postmenopausal women. *J Clin Ultrasound* 1988; **16**: 301–3.

63. AUBERT J M, ROMBAUT C, ARGACHA P, ROMERO F, LEIRA J, GOMEZ-BOLEA F. Simple adnexal cysts in postmenopausal women: conservative management. *Maturitas* 1998; **30**: 51–4.

64. GOLDSTEIN S R, SUBRAMANYAM B, SNYDER J R, BELLER U, RAGHAVENDRA B N, BECKMAN E M. The postmenopausal cystic adnexal mass: the potential role of ultrasound in conservative management. *Obstet Gynecol* 1989; **73**: 8–10.

65. AUSLENDER R, ATLAS I, LISSAK A, BORNSTEIN J, ATAD J, ABRAMOVICI H. Follow-up of small, postmenopausal ovarian cysts using vaginal ultrasound and CA-125 antigen. *J Clin Ultrasound* 1996; **24**: 175–8.

66. BAILEY C L, UELAND F R, LAND G L, DePRIEST P D, GALLION H H, KRYSCIO R J, *et al*. The malignant potential of small cystic ovarian tumors in women over 50 years of age. *Gynecol Oncol* 1998; **69**: 3–7.

67. CONWAY C, ZALUD I, DILENA M, MAULIK D, SCHULMAN H, HALEY J, *et al*. Simple cysts in the postmenopausal patient: detection and management. *J Ultrasound Med* 1998; **17**: 369–72.

68. VALENTIN L, AKRAWI D. The natural history of adnexal cysts incidentally detected at transvaginal ultrasound examination in postmenopausal women. *Ultrasound Obstet Gynecol* 2002; **20**: 174–80.

69. VALENTIN L, SKOOG L, EPSTEIN E. Frequency and type of adnexal lesions in autopsy material from postmenopausal women: ultrasound study with histological correlation. *Ultrasound Obstet Gynecol* 2003; **22**: 284–9.

70. CRAYFORD T J, CAMPBELL S, BOURNE T H, RAWSON H J, COLLINS W P. Benign ovarian cysts and ovarian cancer: a cohort study with implications for screening. *Lancet* 2000; **355**: 1060–3.

71. MINELLI L. Ovarian cysts. *Eur J Obstet Gynecol Reprod Biol* 1996; **65**: 81–9.

72. CANIS M, MAGE G, POULY J L, WATTIEZ A, MANHES H, BRUHAT M A. Laparoscopic diagnosis of adnexal cystic masses: a 12-year experience with long-term follow-up. *Obstet Gynecol* 1994; **83**: 707–12.

73. YUEN PM, ROGERS MS. Laparoscopic management of ovarian masses: the initial experience and learning curve. *Aust N Z J Obstet Gynaecol* 1994;**34**:191–4.

74. REICH H, JOHNS DA, DAVIS G, DIAMOND MP. Laparoscopic oophorectomy. *J Reprod Med* 1993;**38**:497–501.

75. DANIELL JF, KURTZ BR, LEE JY. Laparoscopic oophorectomy: comparative study of ligatures, bipolar coagulation, and automatic stapling devices. *Obstet Gynecol* 1992;**80**:325–28.

76. MAGE G, WATTIEZ A, CANIS M, MANHES H, POULY JL, BRUHAT MA. [Contribution of celioscopy in the early diagnosis of ovarian cancers.] *Ann Chir* 1991;**45**:525–8.

77. CHAPRON C, QUERLEU D, BRUHAT MA, MADELENAT P, FERNANDEZ H, PIERRE F, *et al.* Surgical complications of diagnostic and operative gynaecological laparoscopy: a series of 29,966 cases. *Hum Reprod* 1998;**13**:867–72.

78. AL-TOOK S, PLATT R, TULANDI T. Adhesion-related small-bowel obstruction after gynecologic operations. *Am J Obstet Gynecol* 1999;**180**:313–15.

79. TOAFF R, TOAFF ME, PEYSER MR. Infertility following wedge resection of the ovaries. *Am J Obstet Gynecol* 1976;**124**:92–6.

80. WEINSTEIN D, POLISHUK WZ. The role of wedge resection of the ovary as a cause for mechanical sterility. *Surg Gynecol Obstet* 1975;**141**:417–18.

81. FEVANG BT, FEVANG J, STANGELAND L, SOREIDE O, SVANES K, VISTE A. Complications and death after surgical treatment of small bowel obstruction: a 35-year institutional experience. *Ann Surg* 2000;**231**:529–37.

82. LEWIS S, MENON U. Screening for ovarian cancer. *Expert Rev Anticancer Ther* 2003;**3**:55–62.

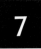

Ultrasound assessment of women with pelvic pain

LIL VALENTIN

Introduction

Pelvic pain is a common gynaecological complaint and ultrasound examination is often performed in an attempt to identify its cause. The ultrasound scan, however, should not be used as a substitute for clinical history and examination. The best use of ultrasound is to confirm or exclude a diagnosis that we suspect on the basis of clinical data.[1] There are several painful conditions that can be seen and diagnosed with ultrasound. This is particularly true of acute painful conditions. However, chronic pelvic pain is a different clinical entity. There is no accepted definition of chronic pelvic pain and there is much controversy about what conditions may explain it.[2] Some conditions that have been suggested to cause chronic pelvic pain, such as neuralgia or irritable bowel syndrome, cannot be visualised by transvaginal ultrasound.

Acute pelvic pain

Adnexal cysts

Adnexal cysts are common incidental ultrasound findings both in pre- and postmenopausal asymptomatic women.[3-5] Cysts larger than 25 mm are found at ultrasound examination in 7% of asymptomatic premenopausal women[5] and cysts larger than 15 mm are found in about 7% of postmenopausal women.[6,7] Thus, if we detect a cyst at ultrasound examination in a woman with pelvic pain, the cyst is not necessarily the cause of her pain. If we can provoke her pain or make it worse by pushing on the cyst with the vaginal ultrasound probe or with our outer free hand, then there is likely to be a relationship between the cyst and the pain. It is not always easy to determine from which organ the pain originates. Peritoneal irritation may make all organs tender. Patient aggravation may also make it difficult to determine which organ causes pain.

Haemorrhagic corpus luteum cysts are common causes of acute pelvic pain in women of fertile age. At ultrasound examination, corpus luteum cysts are characterised by spiderweb-like contents but they may also contain bizarre-looking blood clots.[8] This explains why corpus luteum cysts may sometimes be confused with a malignancy. On Doppler ultrasound examination a corpus luteum cyst is usually richly vascularised. Part of or the whole of its circumference is coloured, and spectral Doppler examination shows high blood flow velocities both in systole and diastole.[9] Typical ultrasound images of corpus luteum cysts are shown in Chapter 6. A haemorrhagic corpus luteum cyst disappears spontaneously and women are often relieved when they are told that their pain is explained by a harmless condition that will resolve spontaneously.

Endometriomas may cause pelvic pain but they are also quite common incidental ultrasound findings. An endometrioma has a thick wall and contains homogenously echogenic material corresponding to its chocolate sauce-like contents.[8] Typical ultrasound images of endometriomas are shown in Chapter 6.

Peritoneal pseudocysts, defined as fluid entrapped between adhesions in the pelvis, often contain an ovary suspended amid the adhesions either in the centre of the cyst or at its periphery.[8, 10, 11] A peritoneal cyst may increase in size at or after ovulation, probably because fluid transudates from the follicle or from the corpus luteum into the pseudocyst. A sudden increase in the amount of fluid in the pseudocyst is probably quite painful. In most cases, acute pain caused by a sudden transudation of fluid resolves spontaneously as the amount of fluid decreases. An ultrasound image of a haemorrhagic corpus luteum cyst entrapped in a peritoneal pseudocyst is shown in Figure 7.1. As in the case of haemorrhagic corpus luteum cysts, women are often relieved when they receive an explanation for their pain and are informed that the condition is not serious and will disappear without intervention. A large peritoneal cyst may cause pain − or at least discomfort − even if there is no sudden transudation of fluid into it. Cyst puncture may be suitable treatment for peritoneal cysts causing pain.[12, 13]

Adnexal torsion

A serious condition that may be more or less painful is torsion of the adnexa. Torsion usually occurs in adnexa containing a lesion, such as an ovarian cyst or a hydrosalpinx, but it may also occur in normal adnexa, especially in prepubertal girls.[14] Although there are some ultrasound findings suggestive of adnexal torsion, this diagnosis cannot be confirmed or excluded with complete certainty by ultrasound examination, even when combined with Doppler assessment of adnexal blood supply.

In adnexal torsion, various degrees of arterial, venous and lymphatic occlusion occur. This causes massive congestion and oedema and later haemorrhagic infarction may occur. This pathophysiology explains the ultrasound findings in cases of adnexal torsion.

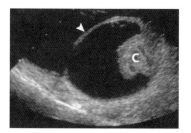

FIGURE 7.1 Haemorrhagic corpus luteum cyst (arrow) entrapped in a peritoneal pseudocyst. The corpus luteum cyst contains a blood clot (c)

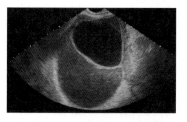

FIGURE 7.2a

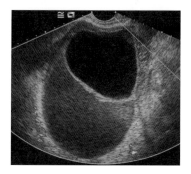

FIGURE 7.2b

Twisted ovarian cyst: **a)** the ultrasound findings are quite inconspicuous: the only ultrasound finding suggesting torsion is the thick wall of the cyst reflecting that it is swollen because of torsion; **b)** no colour (=blood flow) could be detected at colour Doppler examination of this twisted cyst

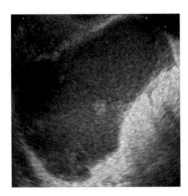

FIGURE 7.3 a

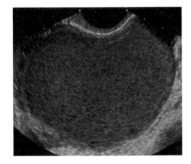

FIGURE 7.3 b

An abscess may be confused with an endometrioma because pus and old chocolate sauce-like blood have similar echogenicity at ultrasound examination: **a)** unilocular thick-walled abscess containing homogenously echogenic material corresponding to pus; **b)** endometrioma

If a normal ovary is involved in the torsion, the oedema causes enlargement of the ovary and the ovary usually loses its oval shape and becomes round or globular. Another feature reported to be typical of ovarian torsion, especially in adolescent girls, is the presence of several round small cysts up to 25 mm in diameter at the periphery of the enlarged ovary.[15] Thus, torsion of a normal ovary in an adolescent girl is characterised by unilateral ovarian enlargement with peripheral, dilated cysts.[15]

If torsion occurs in a hyperstimulated ovary after ovulation induction, the main ultrasound characteristic is a swollen ovarian parenchyma, which makes the diseased ovary look distinctly different from the contralateral one.[15]

If torsion occurs in an ovarian cyst or a hydrosalpinx, the wall, mucosal folds and septa of the lesion look swollen at ultrasound examination.[15–17] If haemorrhagic infarction has occurred, echogenic fluid may be seen in cystic spaces in the tumour. Some fluid, often echogenic and corresponding to blood, in the pouch of Douglas is also a common finding.[15] It may be difficult to detect ultrasound signs of torsion in an ovary containing a dermoid cyst, because of the shadowing typical of these tumours.

Doppler ultrasound examination does not seem to play a decisive role in the diagnosis of adnexal torsion. Colour Doppler signals can be detected either peripherally or centrally in a substantial proportion of twisted adnexa.[18] Doppler findings probably parallel the vascular changes. Persistent arterial flow is compatible with less complete stages of torsion. Therefore, detection of flow using the Doppler technique does not exclude adnexal torsion.

It is important to bear in mind that ultrasound findings may be quite inconspicuous in cases of adnexal torsion (Figure 7.2). Symptoms and clinical findings are at least as important as an ultrasound examination when making a diagnosis of adnexal torsion.

Pelvic inflammatory disease

The ultrasound image of a tubo-ovarian abscess is easily confused with other pelvic tumours and *vice versa*.[19] An abscess may be a unilocular thick-walled cyst containing homogenously echogenic material corresponding to pus, in which case it may be confused with an endometrioma (Figure 7.3). An abscess may also be a multilocular solid tumour, which may be confused with an ovarian cancer (Figure 7.4). However, in some cases of inflammatory process in the tube and adjacent adnexa, it is possible to discern the features of an inflamed tube and so to make a correct diagnosis of pelvic inflammatory disease (Figure 7.5).

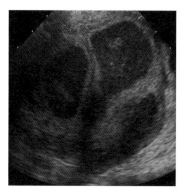

FIGURE 7.4 a

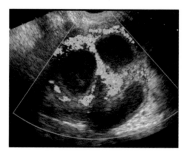

FIGURE 7.4 b

A multilocular solid abscess may easily be confused with ovarian cancer, especially because both inflammatory processes and ovarian malignancies are well-vascularised and contain a large amount of colour Doppler signals at colour Doppler examination: **a)** greyscale ultrasound image; **b)** colour Doppler image

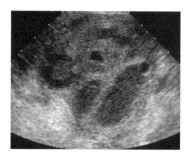

FIGURE 7.5 Pelvic inflammatory disease. The features of an inflamed tube can be recognised. Several transverse sections of a tube with swollen walls containing homogenously echogenic material corresponding to pus can be discerned

A pyosalpinx has a typical appearance at ultrasound examination: it is a thick-walled sausage-shaped cystic structure with swollen mucosal folds protruding into its lumen and it is filled with homogenously echogenic material corresponding to pus (Figure 7.6).[19] However, a pyosalpinx may be confused with a haematosalpinx. It is the clinical history that makes one of the two diagnoses more likely.

In the acute untreated stage, both abscesses and pyosalpinges are richly vascularised at Doppler ultrasound examination but the diagnosis of abscess and pyosalpinx can be made on the basis of the greyscale ultrasound image alone.

In a study from Finland, it was claimed that early acute salpingitis is characterised by a solid homogenous mass with indistinct margins located close to the ovary and richly vascularised at power Doppler ultrasound examination.[20] In an earlier publication, the same research team reported that acute salpingitis is also characterised by a polycystic appearance of the ovaries.[21] The Finnish team claimed that it was possible to distinguish a swollen infected tube from a normal one, if the tube can be seen to float in fluid. However, the evaluation of the degree of tubal swollenness is subjective and a diagnosis of salpingitis made on the basis of subjective findings is likely to be unreliable. The reproducibility of subjective evaluation of the degree of tubal swollenness has not been examined.

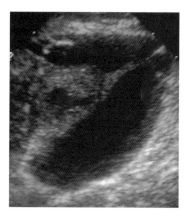

FIGURE 7.6 a

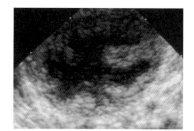

FIGURE 7.6 b

Pyosalpinx: **a)** sausage-shape; **b)** cogwheel appearance explained by swollen mucosal folds protruding into the lumen of the tube

Uterine causes of acute pelvic pain

Uterine fibroids, adenomyosis or haematopyometra may sometimes cause pelvic pain. If pressing on a myoma or on the uterus with the

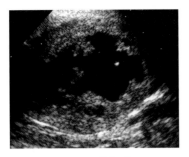

FIGURE 7.7 Myoma with hyaline degeneration

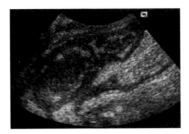

FIGURE 7.8 a

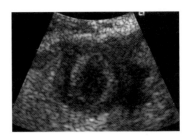

FIGURE 7.8 b

Transvaginal ultrasound image of an acutely inflamed appendix: **a)** sausage-like structure with concentrical layers; **b)** transverse section through the inflamed appendix; the concentrical layers are clearly seen

ultrasound probe or with the free hand does not provoke or worsen the patient's pain, the ultrasound finding is likely to be unrelated to the pain.

Acute fibroid necrosis has been described to yield 'unremarkable' ultrasound findings[22] or to be associated with findings of 'complex heterogeneous internal structures' or with 'internal sonolucent areas'.[23,24] Morphological features of acute fibroid necrosis are usually different form hyaline degeneration (Figure 7.7).

Non-gynaecological conditions that may cause pelvic pain

Gynaecologists should be able to recognise the ultrasound image of some non-gynaecological conditions that may cause pelvic pain, such as appendicitis and diverticulitis. Ultrasound images of these conditions may be encountered when an ultrasound examination is performed because of suspicion of gynaecological disease. An acutely inflamed appendix is a non-compressible sausage-like structure with concentric layers.[25] These concentric layers are best seen on a transverse section of the appendix (Figure 7.8). Hyperechogenic fat close to the appendix or a walled-off fluid collection representing abscess formation are also findings supporting a diagnosis of appendicitis.[26]

Diseased bowel is characterised by increased wall thickness. Because the bowel content is hyperechogenic, diseased bowel may look like a kidney with a hypoechogenic shell and a hyperechogenic core.[27] In acute diverticulitis, the bowel wall is thickened and the inflamed diverticulum may be seen as an outpouching protruding beyond the bowel lumen and beyond the colonic wall. Hyperechogenic fat close to the colon or a walled-off fluid collection representing abscess formation are other findings supporting a diagnosis of sigmoiditis/diverticulitis (Figure 7.9) (also see Chapter 8).[26]

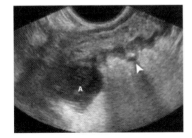

FIGURE 7.9 Transvaginal ultrasound image of acute diverticulitis. The bowel wall is thickened and the inflamed diverticulum is seen as an outpouching protruding beyond the bowel lumen (arrow) and beyond the colonic wall. The walled-off fluid collection represents abscess formation (A) and strongly supports the diagnosis of diverticulitis

Chronic pelvic pain

Whether small endometriotic implants or pelvic adhesions cause pain is controversial [2,28,29] but many consider these two conditions to be possible causes of pelvic pain. However, neither small endometriotic implants nor pelvic adhesions can be confidently diagnosed with transvaginal ultrasound.[30,31] Whether pelvic varicose veins cause pelvic pain is also debatable.[29] Some claim that ultrasound examination can be used to diagnose pelvic congestion syndrome.[32]

Adhesions cannot be seen at ultrasound examination but there are some indirect ultrasound findings suggestive of adhesions. Difficulty with getting a clear image of the adnexa, blurred borders of the ovary [30,31] and fixed adnexa that cannot be made to move when pushed on with the ultrasound transducer [31] suggest the presence of adhesions. So does a large distance (12 mm or more) between the probe and the ovary persisting after abdominal palpation.[31] However, the ultrasound diagnosis of adhesions is not accurate. In one study, the sensitivity was 61% and the specificity 98%.[30] In another study, the sensitivity was 50–80% and the specificity 55–95%, depending on which ultrasound criterion was used to diagnose adhesions.[31]

Using transvaginal ultrasound, an experienced ultrasound examiner can make a confident diagnosis of endometriosis in the uterosacral ligaments, vaginal wall, rectovaginal septum, wall of rectum-sigmoideum and wall of the urinary bladder (positive likelihood ratio 16, negative likelihood ratio 0.1) (Figure 7.10).[33] Rectovaginal endometriosis can also be diagnosed using transrectal ultrasound [34] or by sonovaginography (instillation of saline into the vagina during vaginal scanning).[35] Both methods seem to have good discriminatory capacity.[34,35]

A research team from London have introduced the term 'soft marker' for pelvic pathology, these soft markers being ovarian mobility and site-specific tenderness at transvaginal ultrasound examination.[36] They found that, in women examined with transvaginal ultrasound before a planned laparoscopy for chronic pelvic pain, the presence of soft markers in the absence of what would normally be called abnormal ultrasound findings increased the odds of endometriosis or pelvic adhesions 1.9 times (95% CI 1.2–3.1). This corresponds to a positive likelihood ratio of 3.6 and a negative likelihood ratio of 0.2. Thus, the use of soft markers was not an effective method for predicting or excluding peritoneal endometriosis or adhesions in women with chronic pelvic pain but it could still be useful clinically.

Dilated ovarian and pelvic veins seem to be common in asymptomatic women. In one study [37] where potential renal donors were examined with magnetic resonance imaging, 38% (8/21) of asymptomatic

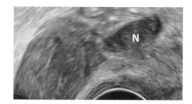

FIGURE 7.10 a

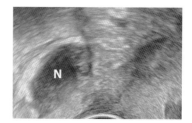

FIGURE 7.10 b

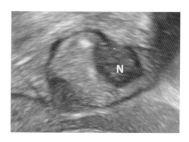

FIGURE 7.10 c

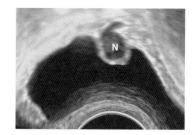

FIGURE 7.10 d

Pelvic endometriosis: **a)** large endometriotic nodule (N) is seen as a solid hypoechoic lesion in the ovarian fossa adjacent to the left ovary; **b)** endometriotic nodule (N) arising from the uterosacral ligament, typically located deep in the pouch of Douglas; **c)** bowel endometriosis with a nodule (N) in the sigmoid colon; **d)** bladder endometriosis with a large nodule (N) at the bladder dome

women had passive reflux from the left renal vein into the left ovarian vein. In another study[38] where potential renal donors were examined with helical computer tomography incompetent and dilated ovarian veins were found in 47% (16/34) of asymptomatic women. The role of ultrasound in the diagnosis of pelvic congestion syndrome – if this represents a true clinical entity – is not clear. Those who have tried to diagnose abnormal pelvic veins with ultrasound have looked either at the ovarian veins and/or at other pelvic veins using greyscale and/or power Doppler ultrasound and have assigned a congestion score to the woman. The diameter of ovarian veins, the flow direction in ovarian veins, the number of pelvic veins, the diameter of pelvic veins and the morphology of pelvic veins (signs of pelvic varicocele) were examined and changes of the Doppler shift waveform during Valsalva manoeuvre were looked for. Results of such studies are variable. In one study,[39] ultrasound results did not differ between women with pelvic congestion syndrome and controls, in another study there was a difference[40] and in a third study[41] there was poor agreement between ultrasound and venographic estimates of congestion.

Clinical implications of normal ultrasound findings in a woman with pelvic pain

In a study comprising 86 (possibly consecutive – this is not clear from the publication) women with pelvic pain and normal ultrasound findings, the pain resolved or improved in 77% (66/86) of the women.[42] Improvement was more common if the pain was acute (less than 2 weeks) or subacute (2 weeks to 6 months) than if it was chronic (more than 6 months): 86% (62/72) versus 50% (7/14). Among the women who underwent further imaging studies or a surgical procedure ($n=20$), significant pathology possibly explaining the pain was found in only five women (endometriosis, adenomyosis, adhesions, pelvic varicosities, diverticulitis), corresponding to 6% of the total study population. This suggests that the risk of significant pelvic pathology is small if the result of a gynaecological ultrasound examination is normal in a woman with pelvic pain. However, the study cited[42] investigated only the negative predictive value of a normal ultrasound result. The negative predictive value depends on the prevalence of pathology in the population studied. Thus, the results of this study are not of general applicability. It is not possible to calculate the sensitivity and specificity with regard to significant pelvic pathology on the basis of the figures published in the article.

It would be difficult to conduct a study to determine with certainty the sensitivity and specificity of pelvic ultrasound for pelvic abnormalities explaining pelvic pain because it would require all women with pelvic pain to undergo an ultrasound examination and then to undergo laparoscopy or laparotomy – even in case of normal ultrasound findings – to confirm the ultrasound findings. Other difficulties would be to define 'normal ultrasound finding' and 'normal findings at laparotomy/laparoscopy' and to determine to what extent an abnormal finding at laparoscopy/laparotomy explained the pain.

Conclusion

Ultrasound examination in a woman with pelvic pain is sometimes useful to confirm or exclude a diagnosis suspected on the basis of symptoms and clinical findings. If ultrasound findings are completely normal with mobile ovaries and no site specific tenderness, the risk of significant pelvic pathology is probably small. When ultrasound findings are abnormal, it is important to thoroughly evaluate whether they explain the pain or if they are merely incidental findings.

Acknowledgements

The studies from the author's institution were supported by grants from the Malmö General Hospital Cancer Foundation, funds administered by the Malmö Health Care Administration, the Faculty of Medicine of Lund University, the Anna-Lisa och Sven-Erik Lundgren Foundation for Medical Research, the Ingabritt and Arne Lundberg Research Foundation, two governmental grants (Landstingsfinansierad regional forskning, Region Skåne, and ALF-medel) and the Swedish Medical Research Council (grant nos. B96-17X-11605-01A, K98-17X-11605-03A, K2001-72X-11605-06A AND K2002-72X-11605-07B).

REFERENCES

1. VALENTIN L. High quality gynecological ultrasound can be highly beneficial, but poor quality gynecological ultrasound can do harm. *Ultrasound Obstet Gynecol* 1999; **13**: 1–7.

2. HOWARD F M. The role of laparoscopy in chronic pelvic pain. *Obstet Gynecol Surv* 1993; **48**: 357–87.

3. SLADKEVICIUS P, VALENTIN L, MARSAL K. Transvaginal gray-scale and Doppler ultrasound examinations of the uterus and ovaries in healthy postmenopausal women. *Ultrasound Obstet Gynecol* 1995; **6**: 81–90.

4. LEVINE D, GOSINK B B, WOLF S I, FELDESMAN M R, PRETORIUS D H. Simple adnexal cyst: the natural history in postmenopausal women. *Radiology* 1992; **184**: 653–9.

5. BORGFELDT C, ANDOLF E. Transvaginal sonographic ovarian findings in a random sample of woman 25–40 years old. *Ultrasound Obstet Gynecol* 1999; **13**: 345–50.

6. CONWAY C, ZALUD I, DILENA M, MAULIK D, SCHULMAN H, HALEY J, *et al*. Simple cyst in the postmenopausal patient: detection and management. *J Ultrasound Med* 1998; **17**: 369–72.

7. AUSLENDER R, ATLAS I, LISSAK A, BORNSTEIN J, ATAD J, ABRAMOVICI H. Follow-up of small, postmenopausal ovarian cysts using vaginal ultrasound and CA-125 antigen. *J Clin Ultrasound* 1996; **24**: 175–8.

8. Grant EG. Benign conditions of the ovary. In: Nyberg D A, Hill L M, Böhm-Velez M, Mendelson E B, editors. *Transvaginal Ultrasound*. St Louis: Mosby Year Book; 1992. p. 187–208.

9. Aleem F, Pennisi J, Zeitoun K, Predanic M. The role of color Doppler in diagnosis of endometriosis. *Ultrasound Obstet Gynecol* 1995;**5**:51–4.

10. Sohaey R, Gardner T L, Woodward P J, Peterson C M. Sonographic diagnosis of peritoneal inclusion cysts. *J Ultrasound Med* 1995;**14**:913–7.

11. Savelli L, de Iaco P, Ghi T, Bovicelli L, Rosati F, Cacciatore B. Transvaginal sonographic appearance of peritoneal pseudocysts. *Ultrasound Obstet Gynecol* 2004;**233**:284–8.

12. Tsai C C, Shen C C, Changchien C C, Hsu T Y, Kung F T, Chang S Y, et al. Ultrasound-guided transvaginal cyst aspiration for the management of pelvic pseudocyst: a preliminary experience. *Chang Gung Med* 2002;**25**:751–7.

13. Jain K A. Imaging of peritoneal inclusion cysts. *Am J Roentgenol* 2000;**174**:1559–63.

14. Nichols D H, Juhlin P J. Torsion of the adnexa. *Clin Obstet Gynecol* 1985;**28**:375–80.

15. Graif M, Shalev J, Strauss J, Engelberg S, Mashiach S, Itzchak Y. Torsion in the ovary: sonographic features. *Am J Roentgenol* 1984;**143**:1331–4.

16. Caspi B, Ben-Galim P, Weissman A, Appleman Z. The engorged fallopian tube: a new sonographic sign for adnexal torsion. *J Clin Ultrasound* 1995;**23**:505–7.

17. Stark J E, Siegel M J. Ovarian torsion in prepubertal and pubertal girls: sonographic findings. *Am J Roentgenol* 1994;**163**:1479–82.

18. Quillin S P, Siegel M J. Transabdominal color Doppler ultrasonography of the painful adolescent ovary. *J Ultrasound Med* 1994;**13**:549–55.

19. Patten R M. The Fallopian tube and pelvic inflammatory disease. In: Nyberg D A, Hill L M, Böhm-Velez M, Mendelson E B, editors. *Transvaginal Ultrasound*. St Louis: Mosby Year Book; 1992. p. 209–21.

20. Molander P, Sjoberg J, Paavonen J, Cacciatore B. Transvaginal power Doppler findings in laparoscopically proven acute pelvic inflammatory disease. *Ultrasound Obstet Gynecol* 2001;**17**:233–8.

21. Cacciatore B, Leminen A, Ingman-Friberg S, Ylostalo P, Paavonen J. Transvaginal sonographic findings in ambulatory patients with suspected pelvic inflammatory disease. *Obstet Gynecol* 1992;**80**:912–6.

22. Chang M Y, Tsai F B, Soong Y K. Infarcted intramural uterine leiomyomata during buserelin acetate treatment. *Chang Gung Med J* 1993;**16**:129–32.

23. Makar A P, Meulyzer P R, Vergote I B, Schatteman E A, Huyghe M L, Meeuwis L A. A case report of unusual complication of myomatous uterus in pregnancy: spontaneous perforation of myoma after red degeneration. *Eur J Obstet Gynecol Reprod Biol* 1989;**31**:289–93.

24. Mayer D P, Shipilov V. Ultrasonography and magnetic resonance imaging of uterine fibroids. *Obstet Gynecol Clin North Am* 1995;**22**:667–725.

25. Puylaert J B, Rioux M, van Oostayen J A. The appendix and small bowel. In: Meire H, Cosgrove D, Dewbury K, Livingstone C, London E, editors. *Abdominal and General Ultrasound: A Comprehensive Text*. 2nd ed. London: Churchill Livingstone; 2001. p. 841–65.

26. Bau A, Atri M. Acute female pelvic pain: ultrasound evaluation. *Semin Ultrasound CT MR* 2000;**21**:78–93.

27. Dubbins P A. The small bowel and colon. In: Meire H, Cosgrove D, Dewbury K, Livingstone C, London E, editors. *Abdominal and General Ultrasound – A Comprehensive Text*. 2nd ed. London: Churchill Livingstone; 2001. p. 765–76.

28. Peters A A, Trimbos-Kemper G C, Admiraal C, Trimbos J B, Hermans J. A randomized clinical trial on the benefit of adhesiolysis in patients with intraperitoneal adhesions and chronic pelvic pain. *Br J Obstet Gynaecol* 1992;**99**:59–62.

29. Thornton J G, Morley S, Lilleyman J, Onwude J L, Currie I, Crompton A C. The relationship between laparoscopic disease, pelvic pain and infertility; an unbiased assessment. *Eur J Obstet Gynecol Reprod Biol* 1997;**74**:57–62.

30. Ubaldi F, Wisanto A, Camus M, Tournaye H, Clasen K, Devroey P. The role of transvaginal ultrasonography in the detection of pelvic pathologies in the infertility workup. *Hum Reprod* 1998;**13**:330–3.

31. Guerriero S, Ajossa S, Lai M P, Mais V, Paoletti A M, Melis G B. Transvaginal ultrasonography in the diagnosis of pelvic adhesions. *Hum Reprod* 1997;**12**:2649–53.

32. Park S J, Lim J W, Ko Y T, Lee D H, Yoon Y, Oh J H, et al. Diagnosis of pelvic congestion syndrome using transabdominal and transvaginal sonography. *Am J Roentgenol* 2004;**182**:683–8.

33. Bazot M, Thomassin I, Hourani R, Cortez A, Darai E. Diagnostic accuracy of transvaginal sonography for deep pelvic endometriosis. *Ultrasound Obstet Gynecol* 2004; **24**:180–5.

34. Fedele L, Bianchi S, Portuese A, Borruto F, Dorta M. Transrectal ultrasonography in the assessment of rectovaginal endometriosis. *Obstet Gynecol* 1998; **91**:444–8.

35. Dessole S, Farina M, Rubattu G, Cosmi E, Ambrosini G, Nardelli G B. Sonovaginography is a new technique for assessing rectovaginal endometriosis. *Fertil Steril* 2003; **79**:1023–7.

36. OKARO E, CONDOUS G, KHALID A, TIMMERMAN D, WANG X, VAN HUFFEL S, et al. The use of ultrasound-based 'soft markers' for the prediction of pelvic pathology in women with chronic pelvic pain: can we reduce the need for laparoscopy? BJOG 2006; 113: 251–6.

37. NASCIMENTO A B, MITCHELL D G, HOLLAND G. Ovarian veins: magnetic resonance imaging findings in an asymptomatic population. J Magn Reson Imaging 2002; 15: 551–6.

38. ROZENBLIT A M, RICCI Z J, TUVIA J, AMIS E S JR. Incompetent and dilated ovarian veins: a common CT finding in asymptomatic parous women. Am J Roentgenol 2001; 176: 119–22.

39. HALLIGAN S, CAMPBELL D, BARTRAM CI, ROGERS V, EL-HADDAD C, PATEL S, et al. Vaginal ultrasound examination of women with and without pelvic venous congestion. Clin Radio 2000; 55: 954–8.

40. PARK S J, LIM J W, KO Y T, LEE D H, YOON Y, OH J H, et al. Diagnosis of pelvic congestion syndrome using transabdominal and transvaginal sonography. Am J Roentgenol 2004; 182: 683–8.

41. CAMPBELL D, HALLIGAN S, BARTRAM C I, ROGERS V, HOLLINGS N, KINGSTON K, et al. Transvaginal power Doppler ultrasound in pelvic congestion. Acta Radiol 2003; 44: 269–74.

42. HARRIS R D, HOLTZMAN S R, POPPE A M. Clinical outcome in female patients with pelvic pain and normal pelvic US findings. Radiology 2000; 216: 440–3.

Ultrasound of non-gynaecological pelvic lesions

MICHAEL JOHN WESTON

Introduction

Ultrasound is a versatile diagnostic tool that is of proven value in the assessment of women with gynaecological complaints. Transvaginal ultrasound has improved the ability of ultrasound to interrogate the pelvic organs with less interference from intervening structures such as gas or fat. However, it is not only the uterus and ovaries that are amenable to ultrasonic inspection. Other pelvic structures such as the bowel, renal tract or pelvic sidewalls are also readily seen. This is fortuitous, as symptoms arising from the pelvis are relatively nonspecific. The gynaecologist may, for instance, need to distinguish between the symptoms caused by pelvic inflammatory disease and those of an inflamed pelvic appendix. An awareness of alternative diagnoses and an appreciation of the normal and abnormal ultrasound appearances of bowel, bladder and other structures will help in achieving the correct diagnosis.

Transvaginal ultrasound, because of the ability to place the probe close to the region of interest, can better enable the diagnosis of pelvic disease. It allows an imaged bimanual palpation to occur, with the movement of tissues relative to each other seen and tender structures found. This can remove doubt so that other imaging modalities such as computed tomography (CT) are not needed. Transvaginal ultrasound also facilitates diagnostic and therapeutic intervention in the pelvis: guided needle biopsies or drainage of collections can all be achieved. This chapter aims to encourage the gynaecologist to look beyond the uterus and ovaries when imaging the pelvis.

Bowel abnormalities

Appendix

NORMAL APPEARANCE

All normal bowel wall shows a typical multilayered appearance of alternating concentric rings of high and low echogenicity. High-resolution scans will show five layers:

▷ an inner bright layer that represents the lumen and mucosa
▷ a dark layer representing lamina propria and muscularis mucosa
▷ a bright layer representing the submucosa
▷ a dark layer representing the muscular wall
▷ a bright layer caused by the serosa that merges with the mesenteric fat.

The normal appendix is found in about 50% of those cases in which it is sought (if the appendix is abnormal it is detected far more readily).[1] Transabdominally, the graded compression technique is used. The probe is placed over the area of interest in the right lower quadrant and pressure gradually applied. This serves to displace or compress normal bowel and to empty the normal bowel of gas and faeces. It also brings the appendix into a closer focal zone of the transducer. Graded compression is usually well tolerated. The appendix appears as a blind-ended tube without peristalsis (Figure 8.1). It typically has an ovoid shape in cross-section;[2] indeed, finding an ovoid shape throughout the length of the appendix is a good criterion to exclude appendicitis. The mural thickness from the lumen to the outer serosa should be less than 3 mm and the outer appendiceal diameter less than 6 mm,[3,4] although there is a wide range. The normal appendix has two patterns: the more common 'collapsed lumen' pattern in which the lumen is empty or can be emptied by compression and the 'rod' pattern in which the thin-walled appendix contains non-compressible hyperechoic material.[1]

If the appendix is not seen at ordinary graded-compression sonography there are additional techniques to aid in its detection. The posterior manual compression technique uses the free hand to apply pressure to the opposite side of the right lower quadrant and to push up towards the probe. This can allow detection of a further 10% of appendices.[5] Children can be given a saline enema to aid in the detection of the ascending colon and caecum: this in turn increases the visualisation of the appendix.[6] Finally, the use of transvaginal ultrasound can find a further 25% of cases with appendicitis in women.[7]

INFLAMMATION

Appendicitis remains the most common cause of acute abdominal pain requiring surgery in the Western world.[8] Surprisingly, there has been no decrease in the rate of misdiagnosis of appendicitis over the past few decades, despite the advent of diagnostic aids such as ultrasound, CT and laparoscopy. Misdiagnosis and unnecessary appendicectomies have even increased among fertile women.[9] Up to one in five women in one series referred to an emergency room because of suspected pelvic inflammatory disease turned out to have acute appendicitis.[10]

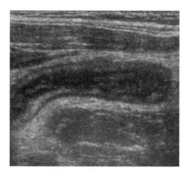

FIGURE 8.1a

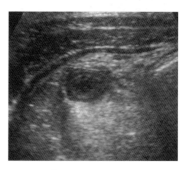

FIGURE 8.1b

The appendix: **a)** longitudinal view: a blind-ended tube with the typical multi-layered pattern of bowel wall is shown. It is noncompressible and has a diameter over 6 mm, in keeping with appendicitis; **b)** transverse view: the appendix shows a rounded rather than an ovoid cross-section. This supports the diagnosis of appendicitis

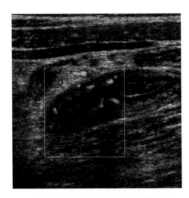

FIGURE 8.2 Longitudinal view of the appendix. There is blood flow shown in the appendix wall on power Doppler. This is a feature of appendicitis

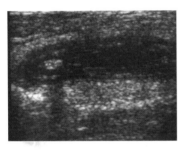

FIGURE 8.3 Longitudinal view of the appendix. An echogenic focus with an acoustic shadow represents an appendicolith within the lumen of the appendix

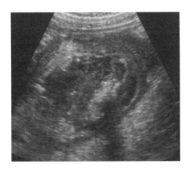

FIGURE 8.4 The appendix is distended with fluid and debris. The layers of the wall are interrupted. This is an appendix abscess in danger of perforation

There are several ultrasound signs to indicate the presence of appendicitis:

▷ an outer diameter of the appendix greater than 6 mm
▷ lack of compressibility
▷ finding blood flow in the wall with colour Doppler (Figure 8.2)
▷ an appendicolith (seen in one-third of cases of appendicitis) (Figure 8.3)
▷ signs of periappendiceal inflammation:
  ■ hyperechoic halo of adjacent fat
  ■ caecal wall thickening over 5 mm
  ■ local lymph nodes of 5 mm diameter or more
  ■ peritoneal fluid.

The most reliable signs are an outer diameter of greater than 6 mm and a periappendiceal halo of inflamed, hyperechoic fat.[11] The overall sensitivity for appendicitis by graded compression sonography is between 77% and 89% with a specificity of up to 96%. Failing to find the appendix has a 90% negative predictive value for appendicitis.

Appendicitis of a pelvic appendix accounts for only 20–25% of cases but this type of appendicitis is most likely to be confused with gynaecological disease. Transvaginal ultrasound is often unable to apply compression to the appendix or to confirm that it joins to the caecum. These limitations are offset by the higher resolution scan afforded by the transvaginal probe. Discontinuity of the echogenic submucosa of the appendix indicates mural necrosis is occurring and that perforation may occur (Figure 8.4). If perforation does occur, a localised periappendiceal collection may be seen.[12] In more advanced cases, there may be a large inflammatory phlegmon of pus and matted-together loops of bowel.

There are alternative methods of imaging the appendix with CT being the most widely accepted. CT has advantages over ultrasound in the patient who is obese and those in great pain or with a retrocaecal appendix. CT is also thought to be less operator-dependent and to provide images that are easier to interpret. Helical CT has been reported to give sensitivities for acute appendicitis of 90–100%. However, at least one comparative study using non-specialist staff in a general hospital showed that ultrasound and CT had a similar accuracy.[13] There has been concern expressed that technology and imaging tools should not detract from proper and timely clinical evaluation. There remains a small risk of perforated acute appendicitis even after normal CT and ultrasound examinations.

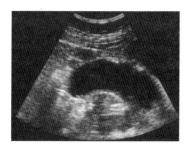

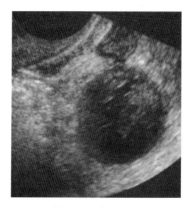

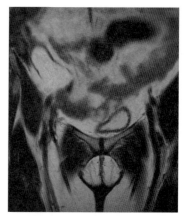

FIGURE 8.5a Ultrasound of mucocele: a thin-walled ovoid structure with apparently anechoic contents is shown behind the right side of the bladder

FIGURE 8.5b Transvaginal ultrasound shows the contents of the lesion to have structure. Mucoceles typically demonstrate an onion-layer appearance to their contents

FIGURE 8.5c Magnetic resonance image of the mucocele demonstrates that is relatively mobile, sitting much higher in the right iliac fossa than it was on the ultrasound

MUCOCELE

Appendiceal mucocele occurs when there is accumulation of mucoid material within the lumen of the appendix distal to an obstruction. It is rare, occurring in only 0.25% of appendicectomies. Approximately 10% of appendiceal mucoceles are due to cystadenocarcinoma; there is also an association with colonic and ovarian carcinoma. Mucoceles occur more commonly in women than men. Preoperative diagnosis is useful to alert the surgeon so that unintended rupture of the mucocele and the development of pseudomyxoma peritonei can be avoided.

Ultrasound can show different patterns, including a cystic structure with thin walls (Figure 8.5), a cyst with septations and, the most common appearance, layered rings of mucus of different echogenicity. Small calcifications can be present in the wall. A mucocele can mimic an ovarian cyst or a hydrosalpinx and can give rise to delay in making the correct diagnosis. Finding a normal ovary separate to the lesion and showing the lesion joins to the caecum are valuable signs.[14, 15]

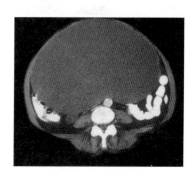

FIGURE 8.5d Computed tomography of the abdomen. A large tumour filling the abdomen is demonstrated. This eventually proved to be a metastatic deposit to the ovary of a mucinous adenocarcinoma of the appendix. Interestingly, in hindsight, the abnormal appendix is visible behind the mass on the right

Diverticulitis

Diverticulosis of the colon affects one-third of the population over the age of 40 years and two-thirds over the age of 85 years. Inflammation develops in 10–25% of those with diverticulosis.[16] Patients with acute diverticulitis typically present with symptoms of pain, fever and leucocytosis. These symptoms are nonspecific and imaging is needed to avoid erroneous clinical diagnosis. However, because diverticulitis affects an older age group there is less potential for confusion with

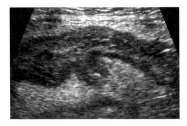

FIGURE 8.6 Longitudinal view of the descending colon showing a mural out-pouching, typical of a diverticulum

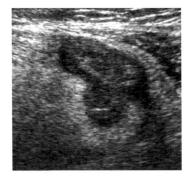

FIGURE 8.7 There is a halo of bright, 'inflamed' fat around the diverticulum, indicating that this is diverticulitis

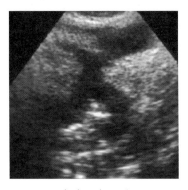

FIGURE 8.8 The bowel seen in cross-section shows a 'pseudokidney' sign. There is a dark track leading from the bowel to a small, superficial fluid collection. This is a localised perforation and could be due to diverticulitis or tumour

acute gynaecological disease. Diverticulosis most commonly affects the sigmoid colon but does also occur in the right colon. If ultrasound is used to assess people with right lower-quadrant abdominal pain, the incidence of right colonic diverticulitis is about one case in 34 appendectomies.[17]

Graded compression sonography is used in a similar fashion to that described for imaging appendicitis. Particular attention needs to be paid to the area of the patient's greatest tenderness. The ultrasound features of diverticulitis are:

▷ direct vision of the diverticulum as an out-pouching from the colonic wall (Figure 8.6)
▷ localised circumferential colonic-wall thickening at the level of the diverticulum
▷ 'bright' inflamed fat around the diverticulum (Figure 8.7); this fat is typically non-compressible
▷ a faecolith in the diverticulum: faecoliths typically cast a clean acoustic shadow with sharp boundaries.

Complications of diverticulitis include bowel obstruction, free perforation and fistula or abscess formation. Extraluminal air may be seen on ultrasound as echogenic foci within the peridiverticular fat or as gas within a fluid collection or abscess. Up to one-third of patients with diverticulitis will show an associated abscess on ultrasound.[18] Most of these abscesses will spontaneously discharge into the colon with conservative management. Intervention and drainage is usually only required for a large abscess with a persistent spiking fever.

Transabdominal ultrasound may often fail to visualise the lower sigmoid colon because this area is hidden by overlying bowel gas. Transvaginal[19] and transrectal[20] ultrasound can access this region. The ultrasound signs are the same as on transabdominal scans. It is not uncommon for previously unsuspected diverticulitis to be diagnosed at transvaginal ultrasound[12] and, as with appendicitis, this occurs because the diseased segment of bowel is deep within the true pelvis.

Differentiation of diverticulitis from colonic carcinoma can be difficult (Figure 8.8). Colonoscopy is advised once the inflammation has settled.[21]

Inflammatory bowel disease

Crohn's disease and ulcerative colitis show different patterns of bowel involvement. Crohn's disease affects the distal small bowel in 20%, the colon in 30% and both small and large bowel in 50%. It typically produces skip lesions with intervening regions of normal bowel. Ulcerative colitis is limited to the colon and involvement is continuous from the rectum more proximally.

Crohn's disease involves all the layers of the bowel wall (Figure 8.9). Sonography shows the transmural pattern with irregular thickening of mucosa and muscularis layers. The unsharpness of the layers suggests an acute phase of the disease.[22] The serosal involvement shows as hypertrophic fat around the bowel, often said to have a frosted glass appearance.[23] Deep ulcers are revealed by discontinuity of the echogenic submucosal ring. This dark track through the submucosa may be seen to extend outside of the bowel as a fistula. Perianal disease is common in Crohn's disease so transvaginal ultrasound in women is a much more comfortable way of examining the rectum than transrectal ultrasound.

Crohn's ileocolitis forms part of the differential diagnosis of right lower quadrant pain. Other causes such as campylobacter and yersinia ileocolitis should be considered if there are enlarged mesenteric lymph nodes.[24]

Ulcerative colitis produces less colonic wall thickening than Crohn's disease and the stratification of the layers is better preserved. Mural inflammation is usually limited to the mucosal layers and the pericolonic fat is normal. Chronic inflammation will lead to loss of the normal haustral pattern.[23] The superficial ulcerations that occur are usually not seen at ultrasound.

Bowel duplication cysts

Mesenteric cysts, duplication cysts and complications of Meckel's diverticulum[25] may all present as pelvic cysts or masses. The diagnosis may not be made until surgery but ultrasound can give the clue to their origin by showing the relationship with bowel and by showing that the gynaecological tract is normal.

Bowel cancer

Ultrasound is not indicated in the search for gastrointestinal tumours but these tumours may be seen serendipitously during pelvic ultrasound. Primary adenocarcinoma, lymphoma and metastasis to the gut can all be shown. The classic appearance of an annular carcinoma is the 'pseudokidney' sign (Figure 8.8). The dark outer margin represents the thickened bowel wall and the white inner region, the bowel lumen.[12] Tumours may however present as focal mural thickenings or as localised rounded intra- or extraluminal masses (Figure 8.10). High-resolu-

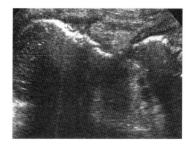

FIGURE 8.9   A large right flank abscess is shown. This eventually proved to be due to Crohn's disease

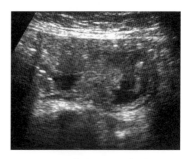

FIGURE 8.10   Colon cancer. A focal intraluminal, rounded mass is shown arising from the posterior colonic wall. There is interruption of the underlying dark ring of the muscular bowel wall layer. This indicates local invasion

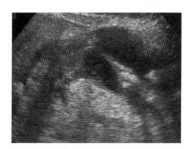

FIGURE 8.11a

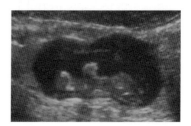

FIGURE 8.11b

Gastric lymphoma: **a)** longitudinal image of gastric antrum and pylorus showing considerable thickening of the gastric wall; **b)** transverse view of the stomach showing the gross mural thickening due to lymphomatous infiltration

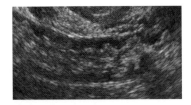

FIGURE 8.12 a Transvaginal scan of normal colon

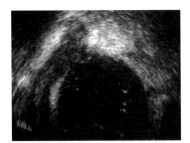

FIGURE 8.12 b Transrectal scan of a long-segment of abnormal, thick-walled colon and a pericolic abscess. A needle has been inserted transrectally and its tip can be seen in the collection

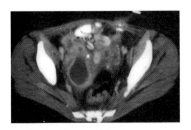

FIGURE 8.12 c Computed tomography scan of a peritoneal dialysis-related pelvic abscess

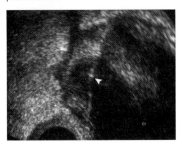

FIGURE 8.12 d Transvaginal scan of a peritoneal dialysis related pelvic abscess. A needle has been inserted into the abscess (arrow)

tion ultrasound to identify which bowel wall layer is involved will help differentiate primary from secondary tumours; adenocarcinoma shows mucosal involvement whereas metastases more typically involve the serosa. Looking at the liver for metastases may help to make the diagnosis of bowel cancer clear. Lymphoma usually obliterates the bowel-wall stratification early on in its course to show massive transmural hypoechogenicity (Figure 8.11).[22]

Many benign and malignant conditions of bowel show similar appearances of bowel-wall thickening. The features that suggest a lesion is malignant are a short (less than 10 cm long) diseased segment, a lack of circumferential involvement and loss of mural stratification.[26] Malignant conditions also tend to give a greater wall thickness than benign conditions. Not all of these features need be present for a diagnosis of malignancy to be made.

Invasive procedures

Abscess drainage

The mortality in undrained abdominal abscesses is high, probably over 45%.[27] Pelvic collections are often not amenable to standard percutaneous drainage because of the interposition of other structures. Transgluteal, transperineal, transrectal and transvaginal routes are all alternative routes of access. The correct route to use depends on the position of the abscess and its aetiology. Bowel disease-related abscesses are better drained transrectally than transvaginally to avoid the development of a colovaginal fistula. Pelvic collections thought not to be related to bowel disease are better approached transvaginally to avoid introducing rectal organisms into a collection that might not be infected. The transperineal route may be required if the patient has had surgery such as an abdominoperineal resection that precludes an endoluminal route.[28] The transgluteal route requires CT guidance to achieve. It is often more painful than the endoluminal approaches, though adopting an infra-piriformis approach is much less painful than a transpiriformis route.[29]

There are numerous publications attesting to the safety and efficacy of both transrectal and transvaginal abscess drainage (Figure 8.12).[30–35] It does not seem to matter if a single-step trocar technique or a Seldinger technique is used.[32] Provided that the abscess is emptied completely, subsequent catheter dislodgement does not affect outcome.[36] This has led some centres to advocate aspiration and lavage as an alternative to drain placement.[35] Appropriate antibiotic therapy is needed for all the techniques.

Tumour biopsy

Patients with peritoneal carcinomatosis do not benefit from surgery if the primary disease is not ovarian. Biopsy of omental cake, peritoneal disease or pelvic mass can allow a site-specific primary diagnosis to be made. Standard haematoxylin and eosin analysis supplemented by immunohistochemical analysis provide the diagnosis in 97%.[37] Transvaginal ultrasound-guided biopsy is a safe way to obtain material if other percutaneous routes are unavailable (Figure 8.13).

The technique is simple and quick to perform. Local anaesthesia is not needed. The mass is identified at transvaginal scan. Gentle pressure is applied with the transducer to stretch the vaginal wall taut and to bring the mass into direct apposition with the vaginal wall. Colour Doppler is used to check that there are no large vessels intervening. A spring-loaded 18-gauge biopsy needle is passed down the transducer guide into the lesion and fired in one smooth motion. Some self-limiting vaginal bleeding will be seen afterwards.

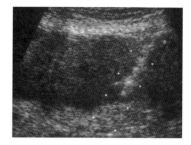

FIGURE 8.13 Tumour biopsy: transabdominal omental cake biopsy; immunohistochemistry confirmed the tumour to be from a breast primary

Renal tract

Ultrasound has well-recognised value in evaluating the kidneys. Views of the kidneys should be part of any ultrasound examination of the pelvis – if only to check that an occult pelvic pathology is not causing a hydronephrosis. Other manifestations of bladder, urethral and distal ureteric disease have to be actively looked for during pelvic sonography.

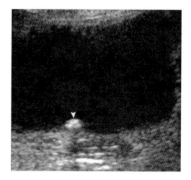

FIGURE 8.14 Transabdominal ultrasound of the bladder: a 9-mm stone is shown impacted at the right vesicoureteric junction (arrow)

Stones

Ultrasound is highly sensitive at detecting calculi in the kidneys. It is less effective at finding ureteric calculi, as the mid-third of the ureter is often hidden behind bowel gas. Their presence can be inferred from unilateral upper tract dilation corresponding to the side of pain, a collapsed distal ureter and ipsilateral reduction of ureteric jets into the bladder. Confirmation of a ureteric stone as the cause requires at least a plain radiograph and probably an intravenous urogram or spiral stone-searching CT. In contrast, the distal ureter and ureterovesical junction are readily visible to ultrasound and stones may be clearly seen (Figure 8.14); indeed transvaginal ultrasound may be best,[38] particularly in women allergic to contrast agents or who are pregnant. Transplant kidneys in the pelvis can suffer from stone disease and ultrasound is sensitive at depicting these. Stones characteristically manifest on ultrasound as a bright focus with sharp acoustic shadowing.

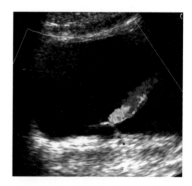

FIGURE 8.15 Colour Doppler shows a jet of urine entering the bladder from the ureteric orifice. A small ureterocele is lifted up and revealed by the jet

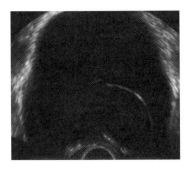

FIGURE 8.16 Transvaginal scan of a large, distended ureterocele

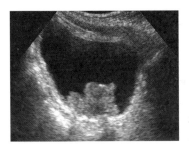

FIGURE 8.17a Polypoidal bladder tumour. A fleck of calcification is seen at its margin

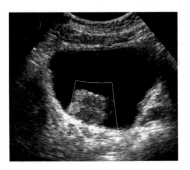

FIGURE 8.17b Colour Doppler, by showing the lesion contains blood flow, confirms that it is not a blood clot

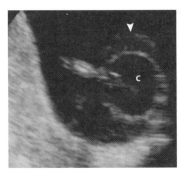

FIGURE 8.17c Blood clot (arrow) is seen adherent around the bladder catheter (c)

Bladder stones are readily visible on ultrasound. Rolling the patient will show the stone to move, though sometimes a stone may be trapped in a bladder diverticulum (diverticula are a relatively blind region at cystoscopy).

Ureterocele

A ureterocele can be clinically silent and without upper tract dilation. The diagnosis may be made for the first time during sonography of the pelvis. The ureterocele may lie collapsed against the bladder wall and only become visible at transabdominal sonography when a jet of urine is passed through the ureterovesical junction (Figure 8.15). This causes the characteristic ballooning of the ureterocele into the bladder lumen.[39] If there is restriction to the flow of urine, the ureterocele may remain distended. Transvaginal sonography demonstrates the dilated distal ureter and ureterocele clearly,[40] only the inexperienced might mistake the appearance for a hydrosalpinx (Figure 8.16). Ureteroceles are associated with ipsilateral renal pathology. The kidney may be duplex or single-system and the ureterocele may be in an ectopic location.

Bladder tumour

Haematuria may be confused with vaginal blood loss by some women. Furthermore, bladder carcinoma is a common disease in the elderly. Consequently, ultrasound views of the bladder should be part of any investigation of postmenopausal bleeding. An ultrasound diagnosis of bladder cancer is specific, up to 99%, but ultrasound is only about 60% sensitive for bladder tumour in the setting of haematuria.[41] The most common appearance of a bladder tumour on ultrasound is a polypoid lesion arising from the trigone,[42] but there is much variation (Figure 8.17). Nearly half will show some calcification. Colour and spectral Doppler are of no help in determining the grade or nature of a bladder tumour but do have value in distinguishing a tumour from a blood clot adherent to the wall.[43] Transvaginal ultrasound is particularly helpful in patients with poor bladder filling as only retention of a small amount of urine in the bladder is needed. Partial withdrawal of the probe and anterior angulation will show the bladder.[12]

Urethra

The female urethra is well-visualised either at transperineal sonography or at transvaginal sonography with the probe withdrawn near to the introitus. There is an undoubted role for transperineal sonography in the assessment of urinary stress incontinence.[44] Paraurethral cysts and abscesses are notoriously difficult to diagnose on conventional imaging. Few operators include the urethra in their standard pelvic ultrasound protocols so the diagnosis may be overlooked. The prevalence of paraurethral cysts in asymptomatic women is about 3%.[45]

Vascular abnormalities

Aneurysms

The use of colour Doppler as part of the assessment of any pelvic mass should reliably prevent the misdiagnosis of aorta and iliac regional vessel aneurysms. True and false aneurysms are usually unexpected findings. Early reports emphasise how the greyscale appearances of aneurysms containing clot can mimic gynaecological lesions.[46,47] Patients with a history of recent trauma, surgery or infection are at risk of vascular injury; colour Doppler is mandatory in their evaluation. A true aneurysm still retains an arterial wall around it, whereas a false aneurysm is an arterial leak to and fro into a temporarily enclosed space. False aneurysms may be surrounded by very large amounts of blood clot so that identifying the relationship of the artery to the mass can require care (Figure 8.18).

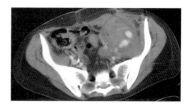

FIGURE 8.18 Computed tomography of a large left pelvic false aneurysm arising from the iliac artery

Deep vein thrombosis

Ultrasound is reliable at detecting thrombus within the femoral and popliteal veins. Ultrasound is much less reliable at detecting the proximal extent of any such thrombus. In one cohort of patients, in whom ultrasound had shown thrombus to extend to the inguinal ligament, magnetic resonance imaging showed that 67% had thrombus into the iliac veins and 22% had clot extension to the cava.[48] Pelvic pathology can alter venous flow and predispose to deep vein thrombus. A swollen leg in the presence of a pelvic mass should prompt the search for a DVT (Figure 8.19).

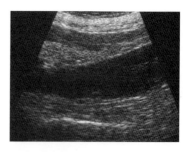

FIGURE 8.19 a

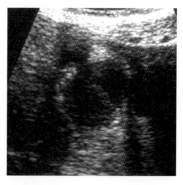

FIGURE 8.19 b

a) Longitudinal section and b) transverse section of an iliac vein containing non-occlusive blood clot

Varicosities and distended pelvic veins

Dilated pelvic veins around the gynaecological apparatus are relatively common findings. They may be mistaken for dilated fallopian tubes. Flow is often slow within them so colour Doppler may not reveal their vascular nature. The Valsalva manoeuvre helps by causing the veins to distend and flow to be seen. Transvaginal ultrasound can be used to apply gentle pressure and show that the varices are compressible. The diagnosis of pelvic congestion syndrome requires far more than just the finding of dilated pelvic veins, as dilated veins are so commonly seen in asymptomatic women.[49] Some believe that a combination of finding a dilated left ovarian vein with reversed caudal flow, a varicocele, dilated arcuate veins crossing the uterine myometrium, polycystic changes of the ovary and alteration of Doppler waveform during Valsalva can make the diagnosis.[50]

Anterior sacral meningocele

This is a congenital condition that usually manifests during the first years of life. It is associated with tethering of the spinal cord and neurogenic bladder problems. It is defined as a spinal fluid-filled sac in the pelvis that communicates with the spinal subarachnoid space through a defect in the anterior sacral wall. Very rarely, an anterior sacral meningocele remains asymptomatic and only presents when the woman becomes pregnant and is scanned for the first time.[51]

Hernia

The real-time nature of ultrasound examination lends itself to examination of musculoskeletal structures. The ability to observe reduction of a hernia during compression with the ultrasound probe and its subsequent prolapse on straining is a great advantage. Both the common groin hernias and less common sites, such as a spigelian hernia between abdominal muscles, can be shown by ultrasound (Figure 8.20).[52,53]

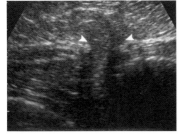

FIGURE 8.20 A small hernia of peritoneal fat is shown (between the arrows) into the anterior abdominal wall

Conclusion

Ultrasound is a powerful tool in the initial investigation of symptoms affecting the pelvis. Gynaecologists need to remember the non-gynaecological causes and be alert to ultrasound signs outside of the uterus and ovaries. Reassuringly, a negative pelvic ultrasound scan has a strong negative predictive value for the presence of significant pathology, particularly in the assessment of pelvic pain.[54]

REFERENCES

1. SIMONOVSKY V. Sonographic detection of normal and abnormal appendix. *Clin Radiol* 1999;**54**:533–9.

2. RETTENBACHER T, HOLLERWEGER A, MACHEINER P, GRITZMANN N, DANIAUX M, SCHWAMBERGER K, et al. Ovoid shape of the vermiform appendix: a criterion to exclude acute appendicitis – evaluation with US. *Radiology* 2003;**226**:95–100.

3. SIMONOVSKY V. Normal appendix: is there any significant difference in the maximal mural thickness at US between pediatric and adult populations? *Radiology* 2002;**224**:333–7.

4. RETTENBACHER T, HOLLERWEGER A, MACHEINER P, RETTENBACHER L, TOMASELLI F, SCHNEIDER B, et al. Outer diameter of the vermiform appendix as a sign of acute appendicitis: evaluation at US. *Radiology* 2001;**218**:757–62.

5. LEE J H, JEONG Y K, HWANG J C, HAM SY, YANG S O. Graded compression sonography with adjuvant use of a posterior manual compression technique in the sonographic diagnosis of acute appendicitis. *AJR Am J Roentgenol* 2002;**178**:863–8.

6. HAN T I. Improved sonographic visualization of the appendix with a saline enema in children with suspected appendicitis. *J Ultrasound Med* 2002;**21**:511–6.

7. CASPI B, ZBAR AP, MAVOR E, HAGAY Z, APPELMAN Z. The contribution of transvaginal ultrasound in the diagnosis of acute appendicitis: an observational study. *Ultrasound Obstet Gynecol* 2003;**21**:273–6.

8. GRAFFEO C S, COUNSELMAN FL. Appendicitis test. *Emerg Med Clin North Am* 1996;**14**:653–71.

9. FLUM D R, MORRIS A, KOEPSELL T, DELLINGER EP. Has misdiagnosis of appendicitis decreased over time? *JAMA* 2001;**286**:1748–53.

10. MOLANDER P, PAAVONEN J, SJOBERG J, SAVELLI L, CACCIATORE B. Transvaginal sonography in the diagnosis of acute appendicitis. *Ultrasound Obstet Gynecol* 2002;**20**:496–501.

11. KESSLER N, CYTEVAL C, GALLIX B, LESNIK A, BLAYAC P M, PUJOL J, et al. Appendicitis: evaluation of sensitivity, specificity, and predictive values of US, Doppler US, and laboratory findings. *Radiology* 2004;**230**:472–8.

12. DAMANI N, WILSON S R. Nongynecologic applications of transvaginal US. *Radiographics* 1999;**19**:S179–200.

13. POORTMAN P, LOHLE PN, SCHOEMAKER C M, OOSTVOGEL H J, TEEPEN H J, ZWINDERMAN KA, et al. Comparison of CT and sonography in the diagnosis of acute appendicitis: A blinded prospective study. *AJR* 2003;**181**:1355–9.

14. DEGANI S, SHAPIRO I, LEIBOVITZ Z, OHEL G. Sonographic appearance of appendiceal mucocele. *Ultrasound Obstet Gynecol* 2002;**19**:99–101.

15. CASPI B, CASSIF E, AUSLENDER R, HERMAN A, HAGAY Z, APPELMAN Z. The onion skin sign. A specific sonographic marker of appendiceal mucocele. *J Ultrasound Med* 2004;**23**:117–21.

16. ROBERTS P, ABEL M, ROSEN L, CIROCCO W, FLESHMAN J, LEFF E, et al. Practice parameters for sigmoid Diverticulitis – supporting documentation. *Dis Colon Rectum* 1995;**38**:126–32.

17. OUDENHOVEN LFIJ, KOUMANS R KJ, PUYLAERT J B C M. Right colonic Diverticulitis: US and CT findings – new insights about frequency and natural history. *Radiology* 1998;**208**:611–8.

18. RIPOLLES T, AGRAMUNT M, MARTINEZ M J, COSTA S, GOMEZ-ABRIL S A, RICHART J. The role of ultrasound in the diagnosis, management and evolutive prognosis of acute left-sided colonic diverticulitis: a review of 208 patients. *Eur Radiol* 2003;**13**:2587–95.

19. BROEKMAN B A M W, PUYLAERT J B C M, VAN DESSEL T. Sigmoid diverticulitis in the female: transvaginal sonographic findings. *J Clin Ultrasound* 1993;**21**:393–5.

20. HOLLERWEGER A, RETTENBACHER T, MACHEINER P, BRUNNER W, GRITZMANN N. Sigmoid diverticulitis: value of transrectal sonography in addition to transabdominal sonography. *AJR Am J Roentgenol* 2000;**175**:1155–60.

21. PUYLAERT J B C M. Ultrasound of acute GI tract conditions. *Eur Radiol* 2001;**11**:1867–77.

22. GRITZMANN N, HOLLERWEGER A, MACHEINER P, RETTENBACHER T. Transabdominal sonography of the gastrointestinal tract. *Eur Radiol* 2002;**12**:1748–61.

23. VALETTE P-J, RIOUX M, PILLEUL F, SAURIN J-C, FOUQUE P, HENRY L. Ultrasonography of chronic inflammatory bowel diseases. *Eur Radiol* 2001;**11**:1859–66.

24. ABU-YOUSEF M M. Ultrasonography of the right lower quadrant. *Ultrasound Q* 2001;**17**:211–25.

25. JOHNSTON AT, KHAN A L, BLEAKNEY R, KEENAN R A. Stromal tumour within a Meckel's diverticulum: CT and ultrasound findings. *Br J Radiol* 2001;**74**:1142–4.

26. TRUONG M, ATRI M, BRET P M, et al. Sonographic appearance of benign and malignant conditions of the colon. *AJR Am J Roentgenol* 1998;**170**:1 451–5.

27. MEN S, AKHAN O, KOROGLU M. Percutaneous drainage of abdominal abscess. *Eur J Radiol* 2002;**43**:204–18.

28. SPERLING D C, NEEDLEMAN L, ESCHELMAN D J, HOVSEPIAN D M, LEV-TOAFF A S. *Radiology* 1998;**208**:111–5.

29. HARISINGHANI M G, GERVAIS D A, MAHER M M, CHO C H, HAHN PF, VARGHESE J, et al. Transgluteal approach for percutaneous drainage of deep pelvic abscesses: 154 cases. *Radiology* 2003;**228**:701–5.

30. van Sonnenberg E, D'Agostino H B, Casola G, Goodacre B W, Sanchez R B, Taylor B. US-guided transvaginal drainage of pelvic abscesses and fluid collections. *Radiology* 1991;**181**:53–6.

31. Feld R, Eschelman D J, Sagerman J E, Segal S, Hovsepian D M, Sullivan K L. Treatment of pelvic abscesses and other fluid collections: efficacy of transvaginal sonographically guided aspiration and drainage. *AJR Am J Roentgenol* 1994;**163**:1141–5.

32. Lee B C, McGahan J F, Bijan B. Single-step transvaginal aspiration and drainage for suspected pelvic abscesses refractory to antibiotic therapy. *J Ultrasound Med* 2002;**21**:731–8.

33. Nelson A L, Sinow R M, Oliak D. Transrectal ultrasonographically guided drainage of gynaecologic pelvic abscesses. *Am J Obstet Gynecol* 2000;**182**:1382–8.

34. Alexander A A, Eschelman D J, Nazarian L N, Bonn J. Transrectal sonographically guided drainage of deep pelvic abscesses. *AJR Am J Roentgenol* 1994;**162**:1227–30.

35. Kuligowska E, Keller E, Ferrucci J T. Treatment of pelvic abscesses: value of one-step sonographically guided transrectal needle aspiration and lavage. *AJR* 1995;**164**:201–6.

36. Ryan R S, McGrath F P, Haslam P J, Varghese J C, Lee M J. Ultrasound-guided endocavitary drainage of pelvic abscesses: technique, results and complications. *Clin Radiol* 2003;**58**:75–9.

37. Spencer J A, Swift S E, Wilkinson N, Boon A P, Lane G, Perren T J. Peritoneal carcinomatosis: image-guided peritoneal core biopsy for tumor type and patient care. *Radiology* 2001;**221**:173–7.

38. Laing F C, Benson C B, DiSalvo D N, Brown D L, Frates M C, Loughlin K R. Distal ureteric calculi: detection with vaginal US. *Radiology* 1994;**192**:545–8.

39. Zerin J M, Baker D R, Casale J A. Single-system ureterocoeles in infants and children: imaging features. *Paediatr Radiol* 2000;**30**:139–46.

40. Shimoya K, Shimizu T, Hashimoto K, Koyama M, Sawamura A, Murata Y. Diagnosis of ureterocoele with transvaginal sonography. *Gynecol Obstet Invest* 2002; **54**:58–60.

41. Datta S N, Allen G M, Evans R, Vaughton K C, Lucas M G. Urinary tract ultrasonography in the evaluation of haematuria – a report of over 1,000 cases. *Ann R Coll Surg Engl* 2002;**84**:203–5.

42. Dibb M J, Noble D J, Peh W C, Lam C H, Yip K H, Li J H, et al. Ultrasonographic analysis of bladder tumors. *Clin Imaging* 2001;**25**:416–20.

43. Horstman W G, McFarland R M, Gorman J D. Color Doppler sonographic findings in patients with transitional cell carcinoma of the bladder and renal pelvis. *J Ultrasound Med* 1995;**14**:129–33.

44. Sendag F, Vidinli H, Kazan M, Italy I M, Asker N, Vidinli B, et al. Role of perineal sonography in the evaluation of patients with stress urinary incontinence. *Aust N Z J Obstet Gynaecol* 2003;**43**:54–7.

45. Cross J J, Fynes M, Berman L, Perera D. Prevalence of cystic paraurethral structures in asymptomatic women at endovaginal and perineal sonography. *Clin Radiol* 2001;**56**:575–8.

46. Baron R L, Banner M P, Pollack H M. Isolated internal iliac artery aneurysms presenting as giant pelvic masses. *AJR Am J Roentgenol* 1983;**140**:784–6.

47. Arenson A M, Graham R, Hamilton P, Mitchell S. Iliac artery aneurysms presenting as large pelvic masses. *Australas Radiol* 1989;**33**:229–32.

48. Borst-Krafek B, Fink A M, Lipp C, Umek H, Kohn H, Steiner A. Proximal extent of pelvic vein thrombosis and its association with pulmonary embolism. *J Vasc Surg* 2003;**37**:518–22.

49. Halligan S, Campbell D, Bartram C I, Rogers V, El-Haddad C, Patel S, et al. Transvaginal ultrasound examination of women with and without pelvic venous congestion. *Clin Radiol* 2000;**55**:954–8.

50. Park S J, Lim J W, Ko Y T, Lee D H, Yoon Y, Oh J H, et al. Diagnosis of pelvic congestion syndrome using transabdominal and transvaginal sonography. *AJR Am J Roentgenol* 2004;**182**:683–8.

51. Hanna A S, Morandi X. Anterior sacral meningocoele in pregnancy. Case report. *J Neurosurg* 2001;**94**:162–4.

52. Bradley M, Morgan D, Pentlow B, Roe A. The groin hernia: an ultrasound diagnosis? *Ann R Coll Surg Engl* 2003;**85**:178–80.

53. Vos D I, Scheltinga M R. Incidence and outcome of surgical repair of spigelian hernia. *Br J Surg* 2004;**91**:640–4.

54. Harris R D, Holtzman S R, Poppe A M. Clinical outcome in female patients with pelvic pain and normal pelvic US findings. *Radiology* 2000;**216**:440–3.

Ultrasound imaging in reproductive medicine

POVILAS SLADKEVICIUS

Introduction

One in six couples seeks help for infertility during their reproductive years.[1] Subfertility investigations should be performed without delays (because female fertility decreases with age) and should be as non-invasive as possible.[2] Many fertility clinics use diagnostic hysteroscopy to assess the uterine cavity and evaluate the tubal ostia. Laparoscopy is also often used to examine internal pelvic organs and to assess tubal patency. However, both hysteroscopy and laparoscopy are invasive and expensive tests which could be replaced by transvaginal ultrasound examination. Simplified ultrasound-based infertility investigation protocols have been described.[3,4] The concept of a 'pivotal' pelvic ultrasound examination includes an examination of the uterus and uterine cavity, endometrium, ovarian morphology and follicular size, blood flow in the uterus and ovaries and hystero-contrast sonography (HyCoSy) to check tubal patency, all performed at the same examination.[3–5] The late preovulatory phase of the menstrual cycle (days 8–12) is usually suggested as the optimal time to perform these examinations. Most studies involving the ultrasound techniques referred to in this chapter are classified as evidence grade B.[6]

The pivotal scan

The aim of the pivotal scan is to assess the uterus, endometrium, fallopian tubes and ovaries.

Uterus

Ultrasound examination is as effective a diagnostic test as hysteroscopy or laparoscopy for the diagnosis of uterine abnormalities.[7] Normal findings at ultrasound examination of the uterus and endometrium are described in Chapter 2. Uterine size and shape may be affected by adenomyosis or fibroids. The shape of the uterus can be also be distorted by congenital uterine anomalies. Ultrasonographic features of uterine pathology are described in Chapter 3. A causal relationship between fibroids or adenomyosis and infertility has not been established,[8] except in cases of submucous fibroids. In women undergoing assisted reproduction, the presence of uterine fibroids affecting the uterine cavity is associated with a reduced chance of clinical pregnancy.[9,10] Surgical treatment of intramural and subserous fibroids does not enhance pregnancy rate in women undergoing assisted reproduction,[11,12] while removal of submucous fibroids is beneficial.[8,9] Studies have shown that the presence of adenomyosis on ultrasound scan has no impact on the rate of embryonic implantation in cycles of *in vitro* fertilisation (IVF).[13]

Three-dimensional ultrasound has been used to assess uterine anatomy and to detect congenital anomalies of the uterus. The ability to visualise both the uterine cavity and the myometrium on a three-dimensional scan facilitates the diagnosis of uterine anomalies and enables easy differentiation between a subseptate and bicornuate uterus. Complete or almost complete agreement (92–100%) between three-dimensional ultrasound scanning and hysterosalpingogram[14,15] and laparoscopy[16] in the assessment of uterine malformations has been reported. The role of surgical correction of uterine anomalies to improve fertility or assisted reproduction outcome is uncertain.[17,18]

Ultrasonographic assessment of the uterus and endometrium is best performed in the late follicular phase of the cycle. Focal lesions in the uterine cavity, such as endometrial polyps, submucous fibroids, foreign bodies and adhesions, may be seen at conventional greyscale imaging. If the findings are not clear, the scan can be supplemented with saline infusion sonography (SIS). This is a simple test which involves injection of 5–15 ml saline through a catheter into the uterine cavity.[19] SIS has been shown to be as effective as diagnostic hysteroscopy for the evaluation of the uterine cavity.[20,21] However, it is less expensive and more acceptable to women than hysteroscopy as it involves the use of very fine catheters and a small amount of fluid to distend the uterine cavity.[22] Therefore, SIS should be performed on all fertility patients if there is a suspicion of an abnormality of the uterine cavity on conventional transvaginal ultrasound examination.

There is little robust evidence to support routine removal of endometrial polyps in infertile women in order to improve reproductive outcomes.[12] However, one randomised controlled trial has shown that hysteroscopic polypectomy doubled the pregnancy rate from 28% to 63% in couples undergoing intrauterine insemination (IUI) treatment.[23] These results are in accordance with two non-randomised studies of polypectomies in women undergoing IVF treatment.[24,25] There seems to be an emerging consensus that, if an endometrial polyp is the only detectable problem in an infertile couple, it is justified to remove it, as spontaneous conceptions frequently occur in the first 3–4 months following surgery.[25,26]

Assessment of the uterine cavity is important in subfertile women who have previously used intrauterine contraceptive devices or have undergone

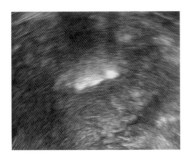

FIGURE 9.1 A longitudinal view of the uterus showing hyperechoic tissue with shadowing adjacent to the internal os, a typical ultrasound finding in women with retained fetal bones within the uterine cavity

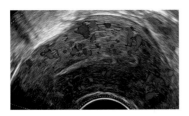

FIGURE 9.2 Uterine vascularity using colour Doppler: a longitudinal view of an anteverted uterus on transvaginal scan demonstrates larger arcuate vessels located subserosally and thin, parallel radial arteries approaching the uterine cavity at right angles

termination of pregnancy. The differential diagnosis in such women includes forgotten intrauterine contraceptive devices,[19,27] fetal bones remaining,[28] osseous metaplasia,[29] calcified submucous fibroids caused by trauma during dilatation and curettage[27] and Asherman syndrome.[30] The presence of foreign bodies within the endometrium may lead to subfertility by preventing implantation of a blastocyst because of increased prostaglandin production (thus changing the milieu of the uterine cavity) or by inducing reactive endometritis.[27] Removal of foreign bodies from the uterine cavity may restore fertility.[28,29] Fetal bones and osseous calcifications are seen within the uterine cavity at transvaginal ultrasound examination as hyperechoic foci or linear echoes with acoustic shadowing (Figure 9.1).

Doppler ultrasound assessment of blood flow in the uterine arteries and their branches plays a role in the monitoring of menstrual cycles. In the follicular phase of the cycle, uterine artery pulsed Doppler waveform is characterised by a high peak systolic velocity, proto-diastolic notch and low end-diastolic velocity, which is typical of high impedance to blood flow. During the luteal phase, the pulsed Doppler waveform in the uterine artery typically shows high peak systolic velocity and high end diastolic flow with no proto-diastolic notch. Impedance to blood flow is significantly lower than in the follicular phase, which might be explained by progesterone induced vasodilatation.[31-33]

Spiral arteries (subendometrial arteries) can be seen within the functional zone of the endometrium, using colour or power Doppler ultrasound (Figure 9.2). Their pulsed Doppler waveform is characterised by much lower velocity and impedance than the main uterine arteries but the changes in resistance follow the same cyclical pattern as observed in the uterine arteries.[31]

A substantial proportion of subfertile women have higher impedance to flow in their uterine circulation (higher pulsatility index in the uterine artery) compared with fertile women.[34,35] Higher impedance to flow in the uterine circulation appears to be associated with reduced conception rate in assisted reproduction cycles. This suggests that uterine impedance to flow may affect uterine receptivity. Women who are infertile and who conceive as a result of assisted reproductive techniques are at higher risk of spontaneous miscarriage, preterm birth and fetal growth restriction than women who are fertile.[36,37] It is plausible that the pre-existing increased uterine impedance to flow and the higher risk of pregnancy complications in women who are infertile are interrelated. However, there is no established treatment to improve blood flow in the uterine arteries and so the value of including measurement of uterine artery blood flow velocities in infertility investigations must be questioned.

Fallopian tubes

Assessment of tubal patency is an integral part of routine fertility investigations. Although healthy tubes are not visible on conventional greyscale ultrasound examination, hydrosalpinx can be seen (see Chapter
6). A finding of hydrosalpinx is significant and indicates tubal blockage.
The presence of hydrosalpinx on transvaginal ultrasound examination
in women undergoing IVF is associated with poor implantation, poor
pregnancy rates and increased early pregnancy loss. There is some evidence to suggest that the presence of a hydrosalpinx affects endometrial
receptivity.[38–40] Before starting IVF treatment, all women with ultrasonographically visible hydrosalpinges should be offered laparoscopic salpingectomy to improves the chance of successful IVF treatment.[12, 41]

Traditionally, tubal patency has been assessed by hysterosalpingography (HSG). This examination can be replaced by HyCoSy, where the
flow of contrast medium from the uterine cavity into the fallopian tubes
is observed using ultrasound.[42] HyCoSy can be incorporated in the pivotal scan. Once learned, it is relatively easy and quick to perform.[43] No
anaesthesia or sedative is needed. The examination begins with a conventional transvaginal scan where the uterine position is determined
and any uterine or adnexal abnormalities are noted. Then the vagina
and cervix are cleansed with chlorhexidine and a balloon catheter is
inserted gently through the cervical canal using a pair of forceps. The
balloon is then inflated with air to fix it in position above the internal
os. Saline is then infused (hydrosonography) to visualise the uterine
cavity. Then a contrast medium is slowly injected during continuous
scanning.[43]

During HyCoSy, the whole tube can rarely be seen in a single scanning plane because of tubal tortuosity. However, by manipulating the
probe, the contrast can be followed from the interstitial part to the
fimbrial end of the tube, where free spill can be observed. Observing
free spill may be difficult, because the contrast agent has the same
echogenicity as the surrounding bowel. The proximal end of the tube,
however, when filled with running contrast medium is almost always
visible. If one can observe moving contrast in the interstitial part of the
tube for 10 seconds and if no hydrosalpinx is seen, the fallopian tube is
almost certainly patent, even if free spill of contrast is not clearly seen
(Figure 9.3).[44]

Three-dimensional ultrasound enables the capture of a volume
including the full length of the tube. Power Doppler, which is sensitive
to slow flow, makes it possible to detect the flow of contrast medium
along the full length of the tube and free spill at the fimbrial end of
the tube at three-dimensional ultrasound examination.[45, 46] Surface ren-

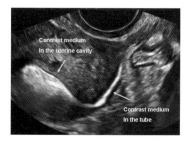

FIGURE 9.3 HyCoSy technique with
hyperechoic contrast visible within the
uterine cavity and proximal section of
the left fallopian tube

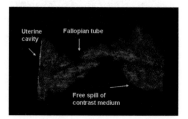

FIGURE 9.4 Tubal patency, using
three-dimensional power Doppler to
demonstrate the flow of contrast within
the entire length of the fallopian tube

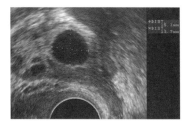

FIGURE 9.5a

Follicle growth and ovulation in a normal cycle: **a)** a 14-mm follicle is seen on day 11 which contains anechoic fluid; its inner wall is smooth and clear; **b)** on day 14, the mean follicle diameter has increased to 20 mm; **c)** on day 15, the follicle is collapsed and Doppler examination shows high vascularity typical of corpus luteum

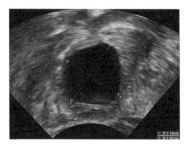

FIGURE 9.5b

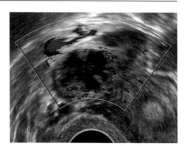

FIGURE 9.5c

dering of power Doppler signals in a three-dimensional volume demonstrates the stream of contrast along the fallopian tubes.[45,46] Despite these obvious advantages, Watermann *et al.*[47] found that the use of three-dimensional power Doppler ultrasound did not significantly contribute to the diagnostic accuracy of HyCoSy (Figure 9.4).

Ovaries

The appearances of normal ovaries on transvaginal ultrasound examination are described in Chapter 2. In the follicular phase of the cycle at least four to six follicles are seen, one of which grows to become the dominant follicle: that is, the ovulating follicle. During the 4–5 days preceding ovulation, the dominant follicle grows at a rate of approximately 2 mm/day. Just before ovulation, the follicle reaches an average diameter of 21 mm, range 17–27 mm.[48] After ovulation it collapses, with a decrease in its size, and it changes into a solid or cystic mass with internal echoes, the corpus luteum. Concurrently, the amount of fluid in the pouch of Douglas increases (Figure 9.5).

POLYCYSTIC OVARIES

Polycystic ovaries are characterised by increased number of antral follicles, prominent ovarian stroma and increased ovarian volume (Figures 9.6, 9.7). They are different from multicystic ovaries, which contain a few follicles larger than 10 mm and no increase in ovarian stroma.[49] In 2003, new guidelines for the diagnosis of polycystic ovary syndrome (PCOS) were produced.[50,51] According to these guidelines, a diagnosis of PCOS should be made when at least two of the following three criteria are met:

▷ hyperandrogenism
▷ chronic anovulation
▷ polycystic ovaries at ultrasound examination.

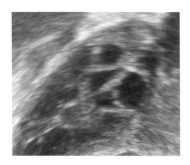

FIGURE 9.6 Polycystic ovaries in a woman with a history of infertility and anovulation; note the large number of small follicles scattered within the ovary; the ovarian volume was 13 ml

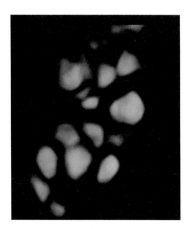

FIGURE 9.7 Three-dimensional image of follicles in a case of polycystic ovaries

Polycystic ovaries should manifest at least one of the following features:

▷ 12 or more follicles measuring 2–9 mm in diameter
▷ increased ovarian volume (greater than 10 cm³).

If there are one or more follicles greater than 10 mm in diameter, volume calculation should be repeated at a time of ovarian quiescence. The presence of one criterion in one ovary is sufficient to provide a diagnosis of polycystic ovaries. The distribution of follicles, characteristics of the ovarian stroma, results of Doppler ultrasound or three-dimensional ultrasound are not required to make a diagnosis of polycystic ovaries.[50,51] Women with polycystic ovaries who have neither hyperandrogenism nor chronic anovulation do not have PCOS. They have only polycystic ovaries. However, polycystic ovaries have the same adverse effects on results of assisted reproduction techniques as PCOS;[52,53] that is, an increased risk of ovarian hyperstimulation syndrome (OHSS) and multiple pregnancy.

ASSESSMENT OF OVARIAN RESERVE

The number of antral follicles decreases between the ages of 22 and 42 years[54,55] and it may be used as a measure of female fertility. Ovarian volume and antral follicle count have been used to assess ovarian reserve at the time of initiation of ovarian stimulation both for IVF treatment and ovulation induction. Baseline FSH levels, number of cycle cancellations and amount of gonadotrophins required for cycle stimulation tend to be significantly higher, while the number of retrieved oocytes is significantly lower in women with small ovaries and only few antral follicles on baseline scan.[56,57] In some studies, there was a significant correlation between the number of antral follicles and the FSH levels on cycle day 3, amount of gonadotrophin used, number of oocytes retrieved, number of fertilised eggs and number of embryos developed in IVF cycles.[58,59] Assessment of ovarian reserve therefore helps in counselling patients about likely success of assisted reproductive techniques and in planning ovarian stimulation with gonadotrophins.

DOPPLER ULTRASOUND EXAMINATION OF OVARIAN CIRCULATION

Angiogenesis, vessel maturation and vessel regression seem to play a critical role in the selection of the dominant follicle, ovulation and corpus luteum formation and function.[60] According to results of colour Doppler ultrasound examinations performed in normal menstrual cycles, blood flow in intraovarian vessels is characterised by low velocity and relatively high resistance in the early follicular phase.[31,32] Dur-

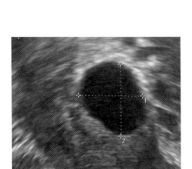

FIGURE 9.8 a

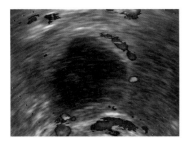

FIGURE 9.8 b

a) An ultrasound scan on day 14 shows a normal 19-mm preovulatory follicle which contains anechoic fluid; **b)** a follow-up scan 48 hours later shows that the follicle has slightly increased in size; its wall has become irregular and the follicular fluid is moderately echogenic; on Doppler examination, the follicle vascularity is only marginally increased. These findings are typical of a luteinised unruptured follicle

ing follicular growth, intraovarian blood flow increases continuously as reflected by an increase in peak systolic velocity in ovarian vessels.[31,61] After the LH surge,[62] peak systolic velocity in the vessels of the dominant follicle rises significantly with almost no change in pulsatility index. A subjective scoring system for assessment of follicular vascularity using power Doppler imaging has been suggested.[63,64] The scoring system consists of assessing the percentage of the follicular circumference with detectable colour Doppler signals. Poor follicular vascularisation seems to be associated with poor pregnancy rates.[63,64]

In a normal luteal phase, a colour or power Doppler image of the dominant ovary shows a colour ring surrounding the corpus luteum. This colour ring reflects the rich vascularisation of the wall of the corpus luteum. High peak systolic velocity in the vessels of the wall of the corpus luteum is supposed to indicate a healthy corpus luteum,[65] whereas low velocity is said to indicate an unruptured luteinised follicle (Figure 9.8).[66] The vascularisation of the corpus luteum increases from ovulation to the mid-luteal phase and then decreases until menstruation. The progesterone concentration changes reflect the pattern of the changes in the vascularisation of the corpus luteum.[33,67]

Adequate ovarian blood circulation is important for normal ovarian function. However, whether Doppler examination of ovarian and follicular vascularisation in a natural menstrual cycle before starting IVF treatment can predict the quality of eggs produced during IVF remains to be clarified. One can only assume that good quality of the eggs in the natural menstrual cycles is predictive of good oocytes during assisted reproduction.

Ovarian stromal blood flow velocity is significantly higher in women with polycystic ovaries than in women with normal ovaries.[68,69] The reason for this increased stromal flow is unknown. It may be related to high levels of angiogenic cytokines in the theca cell layer. It has been shown that women with polycystic ovaries have higher ovarian stromal blood flow velocities and serum concentration of vascular endothelial growth factor (VEGF) than those with normal ovaries.[52] It is well known that women with polycystic ovaries are susceptible to OHSS and increased stromal flow may be associated with increased susceptibility to this condition. VEGF is used to assess ovarian response during infertility treatment. A significant rise in serum VEGF concentration after administration of human chorionic gonadotrophin (hCG) appears to be one of the most important predictors of OHSS.[70]

ADNEXAL TUMOURS

It is not unusual to detect adnexal tumours during the pivotal scan, often ovarian cysts. Several types of adnexal tumours manifest typical ultrasound morphology (see Chapter 6).[71,72] Endometriomas[73] and dermoid cysts[74] are two examples of frequently encountered masses. They account for more than two-thirds of persistent adnexal masses in women of fertile age.[75] Local intrafollicular ovarian inflammation and intraperitoneal inflammation at the time of menstruation are important processes in the biology of endometriosis and may explain reduced oocyte quality, infertility and implantation of menstrual endometrial cells on to the peritoneum.[76,77] Women with large ovarian endometriomas may benefit from laparoscopic surgery.[78] Removal of small endometriomas does not improve the chances of pregnancy in IVF treatment cycles.[79] Treatment of minimal and mild ovarian endometriosis does not enhance the results of assisted reproduction.[12]

It is also possible to diagnose extraovarian endometriosis with ultrasound.[80,81] Surgical ablation or resection of endometriotic lesions seems to provide benefit, even in the absence of correctable anatomic defects. After reconstruction of the fallopian tubes, if needed, or in women with less extensive disease, controlled ovarian stimulation in conjunction with intrauterine insemination may be effective treatment. IVF represents an effective means of bypassing the hostile peritoneal environment and anatomical distortion associated with extraovarian endometriosis.[82]

Ultrasound examination during subfertility treatment

Ultrasound examination is used to monitor endometrial growth and ovarian response to medical treatment. Appropriate endometrial growth indicates good endometrial receptivity. Appropriate ovarian response to gonadotrophin stimulation increases the chances that good quality eggs will be released in ovulation induction cycles and that good embryos will be available for embryo transfer in IVF cycles. Ultrasound is also used to monitor embryo transfer.

Monitoring of the uterus and endometrium

Both greyscale ultrasound examination of the endometrium and Doppler ultrasound examination of the uterine arteries have been used to assess 'endometrial receptivity' in IVF cycles.[63,83–93] As estradiol levels rise as a result of follicles maturing, the endometrial thickness also increases. The preovulatory endometrium on the day of hCG administration should have a triple-layer appearance and should have a thickness of at least 7mm (Figure 9.9).[94]

'Good' uterine endometrial vascularisation is considered to be necessary for successful outcome of IVF and attempts have been made to

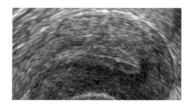

FIGURE 9.9 a

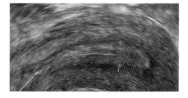

FIGURE 9.9 b

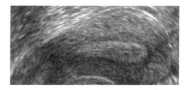

FIGURE 9.9 c

Serial assessment of the endometrium during stimulation of ovulation with clomifene; the endometrium is becoming progressively thicker as the cycle progresses **(a–c)**; the midline echo becomes blurred after ovulation and the endometrial echogenicity is increased

improve uterine perfusion by treating with low-dose aspirin or a nitric oxide donor.[95,96] However, further studies are needed to understand and evaluate the endometrial vascular pattern both in spontaneous and stimulated cycles, as well as the safety of the drugs used to improve endometrial vascularisation.

Results of published studies indicate that endometrial receptivity is only one among several factors that are important for implantation. In oocyte donation programmes, equivalent implantation and pregnancy rates have been found in young women sharing oocytes and their recipients, who were up to 45 years old. This suggests that oocyte quality and embryo quality are the most important factors for successful implantation.[97,98]

Monitoring follicular development

Ultrasound greyscale imaging is regarded as sufficiently accurate to be used alone for monitoring follicular growth during gonadotrophin therapy,[99–101] particularly when GnRH agonists are used for downregulation.[102] An initial scan of the pelvis is mandatory to rule out functional cysts before starting ovulation induction. The first ultrasound scan during therapy is scheduled on day 8 of ovarian stimulation. The results of this scan determine whether the dose of the stimulatory drugs should be increased or reduced and the timing of the next scan. However, even when follicular growth is monitored by ultrasound an estimated 15–30% of ovulation induction cycles are complicated, for example by a spontaneous LH surge, hyperstimulation, cyst formation or poor ovarian response.

Follicular size is expressed as the mean of its two largest orthogonal diameters.[103] Normal follicles increase by 1–3 mm/day until the size of a mature follicle is reached.[103] When the largest follicle is 18–20 mm during gonadotrophin stimulation, ovulation is induced by the administration of hCG. In IVF cycles, once the three largest follicles have attained a diameter of 18 mm or more, hCG is administered and egg collection is scheduled. If a long protocol GnRH analogue schedule is used, the day of hCG administration can be safely delayed by 1–2 days without compromising the treatment results.[104]

For accurate ultrasound monitoring, it is necessary to differentiate ovarian follicles from other anatomical structures with similar appearance. Blood vessels can be recognised by changing the position of the transducer by 90 degrees, whereby a longitudinal view of the vessel is seen as a tubular structure, or by using colour Doppler ultrasound (Figure 9.10). Bowel shows peristalsis. Hydrosalpinges and ovarian cysts do not change in size on serial scans. This is in contrast to follicles, which grow between scans.[105] Persistent cysts, which may appear during ovu-

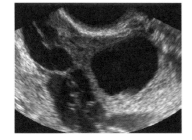

FIGURE 9.10 a

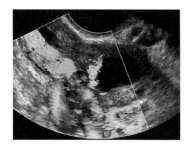

FIGURE 9.10 b

a) Large pelvic veins adjacent to the ovary appear anechoic on B-mode image and are sometimes difficult to differentiate form developing follicles; **b)** the use of colour Doppler facilitates differential diagnosis between follicles which are signal free from abundant Doppler signals within the blood vessels

lation induction or downregulation treatment, can be followed up by ultrasound. Response to cyst treatment by oral contraceptives or by GnRH analogues can be monitored, or puncture and aspiration of the cyst under ultrasound guidance can be performed. Absence of follicles, or growth of only a few follicles despite administration of large doses of gonadotrophin, indicates poor ovarian reserve or even premature ovarian failure. Appearance of more than 35 follicles associated with high serum estradiol levels suggests development of OHSS. In this situation, it is advisable to withhold hCG administration or to administer GnRH analogues. The severity of OHSS is determined by clinical signs (enlarged ovaries, ascites, oedema, pleural effusion, haemoconcentration) and ultrasound findings: ovarian size and the presence of fluid in the peritoneal or pleural cavities. Ultrasound is an important tool in monitoring the course of OHSS and in determining treatment measures (Figure 9.11).[106]

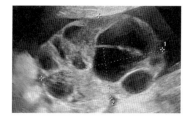

FIGURE 9.11 Ovarian hyperstimulation; note an enlarged ovary with multiple corpus luteum cysts and ascites

There is possibly a relationship between ovarian vascularisation as assessed by Doppler ultrasound and the outcome of IVF treatment, good vascularisation of the follicles being associated with more favourable outcome.[63, 107–110] It has been suggested that evaluation of follicular vascularity by colour or power Doppler ultrasound could be used to determine which follicles contain good eggs resulting in good preimplantation embryos that have good chances to implant and develop into pregnancy.[108–110] Whether measurement of blood flow velocity in follicular vessels[63, 108] is valuable for prediction of outcome of IVF treatment remains to be clarified in randomised trials. Methods of assessing the vascularisation of individual follicles are difficult to practise, because it is difficult to determine exactly from which follicle registered Doppler signals are derived. Moreover, Doppler examination prolongs the egg collection procedure considerably.

Ultrasound-guided IVF procedures

Ultrasound-guided oocyte retrieval

Transvaginal oocyte retrieval does not require general anaesthesia. It is an inexpensive and quick procedure, which is routinely performed in outpatient settings. It is associated with little morbidity and low risk of complications. Adhesions in the pelvis do not hamper ultrasound-guided oocyte retrieval. During transvaginal ultrasound-guided follicle aspiration, it is important to place the tip of the needle precisely within the follicle that is being aspirated. The needle is passed quickly through the vaginal wall and the ovarian capsule into a follicle situated in the middle of the ovary. Puncture of large pelvic vessels must be avoided. Colour Doppler helps to distinguish vessels from cystic structures in the pelvis (Figure 9.10). The follicular fluid is aspirated and the collapsing follicle is observed on the ultrasound screen. The needle is then moved to another follicle by gentle tilting or angling of the transducer but without withdrawal of the needle from the ovarian stroma. All follicles are systematically aspirated. Before the needle is withdrawn from the ovary, those follicles that did not yield an oocyte are re-entered and any remaining fluid is aspirated. In this way, the recovery of oocytes can be maximised. When all follicles in one ovary have been aspirated, the needle is completely withdrawn from that ovary and another puncture is made through the vaginal wall into the other ovary.

Acute pelvic inflammatory disease following oocyte collection is rare (0.6%). Abscess formation after follicle aspiration constitutes only 9% of all complications after ultrasound-guided transvaginal oocyte collection.[111] Pelvic abscesses can be drained by ultrasound-guided puncture using the Seldinger technique.[112] A needle is placed in the abscess under ultrasound guidance. The contents are aspirated before a flexible guidewire is introduced through the needle. The needle is extracted and a plastic catheter with multiple perforations is slid over the guidewire.[112] The guidewire is then removed and the catheter is fixed to the patient's thigh. The patient is treated with antibiotics and is rescanned to confirm the regression of the abscess before catheter removal.

Ultrasound-guided embryo transfer

Ultrasound guidance of embryo transfer seems to improve the outcome of IVF.[113, 114] The explanation may be a reduction in the incidence of difficult transfers that negatively affect clinical pregnancy rate. To reduce the angle between the cervix and the corpus uteri and to facilitate the introduction of the catheter, embryo transfer is performed when the patient has a full urinary bladder. Transabdominal scanning is preferable, although a transvaginal approach has been described.[113] The uterus and endometrial cavity are visualised in a sagittal plane through a full bladder. An assistant holds the probe. Efforts are made to see the catheter as it traverses the cervix and passes through the internal cervical os. Introduction of the catheter is stopped when its tip is 1 cm from the fundus uteri. The transfer volume is gently expelled and the air and fluid surrounding the embryos are seen as bright spots moving through the catheter to be deposited in the uterine fundus (Figure 9.12). Removal of the catheter is followed by ultrasound. The fluid droplets with the embryos should be retained in the fundus. After removal, the catheter is checked under a microscope and flushed for embryos

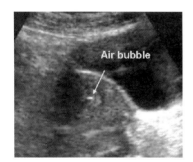

FIGURE 9.12 Ultrasound-guided embryo transfer: the visualisation of the position of the catheter is facilitated by the detection of an air bubble within the uterine cavity on transabdominal scan

remaining within its lumen or adherent to its outside. A catheter with an echodense tip for ultrasound-guided embryo transfer[115] allows good visualisation, even in women who are obese and those with an empty urinary bladder.

Conclusion

Ultrasound plays a dominant role in the diagnostic assessment of the infertile couple, for planning and monitoring fertility treatment. Ultrasound has almost completely eliminated the need for more invasive tests such as hysteroscopy and laparoscopy, which has helped to reduce the cost of investigations and treatment. The use of ultrasound to assess tubal patency has replaced HSG and has eliminated potentially severe risks such as radiation exposure and risk of anaphylactic reaction to iodine contrast. Further work is necessary to establish the role of more complex ultrasound techniques such as Doppler blood flow studies and three-dimensional ultrasound in the assessment of ovarian reserve and endometrial receptivity.

REFERENCES

1. HULL M G, GLAZENER C M, KELLY N J, CONWAY D I, FOSTER P A, HINTON R A, et al. Population study of causes, treatment and outcome of infertility. BMJ (Clin Res Ed) 1985;291:1693–7.

2. CROSIGNANI P, RUBIN B. Guidelines to the prevalence, diagnosis and management of infertility. Hum Reprod 1996;11:1775–807.

3. KELLY S M, SLADKEVICIUS P, CAMPBELL S, NARGUND G. Investigation of the infertile couple: a one-stop ultrasound-based approach. Debate Hum Reprod 2001;16:2481–4.

4. NARGUND G. Time for an ultrasound revolution in reproductive medicine. Ultrasound Obstet Gynecol 2002;20:107–11.

5. SLADKEVICIUS P, CAMPBELL S. Advanced ultrasound examination in the management of subfertility. Curr Opin Obstet Gynecol 2000;12:221–5.

6. SACKETT D L, RICHARDSON W S, ROSENBERG W, HAYNES R B. Evidence-based Medicine. How to Practice and Teach Evidence-based Medicine. Edinburgh: Churchill Livingstone; 1997.

7. HAUGE K, FLO K, RIEDHART M, GRANBERG S. Can ultrasound-based investigations replace laparoscopy and hysteroscopy in infertility? Eur J Obstet Gynecol Reprod Biol 2000;92:167–70.

8. PRITTS E A. Fibroids and infertility: a systematic review of the evidence. Obstet Gynecol Surv 2001;56:483–91.

9. ELDAR-GEVA T, MEAGHER S, HEALY D L, MACLACHLAN V, BREHENY S, WOOD C. Effect of intramural, subserosal and submucosal uterine fibroids on the outcome of assisted reproductive technology treatment. Fertil Steril 1998;70:687–91.

10. DONNEZ J, JADOUL P. What are the implications of myomas on fertility. A need for a debate? Hum Reprod 2002;17:1424–30.

11. VERCELLINI P, MADDALENA S, DE GIORGI O, AIMI G, CROSIGNANI PG. Abdominal myomectomy for infertility: a comprehensive review. Hum Reprod 1998;13:873–9.

12. National Collaborating Centre for Women's and Children's Health. Fertility: Assessment and Treatment for People with Fertility Problems. London: RCOG Press; 2004.

13. CAMARGO F, GAYTAN J, CALIGARA C. SIMON C, PELLICER A, REMOHI J. Impact of ultrasound diagnosis of adenomyosis on recipients of sibling oocytes (abstract). Fertil Steril 2001;76 (Suppl: 1):S150

14. WU M H, HSU C C, HUANG K E. Detection of congenital Mullerian duct anomalies using three-dimensional ultrasound. J Clin Ultrasound 1997;9:487–92.

15. JURKOVIC D, GEIPEL A, GRUBOECK K, JAUNIAUX E, NATUCCI M, CAMPBELL S. Three-dimensional ultrasound for the assessment of uterine anatomy and detection of congenital anomalies: a comparison with hysterosalpingography and two-dimensional sonography. Ultrasound Obstet Gynecol 1995;5:233–7.

16. RAGA F, BONILLA-MUSOLES F, BLANES J, OSBORNE NG. Congenital Mullerian anomalies: diagnostic accuracy of three-dimensional ultrasound. *Fertil Steril* 1996;**65**:523–8.

17. SIMON C, MARTINEZ L, PARDO F, TORTAJADA M, PELLICER A. Mullerian defects in women with normal reproductive outcome. *Fertil Steril* 1991;**56**:1192–3.

18. LIN PC, BHATNAGAR KP, NETTLETON GS, NAKAJIMA ST. Female genital anomalies affecting reproduction. *Fertil Steril* 2002;**78**:899–915.

19. ANDO H, TODA S, HARADA M, YOSHIDA S, KONDO I, MASAHASHI T, et al. Which infertile women should be indicated for sonohysterography? *Ultrasound Obstet Gynecol* 2004;**24**:566–71.

20. WOLMAN I, JAFFA A, HARTOOV J, BAR-AM A, DAVID MP. Sensitivity and specificity of sonohysterography for the evaluation of the uterine cavity in perimenopausal patients. *J Ultrasound Med* 1996;**15**:285–8.

21. SCHWARZLER P, CONCIN H, BOSCH H, BERLINGER A, WOHLGENANNT K, COLLINS WP, et al. An evaluation of sonohysterography and diagnostic hysteroscopy for the assessment of intrauterine pathology. *Ultrasound Obstet Gynecol* 1998;**11**:337–42.

22. TIMMERMAN D, DEPREST J, BOURNE T, VAN DEN BERGHE I, COLLINS WP, VERGOTE I. A randomized trial on the use of ultrasonography or office hysteroscopy for endometrial assessment in postmenopausal patients with breast cancer who were treated with tamoxifen. *Am J Obstet Gynecol* 1998:**179**:62–70.

23. PEREZ-MEDINA T, BAJO-ARENAS J, SALAZAR F, REDONDO T, SANFRUTOS L, ALVAREZ P, et al. Endometrial polyps and their implication in the pregnancy rates of patients undergoing intrauterine insemination: a prospective, randomised study. *Hum Reprod* 2005;**20**:1632–5.

24. MOONEY SB, MILKI AA. Effect of hysteroscopy performed in the cycle preceding controlled ovarian hyperstimulation on the outcome of in vitro fertilization. *Fertil Steril* 2003;**79**:637–8.

25. OLIVEIRA F, ABDELMASSIH VG, DIAMOND MP, DOZORTSEV D, NAGY ZP, ABDELMASSIH R. Uterine cavity findings and hysteroscopic interventions in patients undergoing in vitro fertilization-embryo transfer who repeatedly cannot conceive. *Fertil Steril* 2003;**80**:1371–5.

26. SPIEWANKIEWICZ B, STELMACHOV J, SAWICKI W, CEDROWSKI K, WYPYCH P, SWIDERSKA K. The effectiveness of hysteroscopic polypectomy in cases of female infertility. *Clin Exp Obstet Gynecol* 2003;**30**:23–5.

27. MARCUS SF, BHATTACHARYA J, WILLIAMS G, BRINSDEN P, HAMOU J. Endometrial ossification: a cause of secondary infertility. *Am J Obstet Gynecol* 1994;**170**:1381–3.

28. BASU M, MAMMEN C, OWEN E. Bony fragments in the uterus: an association with secondary subfertility. *Ultrasound Obstet Gynecol* 2003;**22**:402–6.

29. BAHCECI M, DEMIREL LC. Osseous metaplasia of the endometrium: a rare cause of infertility and its hysteroscopic management. *Hum Reprod* 1996;**11**:2537–9.

30. BRONZ L, SUTER T, RUSCA T. The value of transvaginal sonography with and without instillation in the diagnosis of uterine pathology in pre and postmenopausal women with abnormal bleeding or suspect sonographic findings. *Ultrasound Obstet Gynecol* 1997;**9**:53–8.

31. SLADKEVICIUS P, VALENTIN L, MARSAL K. Blood flow velocity in the uterine and ovarian arteries during the normal menstrual cycle. *Ultrasound Obstet Gynecol* 1993;**3**:199–208.

32. TAN SL, ZAIDI J, CAMPBELL S, DOYLE P, COLLINS W. Blood flow changes in the ovarian and uterine arteries during the normal menstrual cycle. *Am J Obstet Gynecol* 1996;**175**:625–31.

33. SLADKEVICIUS P, VALENTIN L, MARSAL K. Blood flow velocity in the uterine and ovarian arteries during menstruation. *Ultrasound Obstet Gynecol* 1994;**4**:421–7.

34. STEER CV, TAN SL, MASON BA, CAMPBELL S. Midluteal-phase vaginal color Doppler assessment of uterine artery impedance in a subfertile population. *Fertil Steril* 1994;**61**:53–8.

35. TINKANEN H, KUJANSUU E, LAIPPALA P. Vascular resistance in uterine and ovarian arteries: its association with infertility and the prognosis of infertility. *Eur J Obstet Gynecol* 1994;**57**:111–15.

36. TAN SL, DOYLE P, CAMPBELL S, BERAL V, RIZK B, BRINSDEN P, et al. Obstetric outcome of in vitro fertilization pregnancies compared with normally conceived pregnancies. *Am J Obstet Gynecol* 1992;**167**:778–84.

37. VERLANEN H, CAMMU H, DERDE MP, AMY JJ. Singleton pregnancy after in vitro fertilization: expectations and outcome. *Obstet Gynecol* 1995;**85**:906–10.

38. STRANDELL A. The influence of hydrosalpinx on IVF and embryo transfer: a review. *Hum Reprod Update* 2000;**6**:387–95.

39. CAMUS E, PONCELET C, GOFFINET F, WAINER B, MERLET F, NISAND I, et al. Pregnancy rates after in-vitro fertilization in cases of tubal infertility with and without hydrosalpinx: a meta-analysis of published comparative studies. *Hum Reprod* 1999;**14**:1243–9.

40. STRANDELL A, WALDENSTRÖM U, NILSSON L, HAMBERGER L. Hydrosalpinges reduces in-vitro fertilization/embryo transfer pregnancy rates. *Hum Reprod* 1994;**9**:861–3.

41. STRANDELL A. Tubal infertility: treatment implications of IVF and surgery regarding hydrosalpinx and ectopic pregnancy [Thesis]. Department of Obstetrics and Gynaecology, Göteborg University, Sweden; 1999 [www.ub.gu.se/sok/dissdatabas/detaljvy.xml?id=4300].

42. CAMPBELL S, BOURNE TH, TAN SL, COLLINS W P. HyCoSy and its future role within the investigation of infertility in Europe. *Ultrasound Obstet Gynecol* 1994;**4**:245–53.

43. SCHULZ W, HOLLIHN K U. *Echovist-200 for tubal patency assessment.* Berlin: Schering Healthcare; 1995.

44. AYIDA G, HARRIS P, KENNEDY S, SEIF M, BARLOW D, CHAMBERLAIN P. Hysterosalpingo-contrast sonography (HyCoSy) using Echovist-200 in the outpatient investigation of infertility patients. *Brit J Radiol* 1996;**69**:910–3.

45. SLADKEVICIUS P, OJHA K, CAMPBELL S, NARGUND G. Three-dimensional power Doppler imaging in the assessment of Fallopian tube patency. *Ultrasound Obstet Gynecol* 2000;**16**:644–7.

46. KIYOKAWA K, MASUDA H, FUYUKI T, KOSEKI M, UCHIDA N, FUKUDA T, et al. Three-dimensional hysterosalpingo-contrast sonography (3-D-HyCoSy) as an outpatient procedure to assess infertile women: a pilot study. *Ultrasound Obstet Gynecol* 2000;**16**:648–54.

47. WATERMANN D, DENSCHLAG D, HANJALIC-BECK A, KECK C, KARCK U, PROMPELER H. Hystero-salpingo-kontrassonographie mit 3-D-ultraschall: eine pilotstudie. *Ultraschall Med* 2004;**25**:367–72.

48. BAKOS O, LUNDKVIST O, WIDE L, BERGH T. Ultrasonographical and hormonal description of the normal ovulatory menstrual cycle. *Acta Obstet Gynecol Scand* 1994;**73**:790–6.

49. ADAMS J, FRANKS S, POLSON D W, MASON H D, ABDULWAHID N, TUCKER M, et al. Multifollicular ovaries: clinical and endocrine features and response to pulsatile gonadotropin releasing hormone. *Lancet* 1985;**(ii)**:1375–9.

50. Revised 2003 consensus on diagnostic criteria and long health risks related to polycystic ovary syndrome (PCOS). The Rotterdam ESHRE/ASRM-sponsored PCOS consensus workshop group. *Hum Reprod* 2004;**19**:41–7.

51. BALEN A H, LAVEN J S E, TAN SL, DEWAILLY D. Ultrasound assessment of the polycystic ovary: international consensus definitions. *Hum Reprod Update* 2003;**9**:505–14.

52. AGRAWAL R, SLADKEVICIUS P, ENGMANN L, CONWAY G S, PAYNE N N, BEKIR J, et al. Serum vascular endothelial growth factor concentrations and ovarian stromal blood flow are increased in women with polycystic ovaries. *Hum Reprod* 1998;**13**:651–5.

53. AGRAWAL R, CONWAY GS, SLADKEVICIUS P, TAN S L, ENGMANN L, PAYNE N, et al. Changes in serum vascular endothelial growth factor (VEGF) and Doppler blood flow velocities in ovarian and uterine blood vessels in IVF: relevance to ovarian hyperstimulation and polycystic ovaries. *Fertil Steril* 1998;**70**:651–8.

54. KLINE J, KINNEY A, KELLY A, REUSS M L, LEVIN B. Predictors of antral follicle count during the reproductive years. *Hum Reprod* 2005;**20**:2179–89.

55. WALLACE W, KELSEY T W. Ovarian reserve and reproductive age may be determined from measurement of ovarian volume by transvaginal ultrasonography. *Hum Reprod* 2004;**19**:1612–17.

56. LASS A, SKULL J, MCVEIGH E, MARGARA R, WINSTON RM. Measurement of ovarian volume by transvaginal sonography before ovulation induction with human menopausal gonadotrophin for in-vitro fertilization can predict poor response. *Hum Reprod* 1997;**12**:294–7.

57. HENDRIKS D J, MOL B W, BANCSI L F, TE VELDI E R, BROEKMANS F J. Antral follicle count in the prediction of poor ovarian response and pregnancy after in vitro fertilization: a meta-analysis and comparison with basal follicle-stimulating hormone level. *Fertil Steril* 2005;**83**:291–301.

58. CHANG M Y, CHIANG C H, HSIEH T T, SOONG Y K, HSU K H. Use of the antral follicle count to predict the outcome of assisted reproductive technologies. *Fertil Steril* 1998;**69**:505–10.

59. ERDEM M, ERDEM A, GURSOY R, BIBEROGLU K. Comparison of basal and clomiphene citrate induced FSH and inhibin B, ovarian volume and antral follicle counts as ovarian reserve tests and predictors of poor ovarian response in IVF. *J Assist Reprod Genet* 2004;**21**:37–45.

60. ABULAFIA O, SHERER D M. Angiogenesis of the ovary. *Am J Obstet Gynecol* 2000;**182**:240–6.

61. BOURNE T, JURKOVIC D, WATERSTONE J, CAMPBELL S, COLLINS W P. Intrafollicular blood flow during human ovulation. *Ultrasound Obstet Gynecol* 1991;**5**:53–9.

62. CAMPBELL S, BOURNE T H, WATERSTONE J, REYNOLDS K M, CRAYFORD T J, JURKOVIC D, et al. Transvaginal color blood flow imaging of the periovulatory follicle. *Fertil Steril* 1993;**60**:433–8.

63. BHAL P S, PUGH N, CHUI D K, GREGORY L, WALKER S M, SHAW R W. The use of transvaginal power Doppler ultrasonography to evaluate the relationship between perifollicular vascularity and outcome in in-vitro fertilization treatment cycles. *Hum Reprod* 1999;**14**:939–45.

64. BHAL P S, PUGH N D, GREGORY L, O'BRIEN S, SHAW R W. Perifollicular vascularity as a potential variable affecting outcome in stimulated intrauterine insemination treatment cycles: a study using transvaginal power Doppler. *Hum Reprod* 2001;**16**:1682–9.

65. BOURNE TH, HAAGSTROM H, HAHLIN M, JOSEFSSON B, GRANBERG S, HELLBERG P, et al. Ultrasound studies of vascular and morphological changes in the human corpus luteum during menstrual cycle. *Fertil Steril* 1996;**65**:753–8.

66. ZAIDI J, JURKOVIC D, CAMPBELL S, COLLINS WP, MCGREGOR A, TAN SL. Luteinized unruptured follicle: morphology, endocrine function and blood flow changes during menstrual cycle. *Hum Reprod* 1995;**10**:44–9.

67. Miyazaki T, Tanaka M, Miyakoshi K, Minegishi K, Kasai K, Yoshimura Y. Power and colour Doppler ultrasonography for the evaluation of the vasculature of the human corpus luteum. *Hum Reprod* 1998;**13**:2836–41.

68. Battaglia C, Artini P G, Salvatori M, Giulini S, Petraglia F, Maxia N, Volpe A. Ultrasonographic patterns of polycystic ovaries: color Doppler and hormonal correlations. *Ultrasound Obstet Gynecol* 1998;**11**:332–6.

69. Zaidi J, Campbell S, Pitroff R, Kyei-Mensah A, Shaker A, Jacobs H S, et al. Ovarian stromal blood flow in women with polycystic ovaries – a possible new marker for diagnosis? *Hum Reprod* 1995;**10**:1992–6.

70. Agrawal R, Tan SL, Wild S, Sladkevicius P, Engmann L, Payne N, et al. Serum vascular endothelial growth factor concentrations in an in vitro fertilization cycles predict the risk of ovarian hyperstimulation syndrome. *Fertil Steril* 1999;**71**:287–93.

71. Valentin L. Pattern recognition of pelvic masses by gray scale ultrasound imaging: the contribution of Doppler ultrasound. *Ultrasound Obstet Gynecol* 1999;**14**:338–47.

72. Valentin L, Hagen B, Tingulstad S, Eik-Nes S. Comparison of 'pattern recognition' and logistic regression models for discrimination between benign and malignant pelvic masses: a prospective cross validation. *Ultrasound Obstet Gynecol* 2001;**18**:357–65.

73. Moore J, Copley S, Morris J, Lindsell D, Golding S, Kennedy S. A systematic review of the accuracy of ultrasound in the diagnosis of endometriosis. *Ultrasound Obstet Gynecol* 2002;**20**:630–4.

74. Mais V, Guerriero S, Ajossa S, Angiolucci M, Paoletti A M, Melis G B. Transvaginal ultrasonography in the diagnosis of cystic teratoma. *Obstet Gynecol* 1995;**85**:48–52.

75. Koonings P P, Campbell K, Mishell D, Grimes D. Relative frequency of ovarian neoplasms: a 10 year review. *Obstet Gynecol* 1989;**74**:921–5.

76. D'Hooghe T M, Debrock S. Endometriosis, retrograde menstruation and peritoneal inflammation in women and in baboons. *Hum Reprod Update* 2002;**8**:84–8.

77. Garrido N, Navarro J, Garcia-Velasco J, Remohi J, Pellicer A, Simon C. The endometrium versus embryonic quality in endometriosis-related infertility. *Hum Reprod Update* 2002;**8**:95–103.

78. Chapron C, Vercellini P, Barakat H, Vieira M, Dubuisson J B. Management of ovarian endometriomas. *Hum Reprod Update* 2002;**8**:591–7.

79. Tinkanen H, Kujansuu E. In vitro fertilization in patients with ovarian endometriomas. *Acta Obstet Gynecol Scand* 2000;**79**:119–22.

80. Fedele L, Bianchi S, Portuese A, Borruto F, Dorta M. Transrectal ultrasonography in the assessment of rectovaginal endometriosis. *Obstet Gynecol* 1998;**91**:444–8.

81. Bazot M, Darai E. Sonography and MR imaging for the assessment of deep pelvic endometriosis. *J Minim Invasive Gynecol* 2005;**12**:178–86.

82. Surrey E S, Schoolcraft W B. Management of endometriosis-associated infertility. *Obstet Gynecol Clin North Am* 2003;**30**:193–208.

83. Steer C V, Campbell S, Tan SL, Crayford T, Mills C, Mason BA, et al. The use of transvaginal color flow imaging after in vitro fertilization to identify optimum uterine conditions before embryo transfer. *Fertil Steril* 1992;**57**:372–6.

84. Coulam CB, Bustillo M, Soenksen DM, Britten S. Ultrasonographic predictors of implantation after assisted reproduction. *Fertil Steril* 1994;**62**:1004–10.

85. Zaidi J, Pitroff R, Shaker A, Kyei-Mensah A, Campbell S, Tan S L. Assessment of uterine artery blood flow on the day of human chorionic gonadotrophin administration by transvaginal colour Doppler ultrasound in an in vitro fertilization program. *Fertil Steril* 1996;**65**:377–81.

86. Coulam C B, Stern J J, Soenksen D M, Britten S, Bustillo M. Comparison of pulsatility indices on the day of oocyte retrieval and embryo transfer. *Hum Reprod* 1995;**10**:82–4.

87. Tekay A, Martikainen H, Jouppila P. Blood flow changes in uterine and ovarian vasculature, and predictive value of transvaginal pulsed colour Doppler ultrasonography in an in-vitro fertilisation programme. *Hum Reprod* 1995;**10**:688–93.

88. Engmann L, Sladkevicius P, Agrawal R, Bekir J, Campbell S, Tan S L. The pattern of changes in ovarian stromal and uterine artery blood flow velocities during in vitro fertilization treatment and its relationship with outcome of the cycle. *Ultrasound Obstet Gynecol* 1999;**13**:26–33.

89. Schild RL, Knobloch C, Dorn C, Fimmers R, van der Ven H, Hansmann M. Endometrial receptivity in an in vitro fertilization program as assessed by spiral artery blood flow, endometrial thickness, endometrial volume, and uterine artery blood flow. *Fertil Steril* 2001;**75**:361–6.

90. Zaidi J, Campbell S, Pitroff R, Tan S L. Endometrial thickness, morphology, vascular penetration and velocimetry in predicting implantation in an in vitro fertilisation programme. *Ultrasound Obstet Gynecol* 1995;**6**:191–8.

91. Applebaum M. The 'steel' or 'Teflon' endometrium – ultrasound visualization of endometrial vascularity in IVF patients and outcome. *Ultrasound Obstet Gynecol* 1993; **3 Suppl 2**:10.

92. Chien LW, Au HK, Chen PL, Xiao J, Tzeng CR. Assessment of uterine receptivity by the endometrial blood flow distribution pattern in women undergoing in vitro fertilization-embryo transfer. *Fertil Steril* 2002;**78**:245–51.

93. Schild R L, Holthaus S, d'Alquen J, Fimmers R, Dom C, van der Ven H, et al. Quantitative assessment of subendometrial blood flow by three-dimensional ultrasound is an important predictive factor of implantation in an in-vitro fertilization programme. *Hum Reprod* 2000;**15**:89–94.

94. Friedler S, Schenker J G, Herman A, Lewin A. The role of ultrasonography in the evaluation of endometrial receptivity following assisted reproductive treatments: a critical review. *Hum Reprod Update* 1996;**2**:323–35.

95. Rubinstein M, Marazzi A, Polak de Fried E. Low-dose aspirin treatment improves ovarian responsiveness, uterine and ovarian blood flow velocity, implantation, and pregnancy rates in patients undergoing in vitro fertilization: a prospective, randomized, double-blind placebo-controlled assay. *Fertil Steril* 1999;**71**:825–9.

96. Cacciatore B, Tiitinen A. Transdermal nitroglycerin administration improves uterine blood flow in infertile women. *J Assist Reprod Genet* 1997;**14 Suppl**:20.

97. Soares S R, Troncoso C, Bosch E, Serra V, Simon C, Remohi J, et al. Age and uterine receptiveness: predicting the outcome of oocyte donation cycles. *J Clin Endocrinol Metab* 2005;**90**:4399–404.

98. Abdalla H I, Wren M E, Thomas A, Korea L. Age of the uterus does not affect pregnancy or implantation rates; a study of egg donation in women of different ages sharing oocytes from the same donor. *Hum Reprod* 1997;**12**:827–9.

99. Balen A H, Braat D D M, West C, Patel A, Jacobs H S. Cumulative conception and livebirth rates after treatment of anovulatory infertility. An analysis of the safety and efficacy of ovulation induction in 200 patients. *Hum Reprod* 1994;**9**:1563–70.

100. Bordt J, Hander J P, Schneider H P G. Ultrasound controlled gonadotrophin therapy of anovulatory infertility. *Fertil Steril* 1986;**46**:818–22.

101. Montzavinos T, Garcia J E, Jones H W. Ultrasound measurement of ovarian follicles stimulated by human gonadotrophins for oocyte recovery and in vitro fertilization. *Fertil Steril* 1983;**40**:461–5.

102. Tan S L, Balen A H, el Hussein E, Mills C, Campbell S, Yovich J, et al. A prospective randomised study of the optimum timing of human chorionic gonadotrophin administration after pituitary desensitisation in in vitro fertilization. *Fertil Steril* 1992;**57**:1259–64.

103. Winfield A C, Wentz A C. *Diagnostic Imaging of Infertility*. Baltimore: Williams & Wilkins; 1987.

104. Tan SL, Balen A, el Hussein E, Mills C, Campbell S, Yovich J, et al. A prospective randomized study of the optimum timing of human chorionic gonadotrophin administration after pituitary desensitization in in vitro fertilization. *Fertil Steril* 1992;**57**:1259–64.

105. Blumenfeld Z, Yoffe N, Brohnstein M. Transvaginal sonography in infertility and assisted reproduction. *Obstet Gynecol Surv* 1990;**46**:36–49.

106. Delvigne A, Rozenberg S. Review of clinical course and treatment of ovarian hyperstimulation syndrome (OHSS). *Hum Reprod Update* 2003;**9**:77–96.

107. Engmann L, Sladkevicius P, Agrawal R, Bekir J S, Campbell S, Tan S L. Value of ovarian stromal blood flow velocity measurement after pituitary suppression in the prediction of ovarian responsiveness and outcome of in vitro fertilization treatment. *Fertil Steril* 1999;**71**:22–9.

108. Nargund G, Bourne T H, Doyle P E, Parsons J H, Cheng W C, Campbell S, et al. Association between ultrasound indices of follicular blood flow, oocyte recovery and pre-implantation embryo quality. *Hum Reprod* 1996;**11**:109–13.

109. Nargund G, Doyle P E, Bourne T H, Parsons J H, Cheng WC, Campbell S, et al. Ultrasound derived indices of follicular blood flow before hCG administration and the prediction of oocyte recovery and pre-implantation embryo quality. *Hum Reprod* 1996;**11**:2512–7.

110. Coulam C B, Goodman C, Rinehart JS. Colour Doppler indices of follicular blood flow as predictors of pregnancy after in-vitro fertilization and embryo transfer. *Hum Reprod* 1999;**14**:1979–82.

111. El-Shawarby S, Margara R, Trew G, Lavery S. A review of complications following transvaginal oocyte retrieval for in-vitro fertilization. *Hum Fertil* (Camb) 2004;**7**:127–33.

112. O'Neill M J, Rafferty E A, Lee S I, Arellano R S, Gervais D A, Hahn P F, et al. Transvaginal interventional procedures: aspiration, biopsy, and catheter drainage. *Radiographics* 2001;**21**:657–72.

113. Anderson R E, Nugent N L, Gregg A T, Nunn S L, Behr B R. Transvaginal ultrasound-guided embryo transfer improves outcome in patients with previous failed in vitro fertilization cycles. *Fertil Steril* 2002;**77**:769–75.

114. Sallam H N, Sadek S S. Ultrasound-guided embryo transfer: a meta-analysis of randomised controlled trials. *Fertil Steril* 2003;**80**:1042–6.

115. Letterie G S. Marshall L, Angle M. A new coaxial system with an echo dense tip for ultrasonographically guided embryo transfer. *Fertil Steril* 1999;**72**:266–8.

10

Ultrasound imaging of the lower urinary tract and uterovaginal prolapse

VIKRAM KHULLAR AND CHARLOTTE CHALIHA

Introduction

For many years, urogynaecologists and urologists have relied on cystometry and urethral function tests to evaluate the female lower urinary tract. However, with the improvements in ultrasound imaging techniques, this diagnostic modality has been increasingly used for the assessment of lower urinary tract dysfunction and pelvic floor disorders. Ultrasound has the advantage of being able to visualise fluid-filled structures without the need for contrast medium. It can also demonstrate soft tissue structures such as the kidney, bladder wall, urethral and anal sphincters and surrounding pelvic floor musculature. It also avoids ionising radiation and can be used safely and repeatedly in women of reproductive age. Most ultrasound equipment is transportable and readily available within a gynaecological department. Operating costs of ultrasound are low and the technique should be readily available in most urogynaecological units.

Ultrasound of the lower urinary tract and pelvis

The bony enclosure of the pelvis around the empty bladder and urethra limits the views obtained by ultrasound imaging. Use of the transabdominal, transvaginal, transrectal and transperineal approaches for ultrasound scanning allows for easy visualisation of different aspects of the lower urinary tract. Perineal and transabdominal probes are usually linear array transducers, while transvaginal and transrectal probes are either linear array or sector scanners. Linear array scanners have the disadvantage of being bulky and having low operating frequencies, whereas sector scanners are smaller, more expensive and operate at a higher frequency producing better image resolution. Higher ultrasound frequency provides better image resolution at the expense of decreased depth of penetration owing to increased attenuation. The 5.0–7.5 MHz frequency probes achieve the best compromise between image resolution and penetration and they are most often used in urogynaecology. With the advent of three-dimensional ultrasound, the lower urinary tract can be simultaneously imaged in more than one plane.

Interpretation of ultrasound images requires care as certain tissues will appear hypoechoic when insonated in one angle and hyperechoic when in the probe is angled in different direction. This occurs when a structure has multiple ordered layers such as collagen and structures where the direction of muscle fibres varies as in the urethral sphincter. This results in muscle appearing hyperechoic when the ultrasound waves pass perpendicular to the long axis of striated muscle fibres and hypoechoic if the waves travel along the long axis of fibres (Figure 10.1a,b).

Transabdominal imaging

The first description of ultrasound imaging of the bladder was by the transabdominal route.[1] Using this approach the transducer is placed on the abdomen and it is aimed caudally below the symphysis. The disadvantage of this approach is that it does not allow visualisation of the bladder neck, which is hidden behind the symphysis. In patients who are obese, images may be difficult to obtain and, as there are no fixed reference points for assessing bladder neck movements, these observations are prone to errors.

MEASUREMENTS OF BLADDER VOLUME

Ultrasound measurement of residual bladder volume eliminates the need for urethral catheterisation with its associated risk of infection. It is indicated in the investigation of women with voiding difficulties, before the initiation of anticholinergic therapy or to check post-void residual after continence surgery.

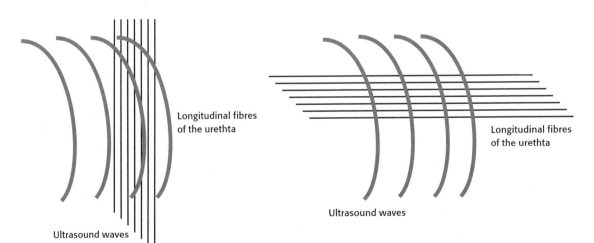

Longitudinal fibres of the urethta

Longitudinal fibres of the urethta

Ultrasound waves

Ultrasound waves

FIGURE 10.1a Ultrasound passes perpendicular to the longitudinal fibres of the urethra and, in this condition, maximal echo is produced so the tissue appears white and hyperechoic

FIGURE 10.1b Ultrasound passes along the longitudinal fibres of the urethra and, in this condition, minimal echo is produced so the tissue appears black and hypoechoic

Volume estimation is performed by scanning the bladder in two perpendicular planes and by measuring three orthogonal bladder diameters. A correction factor is usually applied to account for the fact that the bladder is spherical only when completely full. The most common formula to estimate the residual bladder volume involves multiplication of the three diameters with a factor of 0.7.[2] Using this formula there is a 21% margin of error when compared with the volume of voided urine. Below 50 ml of urine it has been suggested that transvaginal measurement is more accurate,[3] although it may be less acceptable for the patient. At larger residual bladder volumes, transvaginal and transabdominal ultrasound have a similar level of accuracy.[4] Automated bladder scanners have been developed but there are conflicting data in the literature regarding their accuracy. These scanners rely heavily on algorithms fitting the shape of the bladder, and if the shape is different from the anticipated one, the results may be inaccurate. This is important as bladder shape varies pre- and post-voiding. Inaccuracies may also arise by mistaking the uterus for the bladder in the postpartum period and in the presence of large uterine fibroids. Conventional ultrasound imaging is therefore preferable, particularly taking into account wide availability of small portable machines, which are inexpensive and easy to use.[5]

URINARY BLADDER AND URETHRAL ANATOMY

Bladder diverticula are easily visualised with transabdominal ultrasound.[6] Dynamic assessment of the bladder filling is possible, which may show the diverticula filling as the bladder fills, and the diverticula can be seen to empty after micturition. Calculi can develop within diverticula owing to urinary stasis and transitional cell carcinomas have been reported in 5% of cases.[7] Calculi can be distinguished from carcinomas in the bladder as they produce distinct acoustic shadowing, which moves with alterations in posture. Bladder diverticula can be difficult to detect at cystoscopy and ultrasound allows the contents to be checked and observed.

The majority of bladder carcinomas are exophytic and papillary, which facilitates their detection on ultrasound scan. Ultrasound has been considered the method of choice for imaging tumours near or on the trigone and has a role in follow-up of recurrent tumours in preference to cystoscopy.[8,9]

Transvaginal ultrasound

Transvaginal ultrasound allows clearer visualisation of the bladder base, bladder neck, inferior border of the pubic symphysis and periurethral structures.[10] The probe is closer to these structures and thus higher frequencies can be used producing better resolution. Using this approach the urethra is seen as having a hyperechoic core with a hypoechoic rhabdosphincter lateral to it.[11]

Using ultrasound frequencies of 3.5 MHz, the position of the urethra cannot be identified without inserting a urethral catheter. This may interfere with the position and movement of the bladder neck distorting the true anatomical picture. In order to assess bladder neck mobility a fixed reference point is needed to asses its movements accurately during the Valsalva manoeuvre. Compression of the bladder neck should be avoided as the view becomes distorted. Distortion of the posterior urethrovesical angle is seen on both abdominal and transvaginal ultrasound.[12] Distortion by the probe can also alter urethral function. Urethral pressure profilometry studies showed increases in maximum urethral closure pressure and functional urethral length at rest and during stress with a transvaginal probe *in situ*.[13] Care needs to be taken in interpreting functional studies and bladder neck mobility and position when using the transvaginal approach. In women with a large anterior of posterior vaginal wall or vault prolapse probe placement may be difficult and imaging is often poor.

Perineal and translabial ultrasound

This approach uses an abdominal probe covered with a disposable cover, which is placed on the perineal or labial area. This gives a clear view of the bladder neck, urethra or vagina with the urethra appearing hyperechoic and surrounded by a hyperechoic rhabdosphincter. This method is acceptable to women, is less invasive and is easier to perform, especially in women who are obese. There is no distortion of vaginal anatomy or bladder neck and it can be used to assess the position and mobility of the bladder neck.[14] As the probe does not distort the vaginal anatomy it can be used to assess prolapse, as long as the prolapse does not descend caudal to the hymeneal ring, where the probe will impede further movement of the prolapse. Good correlation has been found between quantification of prolapse using translabial ultrasound and the International Continence Society prolapse assessment system.[15]

Bladder neck position and mobility can be reliably assessed by perineal ultrasound using either the central axis of the pubis or its inferior–posterior margin as the point of reference.[16,17] Imaging can be performed with the patient supine or erect and with a full or empty bladder. Measurements are performed at rest and then during a Valsalva manoeuvre. Bladder neck descent is the difference between these two measurements. This measurement has a higher association with urodynamic stress incontinence than other parameters of urethral hypermobility but it is also related to anterior vaginal wall prolapse.[18]

This approach has been suggested as an alternative to video imaging studies to avoid the need for bladder catheterisation. Voiding studies with a translabial probe use the probe fixed in a remote steerable mount that can be controlled by the operator and this is fixed to a specially designed chair.[19] Shaer[20] filled the bladder with Echovist® (Schering Health Care) contrast medium and scanned the bladder at rest and on straining, obtaining clear images of urethral and bladder anatomy. He was also able to observe leakage of urine. However, in the absence of pressure studies to exclude detrusor overactivity the clinical relevance of such detection of leakage is unclear.

Transrectal ultrasound

The transrectal approach was initially developed to study the prostate gland[21] and only later was it used to image the bladder, urethra and anal sphincters. The woman is asked to rest in the supine or left lateral position so as to obtain a sagittal view of the bladder neck. In this position the urethra appears hyperechoic. The surrounding rhabdosphincter appears hypoechoic lateral to the urethra and it is hyperechoic anteriorly. If the rectum is filled with faeces or flatus insertion of the probe may be difficult and the image may contain artefacts.

This approach can be used to measure post-void residuals and image the position of the bladder neck. No restriction of urethrovesical mobility has been reported with a rectal probe in place.[22] However, the probe may move with coughing and, if there is a significant degree of prolapse, this may create artefacts.

The transrectal approach has also been suggested as an alternative to radiological imaging, as the position of the probe does not affect pressure measurements during urodynamics.[22] However, the position of the probe may be more uncomfortable and embarrassing for the patient and this may alter voiding studies in particular.

In patients with spinal cord injury, who lack sensation in the anus and rectum, this method may be of use to image the bladder neck during voiding and urodynamic studies with images similar to those obtained during videocystourethography.[23] It has also been used to diagnose detrusor–sphincter dyssynergia, catheter-induced hyperreflexia, false passages and dilated ureters.[24–27] However, with complete spinal cord transection the sacral cord reflexes may still be intact and insertion of a probe into the anal canal may be difficult and cause alteration in reflex activity of the bladder.

Intraurethral ultrasound

This technique uses high-frequency rotating ultrasound probes within the urethra to give a 360-degree section perpendicular to the plane of the probe. This gives an oblique view through the urethra but it does not give a clear image of the outer border of the rhabdosphincter, nor of the periurethral structures.[28] Also the axis of the probe changes as it is withdrawn down the urethra making interpretation of images more difficult and limits the usefulness of this technique.

Three-dimensional ultrasound

Three-dimensional ultrasound allows images to be obtained from a reconstructed digital volume through a given structure at different angles to the ultrasound beam. This is helpful where images with conventional ultrasound are difficult because of poor access. These images can be reconstructed to allow volume estimations that are more accurate than volume estimations using two-dimensional ultrasound.

Three-dimensional ultrasound has been described as an accurate and reproducible method of assessing urethral sphincter volume in women.[29] Using three-dimensional ultrasound, the images obtained will depend on the approach which was used to record the three-dimensional volume. With the transperineal approach, the rhabdosphincter is a hyperechoic, cylindrical structure around the urethra and the hypoechoic core consists of longitudinal smooth muscle, urethral lumen, urethral epithelium and submucosal plexus. Using a transvaginal or transrectal approach, the ultrasound waves are perpendicular to the long axis of the urethra and the lateral rhabdosphincter therefore appears hypoechoic, while the longitudinal fibres are hyperechoic. These findings have been confirmed with histological examinations of cadaver specimens and electromyographic studies of the striated sphincter muscle.[30,31] There appears to be a good correlation between the volume of the sphincter measured on three-dimensional ultrasound and urethral pressure profilometry. In 19 antenatal women there was a good correlation between sphincter volumes and area under the urethral pressure profile curve, though this relationship was lost following delivery.[32]

Ultrasound for the assessment of urinary incontinence

Ultrasound imaging has been used to define bladder neck anatomy, position and movement in women with stress incontinence. Quinn et al.[10] identified bladder neck opening in women with stress incontinence but the clinical relevance of this is unclear, as an open bladder neck is demonstrated in 21% of continent women.[33]

Creighton[34] used perineal ultrasound to assess bladder neck position and mobility in women with stress incontinence in comparison with continent controls. There was no difference in bladder neck mobility between the two groups. Continent patients were more likely to have higher bladder necks that were more posterior than women with stress incontinence, but there was great overlap between the groups making bladder neck position a test of limited value. Other studies have found a difference in bladder neck mobility between stress incontinence and continent controls but again there is a large degree of overlap between groups.[18,35] It is likely that increased bladder neck mobility reflects uterovaginal prolapse as continent women with uterovaginal prolapse have a higher degree of bladder neck mobility than those without. Also, anterior vaginal wall prolapse correlates well with bladder neck mobility.[13,36,37]

Increased bladder neck mobility during pregnancy has been associated with higher risk of developing postpartum stress incontinence. King and Freeman[38] noted in a group of nulliparous women scanned antenatally and postpartum a tenfold increase in postpartum stress incontinence if the bladder neck moved more than ten degrees with a Valsalva manoeuvre.

Bladder filling, patient position and catheterisation can influence bladder neck mobility and it can be difficult to standardise Valsalva manoeuvres.[39,40] There is also a wide difference in reference measurements for 'normal' bladder descent.[41-43] It is most likely that the aetiology of increased bladder neck mobility is multifactorial and the wide variation of normal values in nulliparous and asymptomatic women indicates that there are congenital, inherited factors that affect bladder neck mobility. This has been suggested in a twin study showing a high degree of heritability for anterior vaginal wall mobility.[44]

Three-dimensional ultrasound allows better definition of the urethral continence mechanism. Khullar et al.[45] used three-dimensional ultrasound to measure urethral sphincter volume and found that those with urodynamic stress incontinence tended to have smaller sphincters than continent controls, though the overlap was large.[45] More recently, colour Doppler studies have been used to demonstrate leakage through the urethra and may be used to demonstrate leak point pressures. This application is still limited to a research tool but is an interesting alternative to conventional video-imaging.[46,47]

Both two- and three-dimensional ultrasound has helped our understanding of the mechanism of success of continence procedures. Richmond and Sutherst[48] assessed 25 continent and 59 incontinent women and found increased bladder neck mobility in those with stress incontinence. In addition, surgery was less successful in those with more mobile bladder necks.[48] Creighton[49] used perineal ultrasound to assess surgical cure after a colposuspension or Raz bladder neck suspension procedure. In those women undergoing colposuspension, bladder neck elevation was not related to cure, whereas in those who underwent the Raz procedure, a lower bladder neck was seen in those whose surgery failed. This suggests that failure of elevation was responsible for failure. Further work using transvaginal ultrasound has shown that successful Burch colposuspension is associated with an increase in the approximation of the bladder neck to the symphysis pubis and decreased descent during Valsalva manoeuvre. Failure of continence surgery has been associated with a return of bladder neck mobility.[50]

The tension-free vaginal tape (TVT) is a relatively new procedure for stress incontinence. Its mechanism of cure is uncertain and though there are changes in voiding parameters,[51-53] the existence of an obstructive effect is disputed by some authors.[54] Dietz and Wilson[55] performed two- and three-dimensional translabial ultrasound in the supine position and after voiding in 141 women who underwent TVT. The TVT was highly echogenic and easily visualised dorsal and lateral to the urethra. This was also seen for other suburethral slings such as the SPARC™ (AMS, Australia, North Parramatta, Australia) and the IVS™ (Tyco Healthcare Ltd, Lane Cove, Australia) tape, though the latter was less echogenic, probably because of its tighter weave. The TVT was found to function by mechanical compression of the urethra between the implant and the symphysis pubis and using three-dimensional ultrasound they found a wide variation in tape placement and movement, which would explain the wide margin of clinical efficacy and safety.

There has been increasing interest in the use of ultrasound to quantify bladder wall thickness as a marker for detrusor overactivity. The rationale is that the detrusor hypertrophies and will therefore be thicker on ultrasound imaging in cases of detrusor overactivity. Measurements

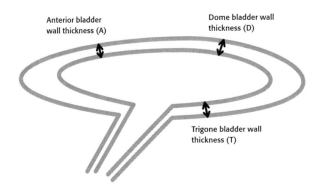

Anterior bladder
wall thickness (A)

Dome bladder wall
thickness (D)

Trigone bladder wall
thickness (T)

FIGURE 10.2 Diagrammatic representation of bladder wall thickness measurement: the bladder wall thickness is calculated as A + D + T / 3

are taken using the transvaginal or translabial approach with the bladder empty and perpendicular to the bladder mucosa at three sites, the anterior wall, trigone and dome of the bladder (Figure 10.2). A mean of all three measurements is then calculated. Using this technique, a mean bladder wall thickness of greater than 5mm was associated with detrusor overactivity.[56] The results of this study compared well to ambulatory urodynamics, as long as women with outflow obstruction were excluded. The method has moderate predictive value for detrusor overactivity but may be more clinically useful when combined with symptoms of the overactive bladder (Figure 10.3).[57] Although the technique has been suggested as a screening test for detrusor overactivity it is not widely used in clinical practice yet. Measuring bladder wall thickness before and after anticholinergic therapy has shown that these drugs reduce the bladder wall thickness.

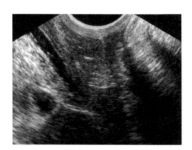

FIGURE 10.3 Ultrasound scan of a bladder containing a small amount of anechoic fluid. The bladder wall thickness is measured from the bladder mucosa to the outermost part of the bladder muscle

Ultrasound for assessment of the pelvic floor and prolapse

Support of the bladder, urethra and pelvic organs is dependent upon the integrity of the paraurethral and paravaginal musculofascial tissues: the pubourethral ligament, pubovesical muscle, paravaginal and endopelvic fascia.[58] Hypermobility of the bladder and prolapse are thought to be due to childbirth-related trauma. The pelvic floor comprises the levator ani, which consists of two parts: the ileococcygeus and the pubococcygeus muscles. The latter is a U-shaped band of muscle extending from the symphysis pubis around the rectum. The medial edge of the pubococcygeus has openings for the urethra, vagina and rectum to pass through and this is termed the levator hiatus.

Transabdominal ultrasound imaging has been used to investigate endopelvic fascial defects but the definition is often poor, owing to the absence of clear reference points and the confounding effect of bladder and rectal filling, uterine position and size and poor visualisation on Valsalva manoeuvre.[59–61] Translabial ultrasound overcomes some of these limitations and has been used to demonstrate uterovaginal prolapse.[62] The inferior border of the symphysis pubis is used as a reference against which descent of the bladder, uterus, rectum and pouch of Douglas can be assessed. This shows good correlation with clinical staging according to criteria developed by the International Continence Society for anterior and central compartment descent but poorer correlation for the posterior compartment.[63]

Three-dimensional ultrasound offers new insights into the pelvic floor as it allows imaging of both the levator ani muscle hiatus and paravaginal support structures in axial and transverse planes. This gives access to transverse planes similar to magnetic resonance imaging. There are two techniques that enable a detailed examination of the pelvic floor: transperineal and transvaginal ultrasound. The former technique can visualise the entire pelvic floor and the pubococcygeus muscle can be clearly visualised as a hyperechoic structure. The vaginal approach identifies the levator ani hiatus by tracing it from its insertion into the inferior body of the pubic symphysis to the anorectal angle posteriorly. This point can be taken as a fixed reference point. The surface area and width of the levator ani can be measured, as well as lateral defects in the vaginal wall (Figure 10.4). The area of the levator hiatus has been found to be larger in women with prolapse compared with healthy controls.[64] However, in women with urodynamic stress incontinence alone, the levator hiatus area is not increased, suggesting that changes in the levator hiatus are important in the pathophysiology of prolapse but not stress incontinence. Further work suggesting the role of the levator hiatus in the genesis of prolapse comes from studies of women before and after delivery. It is well known that childbirth, particularly vaginal delivery, is a significant aetiological factor in the development of prolapse and, interestingly, the levator ani surface area has been found to be increased in women after vaginal delivery.[65]

Another small study investigated the effect of childbirth on the pelvic floor by using two- and three-dimensional translabial ultrasound in a group of 26 nulliparous women in the third trimester of pregnancy.[66] Twenty-three women were seen again at 2–5 months postpartum. Tenting of the vagina (the presence of ventrolateral sulci) was described at three levels: just below the urethral meatus, at the bladder neck and 1.5–2.0 cm above the bladder neck. Antenatally, tenting was visible in 21 of the 26 women but postpartum only five women showed tenting, four of these after vaginal delivery. Loss of tenting did not correlate with changes in bladder neck mobility implying that excess bladder neck mobility may be due to increased fascial compliance rather than disruption of structures. Such stretching is similar to that described above to the levator hiatus. Three-dimensional ultrasound also allows the clear visualisation of the urethra and structures such as paravaginal cysts which can be seen easily and their relationship to the urethra can be studied (Figure 10.5). The urethra itself can be rendered and the ostium for a urethral diverticulum can be identified (Figure 10.6). The information can then be used to determine the relationship of the ostium to the urethral sphincter. This information is important in deciding the surgical approach to a urethral diverticulum.

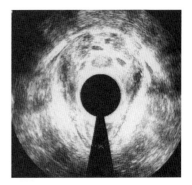

FIGURE 10.4 Transvaginal scan showing a levator ani hiatus surrounded by hypoechoic muscle

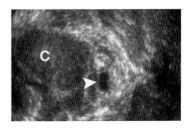

FIGURE 10.5 Three-dimensional scan showing a paravaginal cyst (c) located adjacent to the urethra (arrow)

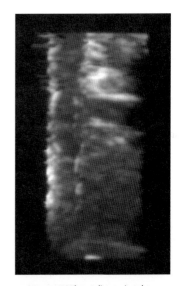

FIGURE 10.6 Three-dimensional reconstruction of the urethra showing a defect in the posterior aspect, which represents the ostium of urethral diverticulum

Conclusions

Ultrasound imaging of the lower urinary tract gives additional insights into the pathophysiology of pelvic floor disorders and can be used as a tool for diagnosis and assessment of treatment. Further work is required in this field to standardise imaging methodology as it presents an acceptable and easily available method that may overcome the invasiveness and morbidity of other traditional investigations.

REFERENCES

1. HOLMES J. Ultrasonic studies of bladder filling and contour. In: Hinman J F, editor. *Hydrodynamics of Micturition*. Illinois: Charles C Thomas; 1971. p. 76–88.

2. POSTON G J, JOSEPH A E A, RIDDLE P R. The accuracy of ultrasound in the measurement of changes in bladder volume. *Br J Ultrasound* 1983; **55**: 361–3.

3. HAYLEN B T, FRAZER M I, SUTHERST J R. WEST C R. Transvaginal ultrasound in the assessment of bladder volumes in women: preliminary report. *Br J Urol* 1989; **63**: 149–51.

4. BAKER K R, CRUTZ H P, LEMIEUX M-C. Limited accuracy of vaginal ultrasound in measuring residual urine volumes. *Int Urogynecol J* 1993; **4**: 138–40.

5. DUDLEY N J, KIRKLAND M, LOVETT J, WATSON A R. Clinical agreement between automated and calculated ultrasound measurements of bladder volume. *Br J Radiol* 2003; **76**: 832–4.

6. GANABATHI K, LEACH G E, ZIMMERN P E, DMOCHOWSKI R. Experience with the management of urethral diverticulum in 63 women. *J Urol* 1994; **152**: 1445–52.

7. FOX M, POWER R F, BRUCE A W. Diverticulum of the bladder-presentation and evaluation in 115 cases. *Br J Urol* 1962; **34**: 286–9.

8. FERNANDEZ A, MAYAYO DEHESA T. Leiomyoma of the urinary bladder floor: diagnosis by transvaginal ultrasound. *Urol Int* 1992; **48**: 99–101.

9. FLANNIGAN G M, GELISTER J S, NOBLE J G, MILROY E J. Rigid versus flexible cystoscopy. A controlled trial of patient tolerance. *Br J Urol* 1988; **62**: 537–40.

10. QUINN M J, BEYNON J, MORTENSEN N J M, SMITH P J. Transvaginal endosonography: a new method to study the lower anatomy of the lower urinary tract in urinary stress incontinence. *Br J Urol* 1988; **62**: 414–8.

11. ATHANSIOU S, KHULLAR V, BOOS K, SALVATORE S, CARDOZO L. Imaging the urethral sphincter with three-dimensional ultrasound. *Obstet Gynecol* 1999; **94**: 295–301.

12. BECO J, LEONARD D, LAMBOTTED R. Study of the artefacts introduced by linear array transvaginal ultrasound scanning in urodynamics. *World J Urol* 1994; **12**: 329–32.

13. WISE B J, BURTON G, CUTNER A, CARDOZO L D. Effect of vaginal probe on lower urinary tract function. *Br J Urol* 1992; **80**: 12–16.

14. CLARK A, CREIGHTON S M, PEARCE M, STANTON S L. Localisation of the bladder neck by perineal ultrasound: methodology and applications. *Neurourol Urodyn* 1990; **9**: 394–5.

15. BUMP R C, MATTIASSON A, BO K, BRUBAKER L P, DELANCEY J O, KLARSKOV P, *et al*. The standardisation of terminology of female pelvic organ prolapse and pelvic floor adjustment. *J Am Obstet Gynecol* 1996; **175**: 10–17.

16. DIETZ H P, WILSON P D. Anatomical assessment of the bladder outlet and proximal urethra using ultrasound and videocystourethrography. *Neurourol Urodyn* 1996; **15**: 212–14.

17. SHAER G N, KOECHLI O R, SCHUESSLER B, HALLER U. Perineal ultrasound for evaluating the bladder neck in urinary stress incontinence. *Obstet Gynecol* 1995; **85**: 220–4.

18. DIETZ H P, CLARKE B, HERBISON P. Bladder neck mobility and urethral closure pressure as predictors of genuine stress incontinence. *Int Urogynecol J Pelvic Floor Dysfunct* 2002; **13**: 289–93.

19. SCHAER G N, SIEGWART R, PERRUCHINI D, DELANCEY J O. Examination of voiding in seated women using remote controlled ultrasound probe. *Obstet Gynecol* 1998; **91**: 297–301.

20. SCHAER G N, KOECHLI O R, SCHUESSLER B, HALLER U. Improvement of perineal sonographic bladder neck imaging with ultrasound contrast medium. *Obstet Gynecol* 1995; **86**: 950–4.

21. WATANABE H, IGARI D, TANAHASI Y. Development and application of new equipment for transrectal ultrasonography. *J Clinical Ultrasound* 1974;**2**:91–8.

22. RICHMOND D H, SUTHERST J. Transrectal ultrasound scanning in urinary incontinence: the effect of the probe on urodynamic parameters. *Br J Urol* 1989;**64**:582–5.

23. RICHMOND D H, SUTHERST J. Clinical application of transrectal ultrasound for the investigation of the incontinent patient. *Br J Urol* 1989;**63**:605–9.

24. SHAPERO L G, FRIEDLAND G W, PERRKASH I. Transrectal sonographic voiding and cystourethrography: studies in neuromuscular bladder dysfunction. *Am J Roentgenol* 1983;**141**:83–90.

25. PERKAASH I, FRIEDLAND G W. Catheter-induced hyperreflexia in spinal cord injury patients: diagnosis by sonographic voiding cystourethrography. *Radiology* 1986;**159**:453–55.

26. SHABSIGH R, FISHMAN I J, KREBS M. The use of transrectal longitudinal real-time ultrasonography in urodynamics. *J Urol* 1987;**138**:1416–19.

27. SHABSIGH R, FISHMAN I J, KREBS M. Combined transrectal ultrasonography and urodynamics in the evaluation of detrusor-sphincter dyssynergia. *Br J Urol* 1988;**62**:326–30.

28. KIRSCHNER-HERMANNS R, KLEIN H M, MULLER U, SCHAFER W, JAKSE G. Intraurethral ultrasound in women with stress incontinence. *Br J Urol* 1994;**74**:315–18.

29. TOOZS-HOBSON P, KHULLAR V, CARDOZO L. Three-dimensional ultrasound: a novel technique for investigating the urethral sphincter in the third trimester of pregnancy. *Ultrasound Obstet Gynecol* 2001;**17**:421–4.

30. KHULLAR V, ATHANASIOU S, CARDOZO L, BOOS K, SALVATORE S, YOUNG M. Histological correlates of the urethral sphincter and surrounding structures with ultrasound imaging. *Int Urogynaecol J* 1996;**7**:164.

31. KHULLAR V, CARDOZO LD, SALVATORE S, HILL S. Ultrasound: a noninvasive screening test for detrusor instability. *Br J Obstet Gynaecol* 1996;**103**:904–8.

32. ROBINSON D, TOOZS-HOBSON P, CARDOZO L, DIGESU A. Correlating structure and function: three-dimensional ultrasound of the urethral sphincter. *Ultrasound Obstet Gynecol* 2004;**23**:272–6.

33. CHAPPLE C R, HELM C W, BLEASE S, MILROY E J G, RIKARDS D, OSBORNE J L. Asymptomatic bladder neck incompetence in nulliparous females. *Br J Urol* 1989;**64**:357–9.

34. CREIGHTON S M. *Innovative techniques in the investigation and management of female urinary incontinence.* MD thesis. University of London; 1989.

35. HOL M, VAN BOLHUIS C, VIERHOUT M E. Vaginal ultrasound studies of bladder neck mobility. *Br J Obstet Gynaecol* 1995;**102**:47–53.

36. BHATIA N N, OSTERGARD D R, McQUOWN D. Ultrasonography in urinary incontinence. *Urology* 1987;**29**:90–4.

37. WISE B G, KHULLAR V, CARDOZO L D. Bladder neck movement during pelvic floor contraction and intravaginal electrical stimulation in women with and without genuine stress incontinence. *Neurourol Urodyn* 1992;**11**:309–11.

38. KING J K, FREEMAN R M. Is antenatal bladder neck mobility a risk factor for stress incontinence? *Br J Obstet Gynaecol* 1998;**105**:1300–7.

39. DIETZ H P, WILSON P D. The influence of bladder volume on the position and mobility of the urethrovesical junction. *Int Urogynecol J* 1999;**10**:3–6.

40. DIETZ H P, CLARKE B. The influence of posture on perineal ultrasound imaging parameters. *Int Urogynecol J* 2001;**12**:104–6.

41. BRANDT F T, ALBUQUERQUE C D, LORENZATO F R, AMARAL FJ. Perineal assessment of urethrovesical junction mobility in young continent females. *Int Urogynecol J* 2002;**12**:S4.

42. PESCHERS U M, FANGER G, SCHAER G N, VODUSEK D B, DELANCEY J O, SCHUESSLER B. Bladder neck mobility in continent nulliparous women. *BJOG* 2001;**108**:320–4.

43. DIETZ H P, ELDRIDGE A, GRACE M, CLARKE B. Normal values for pelvic organ descent in healthy nulligravid young Caucasian women. *Neurourol Urodyn* 2003;**22**:420–21.

44. DIETZ HP, HANSELL N, GRACE M, ELDRIDGE A, CLARKE B. Bladder neck mobility is a heritable trait. *Int Urogynecol* **Suppl 2003**;S74.

45. KHULLAR V, ATHANASIOU S, CARDOZO L D, SALVATORE S, KELLEHER C J. Urinary sphincter volume and urodynamic diagnosis. *Neurourol Urodyn* 1996;**15**:334–6.

46. DIETZ H P, McKNOUGHLTY L, CLARKE B. Translabial color Doppler for imaging in urogynecology: a preliminary report. *Ultrasound Obstet Gynecol* 1999;**14**:144–7.

47. MASATA J, MARTAN A, HALASKA M, KASIKOVA E, OTCENASEK M, VOIGHT R. Detection of Valsalva leak point pressure with color Doppler: a new method for routine use. *Neurourol Urodyn* 2001;**20**:494–6.

48. RICHMOND D H, SUTHERST J R. Burch colposuspension or sling for stress incontinence? A prospective study using transrectal ultrasound. *Br J Urol* 1989;**64**:600–3.

49. CREIGHTON S M, CLARK A, PEARCE J M, STANTON S L. Bladder neck ultrasound: appearance before and after continence surgery. *Ultrasound Obstet Gynecol* 1994;**4**:428.

50. QUINN M J, BEYNON J, MORTENSEN N J, SMITH PJ. Vaginal endosonography in the postoperative assessment of colposuspension. *Br J Urol* 1989;**62**:414–18.

51. DIETZ H P, MOURITSEN L, ELLIS G, WILSON P D. Voiding function after TVT. *Int Urogynecol J Pelvic Floor Dysfunct* 2002;**13**:S21.

52. SANDER P, MOLLER LM, RUDNICKI PM, LOSE G. Does the tension-free vaginal tape procedure affect the voiding phase? Pressure-flow studies before and 1 year after surgery. *BJU Int* 2002;**89**:694–8.

53. VALENTINI FA, FRITEL S, NELSON PP, PIGNE A. Contribution of modelling to understanding of the mode of action of suburethral tape procedure for cure of stress incontinence. *Int Urogynecol J Pelvic Floor Dysfunct* 2002; **13**: S1–3.

54. WANG AC, CHEN MCV. Comparison of tension-free vaginal taping versus modified Burch colposuspension on urethral obstruction: a randomised controlled trial. *Neurourol Urodyn* 2003; **22**: 185–90.

55. DIETZ HP, WILSON PD. The 'iris-effect': how two-dimensional and three dimensional ultrasound can help us understand anti-incontinence procedures. *Ultrasound Obstet Gynecol* 2004; **233**: 267–71.

56. KHULLAR V, CARDOZO LD, SALVATPRE S, HILL S. Ultrasound: a non-invasive screening tests for detrusor instability. *Br J Obstet Gynaecol* 1996; **103**: 904–8.

57. SOLIGO M, KHULLAR V, SALVATORE S, LUPPINO GAVMR. Overactive bladder definition and ultrasound measurements of bladder wall thickness: the right way about urodynamics? *Neurourol Urodyn* 2002; **21**: 284–5.

58. DELANCEY JO. Anatomy. In: Cardozo L, Staskin D, editors. *Textbook of Female Urology and Urogynecology*. London: Isis Medical Media; 2001. p. 112–24.

59. OSTRZENSKI A, OSBORNE NG, OSTRZENSKA K. Method for diagnosing paravaginal defects using contrast ultrasonographic technique. *J Ultrasound Med* 1997; **16**: 673–77.

60. NGUYEN JK, HALL CD, TABER E, BHATIA NN. Sonographic diagnosis of paravaginal defects: a standardisation of technique. *Int Urogynecol J* 2000; **11**: 341–5.

61. MARTAN A, MASATA J, HALASKA M, OTCENASEK M, SABIK K. Ultrasound imaging of paravaginal defects in women with stress incontinence before and after paravaginal defect repair. *Ultrasound Obstet Gynecol* 2002; **19**: 496–500.

62. CREIGHTON SM, PEARCE JM, STANTON SL. Perineal video-ultrasonography in the assessment of vaginal prolapse: early observations. *Br J Obstet Gynaecol* 1992; **99**: 310–13.

63. DIETZ HP, HAYLEN BT, BROOME J. Ultrasound in the quantification of female pelvic organ prolapse. *Ultrasound Obstet Gynecol* 2001; **18**: 511–14.

64. ATHANASIOU S, KHULLAR V, BOOS K, SALVATORE S, CARDOZO L. Imaging the urethral sphincter with three-dimensional ultrasound. *Obstet Gynecol* 1999; **94**: 295–301.

65. TOOZS-HOBSON P, ATHANASIOU S, KHULLAR V, BOOS K, HEXTALL A, CARDOZO L. Does vaginal delivery damage the pelvic floor? *Neurourol Urodyn* 1997; **16**: 385–6.

66. TOOZS-HOBSON P, KHULLAR V, CARDOZO L. Three-dimensional ultrasound: a novel technique for investigating the urethral sphincter in the third trimester of pregnancy. *Ultrasound Obstet Gynecol* 2001; **17**: 421–4.

Ultrasound and diagnosis of obstetric anal sphincter injuries

ABDUL H SULTAN AND RANEE THAKAR

Introduction

Anal endosonography is a relatively recent development in the evolution of diagnostic ultrasound. Following the original description of the technique by Bartram in 1989,[1] Sultan et al.[2,3] clarified and validated the interpretation of images. Subsequently, other approaches were described such as transvaginal[4] and transperineal,[5] allowing imaging of the undisturbed anal sphincter. It is now also possible to obtain three-dimensional ultrasound images as well as magnetic resonance images.[6] Anal endosonography is now regarded as the gold standard investigation in patients presenting with faecal incontinence. It is also useful in the diagnosis of anal pain, anorectal tumours, fistulae, abscesses and anismus.[7] The advent of anal endosonography has enabled considerable research into obstetric related anal sphincter trauma, the major aetiological factor in the development of anal incontinence.[8]

Anatomy of the anorectum

Before any attempt is made to image the anal sphincter it is important to have a clear understanding of the anatomy and normal variation of the anorectal musculature to avoid misinterpretation. However, the precise anatomy of the anal sphincter mechanism has remained controversial and there is still disagreement as to whether the external anal sphincter is composed of one, two or three parts. The three-part classification of the external anal sphincter into deep, superficial and subcutaneous components (Figure 11.1)[7,9] remains the most popular. These subdivisions are difficult to demonstrate during cadaveric dissections, however, and they are certainly not identifiable during surgery. The inconsistency in description can be attributed to considerable inter-individual and intra-individual anatomical variation: such a longitudinal section of the anal canal reveals that the two hemispheres of the same individual are not necessarily identical.[10] As the echogenicity of images is dependent upon fibrous tissue content and direction of muscle fibres, an in-depth knowledge is needed of normal appearances and anatomical variants of the anorectal musculature. To overcome some of these

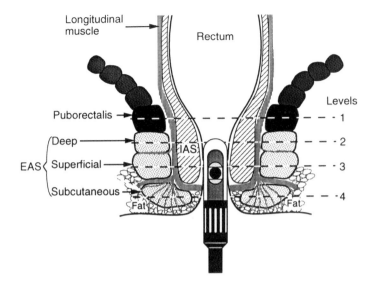

FIGURE 11.1 Schematic representation of the anal canal with the probe in place; level 1 = puborectalis, level 2 = deep (proximal) external anal sphincter (EAS); level 3 = superficial (mid) EAS; level 4 = subcutaneous (distal) EAS (reproduced with permission from Thakar R, Sultan AH. Anal endosonography and its role in assessing the incontinent patient. *Best Pract Res Clin Obstet Gynaecol* 2004; **18**: 157–73)

potential pitfalls, interpretation of dynamic images is essential. Further information regarding contractility of muscle can be obtained by asking the patient to squeeze and strain during the procedure.

Equipment

In 1982, Frentzel-Beyme used the rectal endoprobe (manufactured by B&K Medical, Gentofte, Denmark) with the transducer covered by a fluid-filled balloon to image the prostate gland.[11] In 1986, using the same probe, Beynon et al.[12] clarified the interpretation of endosonic appearances of normal colon and rectum. For the purposes of anal endosonography Law and Bartram modified the tip of the probe by replacing the water-filled balloon with a hard sonolucent plastic cone measuring 17mm in diameter (Figure 11.2).[1] The rotating endoprobe is fitted with a 10 MHz transducer (focal range 5–45mm), which provides a 360-degree cross-sectional image.

Technique

Anal endosonography is performed in the left-lateral position (especially in pregnancy), although some prefer the prone position.[13] The end of the probe is covered with a condom and coupling gel is applied to both sides of the condom. All images are orientated according to convention, such that anterior lies at the top, although earlier descriptions were orientated such that anterior was to the right. The probe is inserted about 6cm into the rectum and, as the probe is withdrawn

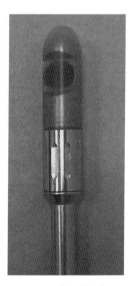

FIGURE 11.2 The original B&K Medical (Gentofte, Denmark) water-filled rotating endoanal ultrasound probe (reproduced with permission from Thakar R, Sultan AH. Anal endosonography and its role in assessing the incontinent patient. *Best Pract Res Clin Obstet Gynaecol* 2004; 18: 57–73)

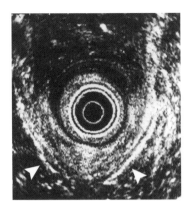

FIGURE 11.3 Sonographic image at level 1 of Figure 11.1 demonstrating the puborectalis muscle (arrow) (reproduced with permission from Thakar R, Sultan A H. Anal endosonography and its role in assessing the incontinent patient. *Best Pract Res Clin Obstet Gynaecol* 2004; **18**: 157–73)

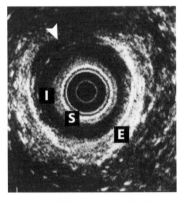

FIGURE 11.4 The deep external anal sphincter (E) at level 2 in Figure 11.1; s = subepithelium, I = internal anal sphincter, E = external anal sphincter. The anterior gap (arrow) shows the sloping and shorter external sphincter in the female (reproduced with permission from Thakar R, Sultan A H. Anal endosonography and its role in assessing the incontinent patient. *Best Pract Res Clin Obstet Gynaecol* 2004; **18**: 157–73)

down the anal canal, images of the puborectalis muscle, the anal epithelium, internal anal sphincter, longitudinal muscle and external anal sphincter become visible (Figure 11.1).

Interpretation

Puborectalis muscle

The puborectalis muscle is the most medial portion of the levator ani muscle and forms a U-shaped sling behind the anorectum. Anteriorly, it attaches to the posterior surface of the symphysis pubis and pubic rami. Sonographically, it appears as a U-shaped hyperechoic band (Figure 11.3).

The anal epithelium (submucosa)

The subepithelial layer, which is composed of connective tissue and smooth muscle, appears hyperechoic (Figures 11.4 and 11.5). The anal cushions, which provide the final seal for the anal canal, are not normally seen during endoluminal examination as they are compressed.

The internal anal sphincter

The internal anal sphincter is a thickened continuation of the circular smooth muscle layer of the bowel and appears homogeneously hypoechoic. It does not extend inferiorly beyond the superficial external sphincter (Figures 11.4, 11.5 and 11.6).

The longitudinal muscle

This layer of smooth muscle appears hyperechoic and is a continuation of the longitudinal muscle of the bowel. It also receives fascial-striated muscle contributions from the puborectalis and the deep external anal sphincter: hence the name 'conjoint' longitudinal muscle. This layer is not always identified by ultrasound as it is often of the same echogenicity as the adjacent external anal sphincter and is distinguishable only in 40% of females (Figure 11.6).[2,3]

The external anal sphincter

The external anal sphincter usually appears hyperechoic but has a heterogeneous appearance. It can appear hypoechoic relative to the

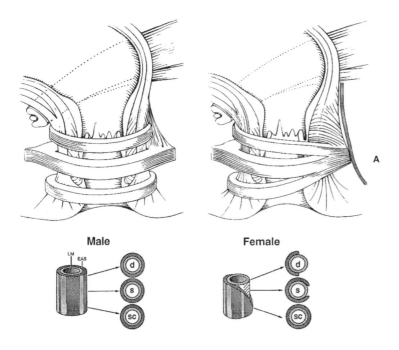

Male   Female

FIGURE 11.5 The anterior anal sphincter is shorter in the female; a cross-sectional scan performed in a woman at the level of the deep (d) external sphincter (EAS) reveals an apparent anterior defect (Figure 11.4), which disappears at the subcutaneous (s). Note that the internal sphincter (IAS) is absent at the level of the subcutaneous (SC) EAS, as shown in Figure 11.8 (A = anterior) (reproduced with permission from Thakar R, Sultan AH. Anal endosonography and its role in assessing the incontinent patient. *Best Pract Res Clin Obstet Gynaecol* 2004; **18**: 157–73)

longitudinal muscle layer, particularly in men (Figure 11.6). The variability in echogenicity is related to variations in the orientation of some fibres of the sphincter.[2,10] Although there is controversy regarding the subdivisions of the external anal sphincter,[10] sonographically, the deep, superficial and subcutaneous components of the external anal sphincter appears as one muscle with variation in shape and echogenicity. Recognition of gender differences are also important.[3,10] Unlike men, 98% of women have a shorter external anal sphincter anteriorly than posteriorly (Figure 11.7).[3,6] In cross-sectional imaging, the sloping fibres produce an apparent anterior defect so this must not be confused with a true sphincter defect. The deficiency of the external anal sphincter at this level may explain the vulnerability of the internal anal sphincter to obstetric damage in the presence of an intact external anal sphincter.

THE DEEP EXTERNAL ANAL SPHINCTER

The deep external anal sphincter does not appear sonographically separate from the puborectalis muscle posteriorly. It is annular and usually has no attachment to the coccyx. In the female, the external anal sphincter is shorter anteriorly and therefore the deep external anal sphincter slopes inferiorly and forwards bilaterally to unite anteriorly. An ultrasound image at this level could easily be misinterpreted as an anterior sphincter defect (Figure 11.4).

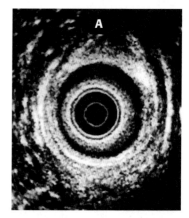

FIGURE 11.6 Image at level 3 (Figure 11.2) illustrates the change from the annular deep external anal sphincter (EAS) to the elliptical superficial EAS. The ellipse is created by anterior attachments to the perineal body and posteriorly to the anococcygeal ligament (A = anterior) (reproduced with permission from Thakar R, Sultan AH. Anal endosonography and its role in assessing the incontinent patient. *Best Pract Res Clin Obstet Gynaecol* 2004; **18**: 157–73)

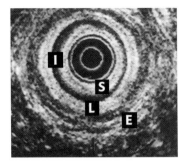

FIGURE 11.7 Image taken from a male patient demonstrating the prominent longitudinal muscle (L) which is only discernible in 40% of females (s = subepithelium, I = internal anal sphincter, E = external anal sphincter) (reproduced with permission from Thakar R, Sultan AH. Anal endosonography and its role in assessing the incontinent patient. *Best Pract Res Clin Obstet Gynaecol* 2004; 18: 157–73)

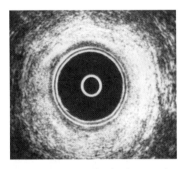

FIGURE 11.8 Image at level 4 demonstrating a conical subcutaneous external anal sphincter. Note that the internal anal sphincter is absent at this level

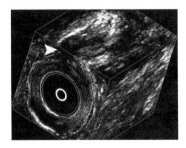

FIGURE 11.9 Three-dimensional image demonstrating an external sphincter defect in the radial and longitudinal dimension (arrow) (reproduced with permission from Thakar R, Sultan AH. Anal endosonography and its role in assessing the incontinent patient. *Best Pract Res Clin Obstet Gynaecol* 2004; 18: 157–73)

THE SUPERFICIAL EXTERNAL ANAL SPHINCTER

The superficial external anal sphincter (Figure 11.5) is more elliptical, with an anterior attachment to the perineal body and posteriorly it tapers to form the anococcygeal ligament.

THE SUBCUTANEOUS EXTERNAL ANAL SPHINCTER

The subcutaneous external anal sphincter (Figure 11.8) is the distal component of the external anal sphincter and is easily distinguishable endosonographically because it lies below the level of the hypoechoic internal anal sphincter ring (Figure 11.5). It is traversed by the terminal strands of longitudinal muscle and appears densely hyperechoic.

Perianal and ischiorectal fat

This hyperechoic layer has a striated heterogeneous appearance owing to fibrous septa (Figure 11.6).

Other imaging techniques and modalities

Three-dimensional endosonography

Three-dimensional endosonography has now been introduced, allowing for computer-aided multi-planar reconstruction of the anal canal (Figure 11.9),[6] so that sagittal images may be combined with longitudinal pressure measurements and the structure may be compared directly with function.[14] Images are obtained using the same probe that is used for two-dimensional imaging. In a prospective study of 45 primiparae who had three-dimensional endoanal scan performed before and after vaginal delivery, Williams *et al.* reported perineal trauma in 29% of women (external sphincter defect 11%, puboanalis defect 20%, transverse perineal muscle defect 7%).[15] The full diagnostic potential of three-dimensional imaging has yet to be realised, although it may aid the interpretation of obstetric tears and fistulae that are difficult to interpret with axial imaging.[16]

Magnetic resonance imaging

Magnetic resonance imaging (MRI) defines the striated components of the sphincter with greater clarity, especially with the endocoil.[17] In a small retrospective study of 22 patients,[18] external sphincter defects were detected in 16 (73%) with sonography and 20 (91%) with endoanal MRI and internal sphincter defects in 15 (68%) and 17 (77%), respectively. However, in a larger prospective study of 52 consecutive patients with faecal incontinence, endosonography was comparable with endoanal MRI in the diagnosis of external sphincter defects.[19] Endoanal MRI is useful in diagnosing external sphincter atrophy, which is an important prognostic factor in the outcome of sphincter repair.[20,21]

Vaginal endosonography

In 1994, Sultan et al.[4] first described transvaginal endosonography to image the anal sphincters at rest with a rotating probe. When compared with endoanal images, the internal sphincter appeared thicker on vaginal endosonography and this was attributed to the lack of anal distension with the endoanal probe. Frudinger et al.[23] reported that the transvaginal technique was inaccurate while Stewart and Wilson[24] found the transvaginal approach reliable and as accurate as endoanal sonography. More recently, Timor-Tritsch et al.[25] used a conventional transvaginal probe (5–9 MHz), with the footprint placed in the fourchette pointing backwards, and showed abnormal sphincter anatomy in symptomatic patients. However the images were not compared with the gold standard technique of endoanal ultrasound.

Transperineal ultrasound

In 1997, Peschers et al.[5] used the conventional convex transducer placed on the perineum to visualise the anal sphincters. In a prospective, single blind study of 55 patients with faecal incontinence and 43 who had no bowel symptoms, there was a 100% intra-observer agreement among researchers on internal anal sphincter lesions as confirmed by surgery. In the external anal sphincter group there was only one discordant result.[5] Another prospective study reported a sensitivity of 50% and the specificity is 84% in diagnosing sphincter defects.[26] It is not useful in visualising the internal anal sphincter in the immediate postpartum period.[27] Roche et al.[28] have suggested that perineal sonography might be more useful in incontinence screening but endoanal scans provide clearer images of the anal sphincter.

Degree	Definition
1	Laceration of the vaginal epithelium or perineal skin only
2	Involvement of the perineal muscles but not the anal sphincter
3	Disruption of the anal sphincter muscles:
a	<50% thickness of external sphincter torn
b	>50% thickness of external sphincter torn
c	Internal sphincter also torn
4	A third-degree tear with disruption of the anal epithelium

TABLE 11.1 Classification of perineal tears[38]

Obstetric anal sphincter injury

Occult anal sphincter trauma

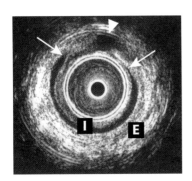

FIGURE 11.10 A persistent anterior defect of the external (arrowhead) and internal sphincter (arrows) (I = internal anal sphincter, E = external anal sphincter) (reproduced with permission from Thakar R, Sultan AH. Anal endosonography and its role in assessing the incontinent patient. *Best Pract Res Clin Obstet Gynaecol* 2004; **18**: 157–73)

The development of anal endosonography in 1989[1] added a new dimension to understanding the pathogenesis of anal incontinence and the diagnosis of obstetric anal sphincter injuries. Until then, the development of anal incontinence was attributed largely to pelvic neuropathy.[28,29] It was subsequently shown that mechanical injury to the anal sphincter (Figure 11.10) is a major aetiological factor.[8,30,31] There have been at least ten prospective studies before and after childbirth indicating that on average about 27% (range 19%[32] to 41%[33]) of women undergoing their first vaginal delivery develop 'occult' sphincter injury. However, as only 33% of these women develop defaecatory symptoms within 2 months of delivery,[8] it remains to be established whether the remaining women with 'occult' defects are at increased risk of developing incontinence later in life.

Although the risk of new recognised anal sphincter injury occurring in subsequent deliveries is small (5%), symptoms of incontinence may be precipitated for the first time following a subsequent delivery[8,34] or later in life. The reasons for this are not clear, as mechanisms that maintain continence are complex but include factors such as ageing, pudendal neuropathy, menopause, anorectal surgery, irritable bowel syndrome and change in diet and bowel habits. Furthermore, because anal incontinence is embarrassing, women delay seeking help. When multiparous women present with anal incontinence it is more likely that significant 'occult' injury had been sustained during the first vaginal delivery.[8,34]

In a study at Queen Charlotte's Hospital, London,[35] a clinical research fellow re-examined women who had sustained obstetric perineal lacerations and found that 40% of obstetric anal sphincter injuries were being missed. When Andrews *at al.*[36] re-examined 241 women following vaginal delivery, they found that the detection rate of obstetric anal sphincter injuries doubled. Endoanal ultrasound was also performed immediately after delivery and repeated at 3 months postpartum. Interestingly, all clinically diagnosed obstetric anal sphincter injuries were identified by endoanal ultrasound. In three women, defects were identified by endoanal ultrasound but not seen clinically. Two of these were isolated internal anal sphincter injuries. In practice, isolated internal anal sphincter injuries would not normally be clinically apparent, as the external anal sphincter would need to be torn as well. There was only one anal sphincter injury diagnosed by scan that was not recognised at delivery (involving both the internal and external anal sphincters). This may therefore represent a genuine occult sphincter injury. No new defects were identified by ultrasound at follow-up that were not seen on the first scan performed immediately after delivery, indicating that all anal sphincter injuries occur at the time of birth and not in the puerperium. However, more importantly this study demonstrates that genuine occult sphincter injuries are a rare occurrence and therefore almost all 'occult' sphincter injuries described previously probably represent unidentified or under-reported anal sphincter tears. There are several plausible explanations for this. Firstly, as obstetric anal sphincter injuries are regarded as triggers for risk management, there is a great disincentive to accurate reporting. Secondly, as alluded to above, a large number of obstetric anal sphincter injuries that are attributed to 'occult' injuries are missed at delivery. Thirdly, owing to a lack of consistency in the classification of obstetric anal sphincter injuries,[37] a number of obstetric anal

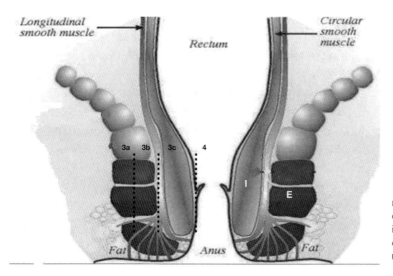

FIGURE 11.11 Schematic representation[45] of the new classification of anal sphincter injuries into 3a, 3b, 3c and fourth-degree[38,39,40] (I = internal anal sphincter, E = external anal sphincter)

sphincter injuries are wrongly classified as second degree. In 2002, 672 practising consultant obstetricians were surveyed and 33% classified a complete or partial external sphincter tear as 'second degree'.[38]

In order to standardise the classification of perineal tears, Sultan proposed the following grading system,[39] (Figure 11.11) which has now been adopted by the Royal College of Obstetricians and Gynaecologists[40] and internationally (Table 11.1).[41] Isolated tears of the anal epithelium[42] without involvement of the anal sphincters (buttonhole) are rare. To avoid confusion they are not included in the classification in Table 11.1.

These injuries that have previously been classified as 'occult' do have clinical relevance as it has been shown that 42% of women who have asymptomatic 'occult' anal sphincter defects after their first vaginal delivery develop faecal incontinence after a subsequent vaginal delivery.[34] It is therefore important that doctors and midwives undergo more focused and intensive training to recognise these tears at delivery. Innovations such as using a specially designed latex model and fresh animal anal sphincters[42] in dedicated hands-on workshops[43] have been shown to change the clinical practice of doctors[44] and midwives.[45] Consequently, a three-fold change of practice was noted among midwives who began performing rectal examinations before and after perineal repair.[46]

Diagnosis of acute obstetric anal sphincter tears

The most accurate method of diagnosing anal sphincter tears is when clinical examination is performed by an experienced person.[35,36] It is our opinion that every woman who has a vaginal delivery, especially if an episiotomy was performed or if a perineal tear occurred, should have a rectal examination to exclude rectal or anal sphincter injury. Any first- or second-degree perineal tear that extends to the anal verge must be assumed to be a third-degree tear until verified by an experienced doctor or midwife. However, even 'buttonhole' tears between the rectum and vagina can occur in isolation with an intact perineum.[42]

The perineum should be examined[46] after adequate exposure and only in the presence of good lighting. The lithotomy position may be useful if exposure is not adequate. A rectal examination should then be performed to exclude injury to the anorectal mucosa and anal sphincter. Diagnosis of anal sphincter disruption requires clear visualisation and confirmation by palpation. The anal sphincter can be palpated by performing a pill-rolling motion with the index finger in the anal canal and the thumb in the vagina. The woman could also be asked to contract her anal sphincter and, if the anal sphincter is disrupted, there will be a distinct gap felt anteriorly (in the absence of an epidural). If the perineal skin is intact, there will be absence of puckering on the peri-anal skin anteriorly. As the external anal sphincter is in a state of tonic contraction, disruption results in retraction of the sphincter ends, so the sphincter ends need to be grasped and retrieved. The internal sphincter is a circular muscle and appears paler than the external sphincter.[42, 44] Under normal circumstances, the distal end of the internal sphincter lies a few millimetres proximal to the distal end of the external sphincter. However, if the external sphincter is relaxed following regional or general anaesthesia, the distal end of the internal sphincter will appear to be at a lower level.

Although postpartum ultrasound has been shown to increase detection of acute anal sphincter injuries, it also increases the false positive rate and consequently unnecessary intervention.[47] It is our opinion that, with improvement in clinical diagnostic skills, detection of obstetric anal sphincter injuries immediately after delivery can be significantly improved[44, 45] and, in practice, postpartum anal endosonography is of limited value.

Conclusions

Anal endosonography is now regarded as an essential investigation in the management of anal incontinence. However, expertise is required in interpretation of images as there are considerable variations in anat-omy. New imaging techniques such as three-dimensional scanning and MRI have provided further insight. Although anal endosonography is a useful investigative tool in the diagnosis of anorectal tumours, fistulae (Figure 11.12), abscesses and anismus, its major contribution is in the improved understanding of obstetric anal sphincter trauma, a major aetiological factor in the development of faecal incontinence.

In acute injuries there is no substitute for accurate clinical assess-ment. Unfortunately, education and training in identifying anal sphinc-ter injuries have been suboptimal; however, the advent of hands-on workshops using models and fresh animal tissue is improving the understanding and management of obstetric anal sphincter injuries.

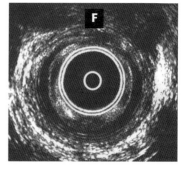

FIGURE 11.12 A rectovaginal fistula tract (F)

REFERENCES

1. LAW PJ, BARTRAM C I. Anal endosonography: technique and normal anatomy. *Gastrointest Radiol* 1989; **14**:349–53.

2. SULTAN A H, NICHOLLS RJ, KAMM M A, HUDSON C N, BEYNON J, BARTRAM C I. Anal endosonography and correlation with in vitro and in vivo anatomy. *Br J Surg* 1993; **80**:508–11.

3. SULTAN A H, KAMM M A, HUDSON C N, NICHOLLS RJ, BARTRAM CI. Endosonography of the anal sphincters: normal anatomy and comparison with manometry. *Clin Radiol* 1994; **49**:368–74.

4. SULTAN A H, LODER P B, BARTRAM C, KAMM M A, HUDSON CN. Vaginal endosonography: a new technique to image the undisturbed anal sphincter. *Dis Colon Rectum* 1994; **37**:1296–9.

5. PESCHERS U M, DeLANCEY J O L, SCHAER G N, SCHUESSLER B. Exoanal ultrasound of the anal sphincter. *Br J Obstet Gynaecol* 1997; **104**:999–1003.

6. GOLD D M, BARTRAM C I, HALLIGAN S, HUMPHRIES K N, KAMM M A, KMIOT W A. Three-dimensional endoanal sonography in assessing anal canal injury. *Br J Surg* 1999; **86**:365–70.

7. THAKAR R, SULTAN A H. Anal endosonography and its role in assessing the incontinent patient. *Best Pract Res Clin Obstet Gynaecol* 2004; **18**:157–73.

8. SULTAN A H, KAMM M A, HUDSON C N, THOMAS J M, BARTRAM C I. Anal sphincter disruption during vaginal delivery. *New Engl J Med* 1993; **329**:1905–11.

9. THAKAR R, SULTAN A H. Management of obstetric anal sphincter injury. *The Obstetrician and Gynaecologist* 2003; **5**:72–7.

10. SULTAN A H. The effect of childbirth on the anal sphincter as demonstrated by anal endosonography and anorectal physiology. MD thesis. University of Natal, South Africa; 1995.

11. FRENTZEL-BEYME B, SCHWARTZ J, AURICH B. [Transrectal prostatic sonography (TPS).] *Computertomographie* 1982; **2**:68–75. [In German.]

12. BEYNON J, FOY D M A, TEMPLE L N, CHANNER J L, VIRJEE J, MORTENSEN J N. The endoscopic appearances of the normal colon and rectum. *Dis Colon Rectum* 1986; **29**:810–13.

13. FRUDINGER A, BARTRAM C I, HALLIGAN S, KAMM M. Examination techniques for endosonography of the anal canal. *Abdom Imaging* 1998; **23**:301–3.

14. WILLIAMS A B, CHEETHAM M J, BARTRAM C I, HALLIGAN S, KAMM M A, NICHOLLS RJ, KMIOT W A. Gender differences in the longitudinal pressure profile of the anal canal related to anatomical structure as demonstrated on three-dimensional anal endosonography. *Br J Surg* 2000; **87**:1674–9.

15. WILLIAMS A B, BARTRAM C I, HALLIGAN S, SPENCER J A, NICHOLS RJ, KMIOT W A. Anal sphincter damage after vaginal delivery using three-dimensional endosonography. *Obstet Gynaecol* 2001; **97**:770–5.

16. BARTRAM C I, SULTAN A H. Imaging of the anal sphincter. In: Sultan A H, Thakar R, Fenner D. *Perineal and anal sphincter trauma*. London: Springer 2007. p.123–32.

17. STOKER J, HUSSAIN S M, LAMERIS J S. Endoanal magnetic resonance imaging versus endosonography. *La Radiologica Medica* 1996; **92**:38–41.

18. ROCIU E, STOKER J, EIJKEMANS M J C, SCHOUTEN W R, LAMERIS J S. Faecal incontinence: endoanal US versus endoanal MR imaging. *Radiology* 1999; **212**:453–8.

19. MALOUF A J, WILLIAMS A B, HALLIGAN S, BARTRAM C I, DHILLON S, KAMM M A. Prospective assessment of accuracy of endoanal MR imaging and endosonography in patients with fecal incontinence. *Am J Roentgenol* 2000; **175**:741–5.

20. BRIEL J W, STOKER J, ROCIU E, LAMERIS J S, HOP W C J, SCHOUTEN W R. External anal sphincter atrophy on endoanal magnetic resonance imaging adversely affects continence after sphincteroplasty. *Br J Surg* 1999; **86**:1322–7.

21. BRIEL J W, ZIMMERMAN D, STOKER J, ROCIU E, LAMERIS J S, MOOI W J, *et al*. Relationship between sphincter morphology on endoanal MRI and histopathological aspects of the external sphincter. *Int J Colorect Dis* 2000; **15**:87–90.

22. WILLIAMS A B, BARTRAM C I, MODWADIA D, NICHOLS T, HALLIGAN S, KAMM M A, *et al*. Endocoil magnetic resonance imaging quantification of external sphincter atrophy. *Br J Surg* 2001; **88**:853–9.

23. FRUDINGER A, BARTRAM C I, KAMM M A. Transvaginal versus anal endosonography for detecting damage to the anal sphincter. *Am J Roentgenol* 1997; **168**:1435–8.

24. STEWART L K, WILSON S R. Transvaginal sonography of the anal sphincter: reliable or not? *Am J Roentgenol* 1999; **173**:179–85.

25. TIMOR-TRITSCH I E, MONTEAGUDO A, SMILEN S W, PORGES R F, AVIZOVA E. Simple ultrasound evaluation of the anal sphincter in female patients using a transvaginal transducer. *Ultrasound Obstet Gynecol* 2005; **25**:177–83.

26. LOHSE C, BRETONES S, BOULVAIN M, WEIL A, KRAUER F. Trans-perineal versus endo-anal ultrasound in the detection of anal sphincter defects. *Eur J Obstet Gynecol Reprod Biol* 2002; **103**:79–82.

27. SHOBEIRI S A, NOLAN T E, YORDAN-JOVET R, ECHOLS K T, CHESSON R R. Digital examination compared to trans-perineal ultrasound for the evaluation of anal sphincter repair. *Int J Gynecol Obstet* 2002; **78**:31–6.

28. ROCHE B, DELEAVAL J, FRANSIOLI A, MARTI M C. Comparison of transanal and external perineal ultrasound. *Eur Radiol* 2002; **11**:1165–70.

29. SNOOKS S J, SWASH M, SETCHELL M, HENRY M M. Injury to innervation of pelvic floor sphincter musculature in childbirth. *Lancet* 1984; **ii**:546–50.

30. ALLEN R E, HOSKER G L, SMITH A R B, WARRELL D W. Pelvic floor damage and childbirth: a neurophysiological study. *Br J Obstet Gynaecol* 1990; **97**:770–9.

31. DONNELLY V S, FYNES M, CAMPBELL D, JOHNSON H, O'CONNELL P R, O'HERLIHY C. Obstetric events leading to anal sphincter damage. *Obstet Gynecol* 1998; **92**:955–61.

32. NAZIR M, CARLSEN E, NESHEIM B. Do occult anal sphincter injuries, vector volume manometry and delivery variables have any predictive value for bowel symptoms after first time vaginal delivery without third and fourth degree rupture? A prospective study. *Acta Obstet Gynecol Scand* 2002; **81**:720–6.

33. RIEGER N, SCHLOITHE A, SACCONE G, WATTCHOW D. A prospective study of anal sphincter injury due to childbirth. *Scand J Gastroenterol* 1998; **33**:950–5.

34. FYNES M, DONNELLY V, BEHAN M, O'CONNELL P R, O'HERLIHY C. Effect of second vaginal delivery on anorectal physiology and faecal incontinence: a prospective study. *Lancet* 1999; **354**:983–6.

35. GROOM K M, PATERSON-BROWN S. Can we improve the diagnosis of third degree tears? *Eur J Obstet Gynecol Reprod Biol* 2002; **101**:19–21.

36. ANDREWS V, SULTAN A H, THAKAR R, JONES P W. Occult anal sphincter injuries – myth or reality? *BJOG* 2006; **113**:95–200.

37. SULTAN A H, THAKAR R. Lower genital tract and anal sphincter trauma. *Best Pract Res Clin Obstet Gynaecol* 2002; **16(1)**:99–116.

38. FERNANDO R J, SULTAN A H, RADLEY S, JONES P W, JOHANSON R B. Management of obstetric anal sphincter injury: a systematic review and national practice survey. *BMC Health Serv Res* 2002; **2**:9.

39. SULTAN A H. Obstetric perineal injury and anal incontinence. *Clin Risk* 1999; **5**:193–6.

40. Royal College of Obstetricians and Gynaecologists. *The Management of Third – and Fourth-degree Perineal Tears.* RCOG Guideline No. 29. London: RCOG; 2001.

41. NORTON C, CHRISTIANSEN J, BUTLER U, HARARI D, NELSON RL, PEMBERTON J, *et al.*, editors. *Incontinence.* 2nd ed. Plymouth: Health Publication Ltd; 2002. p. 985–1044.

42. SULTAN A H, THAKAR R. Third and fourth degree tears. In: Sultan A H, Thakar R, Fenner D. *Perineal and Anal Sphincter Trauma.* London: Springer; 2007. p. 33–51.

43. See, for example: Mayday Hospital Urogynaecology and Pelvic Floor Reconstruction Unit courses at: www.perineum.net.

44. THAKAR R, SULTAN A H, FERNANDO R, MONGA A, STANTON S L. Can workshops on obstetric anal sphincter rupture change practice? *Int Urogynecol J Pelvic Floor Dysfunct* 2001: **12(3)**:S5.

45. ANDREWS V, THAKAR R, SULTAN A H, KETTLE C. Can hands-on perineal repair courses affect clinical practice? *Br J Midwifery* 2005; **13**:562–5.

46. SULTAN A H, KETTLE C. Diagnosis of perineal trauma. In: SULTAN A H, THAKAR R, FENNER D. *Perineal and Anal Sphincter Trauma.* London: Springer; 2007. p. 13–19.

47. FALTIN D L, BOULVAIN M, FLORIS L A, IRION O. Diagnosis of anal sphincter tears to prevent fecal incontinence: a randomized controlled trial. *Obstet Gynecol* 2005; **106**:6–13.

12

Organisation of the early pregnancy unit

EMMA SAWYER AND DAVOR JURKOVIC

Introduction

Early pregnancy complications are one of the most common reasons for women of reproductive age seeking medical help. Many pregnancies are complicated by pain and/or bleeding, which often causes concern because of a perceived risk of miscarriage or ectopic pregnancy. Around 40% of biochemical and clinical pregnancies may result in miscarriage and bleeding complicates around 21% of clinically detected pregnancies.[1] There are many other symptoms which may also cause concern to pregnant women, such as hyperemesis, loss of pregnancy symptoms and gastrointestinal problems.

In the past, a woman with early pregnancy complications would first have to seek advice from her general practitioner or self refer to the accident and emergency (A&E) department in a local hospital. In A&E, early pregnancy problems would often be treated as a low priority and it was not unusual for women to spend many hours waiting to be treated.[1] A&E departments have limited access to diagnostic and laboratory services and many women in the past had been admitted for inpatient investigations.

A significant change has occurred in the management approach to early pregnancy complications. In the past, surgery was considered necessary for both the diagnosis and treatment of early pregnancy complications. It has now been recognised that the majority of miscarriages and a significant proportion of ectopic pregnancies could be managed conservatively.[2,3] Conservative management, however, requires sophisticated diagnostic facilities and a robust follow-up structure, which is not available in emergency departments.

Failings of the traditional approach to early pregnancy complications have been recognised both by women and health providers, which has led to the formation of early pregnancy units.[4] The aim of early pregnancy units is to provide women with rapid and easy access to health professionals dedicated to management of early pregnancy complications. They offer a comprehensive package of care, which includes diagnostic workup, implementation of the appropriate management plan, follow-up, counselling and emotional support.

Facilities for ultrasound examination are an integral part of the early pregnancy unit. The ultrasound scan itself provides a non-invasive diagnosis of normal and abnormal early pregnancy. Transvaginal sonography was introduced in the late 1980s and this, combined with decreased costs and wider availability of equipment, has meant that ultrasound examination has become the mainstay of early pregnancy diagnosis. The demand for ultrasound has been increasing steadily and, to accommodate this, early pregnancy units were set up in the UK in the early 1990s. Although early pregnancy units are nowadays available in most acute hospitals within the UK, they are not organised in a uniform way and there is no agreement about which health professionals should be running the unit, what facilities should be available and who takes overall responsibility for patient care.

Aims of early pregnancy units

Symptoms of miscarriage can be dramatic and frightening for a pregnant woman. A comprehensive service with easy and fast access needs to be provided for women in early pregnancy. An initial assessment to reach a correct diagnosis and plan her treatment is carried out and diagnostic tests instigated. Follow-up is vital and, for those women who have suffered pregnancy loss, offering counselling and support is another important role for an early pregnancy unit.[5] Other benefits to women include continuity of care, continuing support and a point of contact for any queries or emergencies.

From a clinical perspective, the aim of the early pregnancy unit is to provide diagnosis and treatment on an outpatient basis and, following on from this, to maximise the use of expectant management. This has been highlighted by the decrease in the length of admissions and time to diagnosis in women with early pregnancy complications. Before the early pregnancy unit was established, the average time for diagnosis of early pregnancy complications was over 30 hours; since the advent of the early pregnancy unit this has fallen to just 2 hours. By avoiding the protracted channels of A&E, women can be seen, diagnosed and management instigated in a fraction of the time (Figure 12.1).[6]

Similarly, before the opening of early pregnancy units, time from diagnosis to treatment was longer and women with early pregnancy complications stayed in hospital for an average of 1.5 days (range 0.5–3.0 days). The duration of stay for those women requiring evacuation of retained products of conception (ERPC) was longer, at 3 days (range 1.5–5.0 days).[6] Women would have to stay longer than necessary if ultrasonography was not available, for example at weekends or during public holidays.

From a financial perspective, the aim is to run a cost-efficient unit. Savings arise with fewer admissions for ERPC, fewer women needing

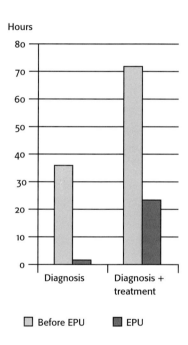

FIGURE 12.1 The effect of opening an early pregnancy unit on the length of time required to complete diagnostic process and management in women with early pregnancy complications (based on data from Bigrigg and Read[6])

laparotomy to treat ectopic pregnancies and, ideally, fewer complaints. Most women can now be treated as day cases and the maximum stay is reduced. In one hospital with a newly established early pregnancy unit, the reduction in length of stay for ERPC from 3 days to 1 day led to a saving of 466 bed days.[6] The cost of an ERPC as a day case gives a saving of £50/case and a saving of approximately £110,000/year is gained through women not being admitted unnecessarily.[6] Of course, funds are required initially in the setting up of a unit.

The gestational age up to which an early pregnancy unit will admit women with early pregnancy complications may vary between units, as there may be a crossover period between early pregnancy and obstetric scanning. The technical aspects of early pregnancy and obstetric scanning differ and this needs to be taken into account, while also being aware of the skills of the sonographers within the unit. Some women presenting to the early pregnancy unit will be uncertain of the date of their last menstrual period or expected gestation. In these cases, the woman should be scanned but then referred on, if necessary, to an obstetric unit for a more detailed scan, if the gestation is beyond that in the early pregnancy unit's protocol. Similarly, the obstetric unit might refer a woman to the early pregnancy unit if the nuchal or dating scan reveals a suspected miscarriage or if findings are smaller than expected for dates. Thus, a good working relationship with the obstetric sonographers is important.

Indications for assessment

Women will attend the unit for a variety of reasons:

▷ symptoms of pregnancy failure: probably the most common reason for women to attend an early pregnancy unit and the majority of women present with bleeding and/or pain
▷ loss of pregnancy symptoms
▷ high risk of ectopic pregnancy
▷ hyperemesis: to diagnose a multiple pregnancy and to exclude a molar pregnancy
▷ dating scans
▷ past history of first-trimester loss and/or recurrent miscarriage (a specialist recurrent miscarriage clinic is ideally located within the early pregnancy unit. From here, investigations can be coordinated and, on conceiving again, the woman has already had contact with the early pregnancy unit and can self-refer for an early scan and then be seen fortnightly throughout the first trimester to monitor development)

▷ high-risk groups, including those women who have had previous caesarean sections; the aim of the early scan in these cases is to exclude a caesarean scar pregnancy
▷ inconclusive scans in women attending termination clinics or family planning clinics to confirm diagnosis.

Source of referrals

The source of referrals varies. Firstly, an option for self-referral is beneficial so women can avoid having to wait for an appointment to be made and sent out. A walk-in service can accommodate self-referrals. Practitioners in primary care are a major source of referrals, as are A&E departments and family planning clinics. Midwives may detect complications in some women who are booked early in pregnancy and need to refer to early pregnancy unit.

The early pregnancy unit should be an accessible service for women and many make it their first point of contact if they are experiencing early pregnancy problems.

Location

Wherever an early pregnancy unit is located, access to other facilities is vital. A pregnancy scan cannot be carried out in isolation, as women might require follow-up, counselling and possible intervention. The unit could be incorporated into the gynaecology ward or outpatient clinic, or even within the antenatal clinic if facilities allow. This, however, may not be the most appropriate setting because of the distress caused by being around women with healthy pregnancies if a scan has shown a miscarriage or ectopic pregnancy.

Scans may be performed within the radiology department but if this is the case, a separate location is required for subsequent follow-up and care. A woman with a distressing scan result would not appreciate being sent to A&E after her scan nor having to wait to be reviewed by the gynaecology team on call.

Undoubtedly, the optimum choice is to have a self-contained unit with adequate facilities and dedicated, appropriately trained staff to run an early pregnancy clinic independently but with ready access to services such as laboratories, wards and operating theatres.

General facilities

A dedicated early pregnancy unit with a walk-in facility in a busy hospital could potentially see 20 women, if not more, during a morning session.

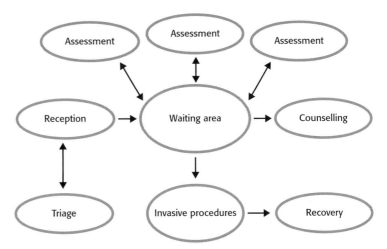

FIGURE 12.2 Organisational structure of the early pregnancy unit

Facilities therefore would need to take this into account (Figure 12.2).

A reception area is the first point of contact for the women and also acts as a filter in cases of inappropriate referral. Alongside this, there is scope for nurse triage, again to redirect women in case of inappropriate referrals or to fast track those women who are unwell. When women arrive, a urine specimen should be requested and a pregnancy test performed; this requires toilet and sluice facilities. An adequate waiting area, with possibly a quieter waiting room is essential, to provide privacy. Other requirements include assessment rooms, counselling rooms and a procedure room and recovery area with resuscitation facilities. Supportive care in early pregnancy confers a significant positive effect on pregnancy outcome in women who have suffered recurrent miscarriage of unknown aetiology.[7]

As previously mentioned, other facilities that are required but do not necessarily need to be within the early pregnancy unit include laboratories and venepuncture, pharmacy, wards and operating theatres.

Direct telephone access to the unit is useful, as many women may require telephone advice, or reassurance, which can be given without the need for them to attend in person.

Technical facilities

An ultrasound machine which produces high-quality images is vital; a mid-range ultrasound machine will probably cost in the region of £30,000–40,000. The transvaginal transducer should transmit at frequencies in the 4.0–7.5 MHz range to obtain high-quality images and the field of view should be more than 90 degrees.

It is sensible to have machines that are not too cumbersome so they can be moved to alternative sites to scan women who may be too unwell to attend the early pregnancy unit itself. Both a transvaginal and transabdominal probe will be used in the early pregnancy unit setting and this should be taken into account when choosing a machine. Transvaginal scan, however, should be used in most cases, as it is more suitable for the examination of very early pregnancies; the images are clearer and it can be performed instantly, as the woman does not need to spent time waiting for her bladder to fill. However, some women may feel that it is an unnecessary intrusion and they may request a transabdominal scan to be performed instead. With an abdominal scan, up to 42% of women will require a vaginal scan because the bladder is not full enough or the scan is inconclusive.[8] In one study, transvaginal scan was superior to abdominal scans at gestations less than 10 weeks in women with retroverted uteri or who were overweight.[9]

A questionnaire-based study of 107 women who underwent transvaginal scan showed that 99% of them would agree to have a similar procedure in the future. This suggests that women attending an early pregnancy unit with early pregnancy problems find transvaginal scanning acceptable.[10]

A probe with a small head and thin shaft is preferable for patient comfort. The probe is disinfected thoroughly at the beginning and end of each scan and a probe cover must be used and removed immediately at the end of the scan.[11] Alternative options for women who have a latex allergy also need to be considered.

Administration

With the advent of computer databases, a paperless clinic can be a key element in the efficient running of an early pregnancy unit. On attending the unit, each woman will have her own identification number; this may correspond to her hospital number or may be a number specific to the unit. All attendances can therefore be reviewed at each new visit, past information obtained without the need for pulling notes from medical records and data and images saved for future reference. Image capture is an essential part of data storage for ultrasound scanning, as it is a visual specialty.

Another advantage of a paperless clinic is the ability to write and send reports as soon as the examination is complete. Computer programs are available specifically for gynaecology and early pregnancy and, with such programs, normal values and ranges can be incorporated to aid diagnosis, for example in early pregnancy dating. Drop-down menus provide continuity of documentation, such as indication for referral and overall diagnosis. This will be of benefit during audits or carrying out database search for research purposes.

A specific database can incorporate the appointment booking and clinic scheduler so that all personnel can gain access from any assessment room and be able to make follow-up appointments when needed.

Issues

As an early pregnancy unit becomes established, the demand for the service will increase and facilities have to meet demand. Patient numbers will undoubtedly rise, as will women's expectations and those of other colleagues within the hospital. Women may expect a scan immediately, which may not be feasible at night or for the whole weekend for example. In an ideal world, the early pregnancy unit should be open for more than 8 hours a day and, ideally, open throughout the weekend too.

It has been realised that most women who attend with bleeding in early pregnancy have continuing pregnancies.[12] As a consequence, the early pregnancy unit provides a service for a large number of women who do not necessarily need further treatment and who in the past would have been managed in the community.

The advent of transvaginal scans has also led to some new problems. The number of inconclusive scans has risen, for example. This may be for a variety of reasons. Firstly, women attend earlier in the pregnancy and it may be too early to see a gestation sac if the β-hCG level is below 1000 iu/l the so-called 'discriminatory zone'.[13] Secondly, a woman may attend following an episode of heavy bleeding, which may represent a miscarriage. The uterus on scan may appear empty but, as no intrauterine gestation sac has been seen previously, one cannot assume this is the explanation for the ultrasound appearance. In these situations, biochemical parameters may have to be incorporated for accurate diagnosis.

Before the early pregnancy unit at Leeds Royal Infirmary was established, a non-viable pregnancy was the most common diagnosis in women presenting with early pregnancy complications. This diagnosis accounted for more than 60% of women presenting. Since the early pregnancy unit has been established, the percentage of women diagnosed with non-viable pregnancies has fallen to just 20%. Conversely, the number of women diagnosed with a viable pregnancy has increased to nearly 50%. Before the existence of the early pregnancy unit, just 20% of women presenting with early pregnancy complications were diagnosed with a viable pregnancy (Figure 12.3).[4]

Once an early pregnancy unit is established, there will undoubtedly be a tendency to refer early. Therefore, the number of women requiring rescans may increase, as it may not be possible to confirm the loca-

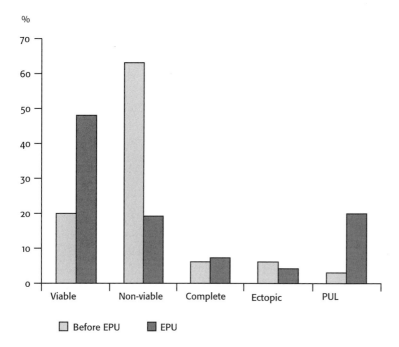

FIGURE 12.3 Final outcomes before and after opening an early pregnancy unit (PUL = pregnancy of unknown location) (modified from Walker and Shilito[4])

tion and viability of a pregnancy in 8–31% of cases at the first visit.[14] It is likely also that there will be more women referred who have had a miscarriage and who would have been managed at home in the past. Inappropriate referrals will also add to the workload.

A study by Haider et al.[15] examined the impact of ultrasound provision after hours on the management of women with suspected early pregnancy complications. They confirmed that the availability of ultrasound facilitates the use of conservative management strategies and decreased the need for admissions. However, their study also showed that many women with low clinical suspicion of having an ectopic pregnancy are classified as being at high risk of ectopic following an inconclusive ultrasound scan. These findings emphasise the need to continue developing effective and safe clinical algorithms for the management of women with non-diagnostic ultrasound scans. The purpose of performing ultrasound scans in early pregnancy units should be better defined. The main objective of performing a scan should be assessment of the early pregnancy viability, rather than screening for an ectopic pregnancy in asymptomatic women. The key issue, however, is to recognise that ultrasound findings are helpful only if interpreted in the clinical context.

Conclusions

The early pregnancy unit provides an easy and fast access point for women with early pregnancy complications and also provides continuity of care and follow-up. In an ideal world, the unit would be open 7 days a week. Women will present for a variety of reasons and will have varying symptoms of varying severity. It is important that the unit has multidisciplinary staff trained to an appropriate level, access to laboratory tests, a gynaecology ward and operating theatre, in case of direct admissions, and facilities for resuscitation. A well-run unit will be cost efficient for the hospital and hopefully ease the burden on over stretched inpatient resources.

REFERENCES

1. GILLING-SMITH C. TOOSZ-HOBSON P, POTTS D J, TOUQUET R, BEARD R W. Management of bleeding in early pregnancy in accident and emergency department. *Br Med J* 1994; **309**: 574–5.

2. NIELSEN S, HAHLIN M. Expectant management of first trimester spontaneous abortion. *Lancet* 1995; **345**: 84–6.

3. CACCIATORE B, KORHONEN J, STENMAN U H, YLOSTALO P. Transvaginal sonography and serum hCG in monitoring of presumed ectopic pregnancies selected for expectant management. *Ultrasound Obstet Gynecol* 1995; **5**: 297–3.

4. WALKER J J, SHILITO J. Early pregnancy units: service and organisational aspects. In: Grudzinkas J G, O'Brien P M S, editors. *Problems in Early Pregnancy: Advances in Diagnosis and Management.* London: RCOG Press; 1997. p. 160–73.

5. MACLEAN M A, CUMMING G P. Providing for women following miscarriage. *Scott Med J* 1993; **38**: 5–7.

6. BIGRIGG M A, READ M D. Management of women referred to early pregnancy assessment unit: care and cost effectiveness. *BMJ* 1991; **302**: 577–9.

7. CLIFFORD K, RAI R, REGAN L. Future pregnancy outcome in unexplained recurrent first trimester miscarriage. *Hum Reprod* 1997; **12**: 387–9.

8. SHILITO J, WALKER J J. Early pregnancy assessment units. *Br J Hosp Med* 1997; **58**: 505–9.

9. CULLEN M T, GREEN J J, REECE E S, HOBBINS J C. A comparison of transvaginal and abdominal ultrasound in visualising the first trimester conceptus. *J Ultrasound Med* 1989; **8**: 565–9.

10. DUTTA R L, ECONOMIDES D L. Patient acceptance of transvaginal sonography in the early pregnancy unit setting. *Ultrasound Obstet Gynecol* 2003; **22**: 503–7.

11. GOLDSTEIN S R. Reprocessing of the vaginal probe between patients. *Ultrasound Obstet Gynecol* 1996; **7**: 92–3.

12. ELSON J, SALIM R, TAILOR A, BANERJEE S, ZOSMER N, JURKOVIC D. Prediction of early pregnancy viability in the absence of an ultrasonically detectable embryo. *Ultrasound Obstet Gynecol* 2003; **21**: 57–61.

13 CACCIATORE B, STENMAN U-H, YLOSTALO P. Diagnosis of ectopic pregnancy by vaginal ultrasonography in combination with a discriminatory serum hCG level of 1000 iu/l (IRP). *Br J Obstet Gynaecol* 1990; **97**: 904–8.

14. CONDOUS G, OKARO E, BOURNE T. Pregnancies of unknown location: diagnostic dilemmas and management. *Curr Opin Obstet Gynecol* 2005; **17**: 568–73.

15. HAIDER Z, CONDOUS G, KHALID A, KIRK E, MUKRI F, VAN CALSTER B, et al. Impact of the availability of sonography in the acute gynaecology unit. *Ultrasound Obstet Gynecol* 2006; **28**: 207–13.

Sonoembryology: ultrasound examination of early pregnancy

Harm-Gerd Karl Blaas and Sturla H Eik-Nes

Introduction

The introduction of diagnostic ultrasound into clinical practice 40 years ago provided a new safe and non-invasive method for in vivo studies of early pregnancy development.[1,2] The initial studies primarily focused on biometrical descriptions of early pregnancy,[3–6] while later work was more concerned with normal and abnormal morphological features of embryos and early fetuses.[7–11] Major improvement in the ultrasound assessment of early pregnancy came with the introduction of transvaginal ultrasound at the end of the 1980s.[12] High-frequency transvaginal transducers improved the image quality to such an extent that a detailed description of the embryonic morphology became possible with in-depth anatomical studies of the brain compartments, the spine, the heart, the stomach, the midgut herniation and the limbs.[13–22]

Ultrasound examination of the embryo and early fetus

There are three main characteristics that mark the early human conceptus: its small size, its rapidly changing anatomical appearance and its uniform development and constant growth (Figure 13.1). The size of the young human conceptus in the first trimester puts high demands on image resolution. It is therefore important to get as close as possible to the target: use the transvaginal approach instead of the transabdominal route and use high-frequency transducers such as 7.5 MHz or more. With the transvaginal approach, acoustic noise (phase front aberrations and reverberations) and attenuation are reduced, thus improving the image resolution.

Standardisation of the orientation of the images is an important process in improving the diagnostic quality. To distinguish between transabdominal and transvaginal ultrasound, and not least to respect the correct anatomic orientation, the ultrasound image obtained by the transvaginal approach should be presented with the 'apex down'.[19,23]

Definitions of age

Embryologists use the Carnegie staging system to divide the human embryonic period into 23 developmental stages,[24] commencing with fertilisation at stage 1, continuing into the fetal period with the onset of marrow formation in the humerus after stage 23, which takes place at 56–57 days post-ovulation,[25] and the designation 'embryo' is replaced by 'fetus'. This corresponds to approximately 10 weeks and 0–1 days menstrual age.

Before the era of ultrasound, information about the developmental stage of the early conceptus was imprecise and age statements like 'months' or 'trimester' were used. Today, the term 'first trimester' is still applied but there are varying definitions of trimester, which means '3 months', based on, for example, a calendar month (28–31 days), a lunar month (28 days), an anomalistic month (27.5 days) or a synodic month (29.5 days). Since the borders between the trimesters do not mark specific developmental steps,[26] we should consider other time categories, such as completed weeks and days. The completion of the midgut herniation marks the end of early pregnancy at approximately 12 weeks 0 days.[19]

FIGURE 13.1 Changes in crown–rump length, biparietal diameter, yolk sac and amniotic sac in normal first trimester pregnancies showing that healthy normal embryos grow at a constant rate. Growth of the yolk sac, however, stops at 9 weeks of gestation (arrow), which coincides with the cessation of its physiological function (modified from Blaas *et al.*, 1998);[15] LMP = last menstural period

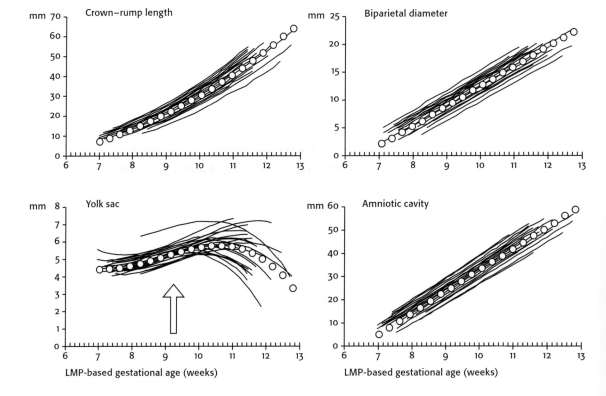

Stage (Weeks+days)	Development event
$4^{+3} - 4^{+6}$	A small gestation sac (2–5 mm) is seen within the endometrium. The sac is spherical, regular in outline and eccentrically situated towards the fundus. It is implanted just below the surface of the endometrium (midline echo) and is surrounded by echogenic trophoblast
$5^{+0} - 5^{+6}$	Yolk sac becomes visible within the chorionic cavity. This should be seen in all pregnancies with a mean gestational sac diameter of >12 mm. The embryonic pole becomes visible at the end of this week and it measures 2–3 mm in length. Heart action is also detectable
$6^{+0} - 6^{+6}$	The embryo changes from being a straight line at the top of the yolk sac to being kidney bean-shaped, with the yolk sac separated from the embryo by the vitelline duct. The crown–rump length measures 4–8 mm. If the heart rate is not detectable, the diagnosis of missed miscarriage is almost certain
$7^{+0} - 7^{+6}$	The crown–rump length measures 9–14 mm. The rhombencephalon becomes distinguishable as a diamond shaped cavity, enabling distinction of cephalad and caudal. The spine is seen as double echogenic parallel lines. The amniotic membrane becomes visible defining the amniotic cavity from the chorionic cavity. The umbilical cord can also be seen
$8^{+0} - 8^{+6}$	Crown–rump length 15–22 mm. Forebrain, midbrain, hindbrain and skull are distinguishable. Limb buds are also visible. Midgut hernia is present. The amniotic cavity expands and the umbilical cord and vitelline duct lengthens
$9^{+0} - 9^{+6}$	Crown–rump length 23–32 mm. The limbs lengthen and hands and feet are seen. Embryonic heart rate peaks at 170–180 beats/minute

TABLE 13.1 Key developmental events in early pregnancy that can be observed on ultrasound

In the following overview of early pregnancy development, all statements of time are based on the last menstrual period, expressed in completed weeks and completed days, assuming a regular cycle with ovulation at 2 weeks and 0 days. This applies also for the embryonic age, simplifying the comparison of embryonic development with first-trimester ultrasound findings. For example, 'during week 7' means 7 completed weeks plus 0–6 days, and 'at the end of week 9' means 9 completed weeks plus 5–6 days.

Normal early embryological development

Data from sonographic studies of embryos and fetuses using high frequency transvaginal probes and a review of the literature are the basis of this chapter (Table 13.1).[13, 19–21, 24, 27]

Gestational age 4 weeks and 0–6 days

EMBRYOLOGY

The occurrence of the primitive streak in the epiblast of the two-cellular layer embryonic disc at stage 6 initiates the developmental phase 'gastrulation', transforming the embryo into the trilaminar disc (ectoderm, mesoderm and endoderm). At the same stage, neurulation begins. This is a process that converts the neural plate via the neural folds into the hollow neural tube. The primitive heart tube appears at the end of week 4.

ULTRASOUND

After 4.5 weeks, the pregnancy becomes detectable as a ring-like structure with a diameter of 2–3 mm lying within the decidua (Figure 13.2).

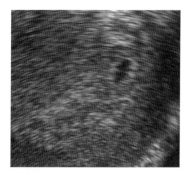

FIGURE 13.2 Longitudinal section through the uterus at 4^{+4} weeks of gestation demonstrating a 2.5 mm gestational sac at the fundal aspect of the uterine cavity

Gestational age 5 weeks and 0–6 days

EMBRYOLOGY

The primordium of the central nervous system, the neural tube, develops from this ectodermal neural plate after a transitional stage of neuroectodermal folding. The closure of the caudal neuropore, creating the ventricular system, takes place at Carnegie stage 12; that is, around 5 weeks and 6 days.[27] The embryonic disc folds cephalocaudally and laterally forming the three-dimensional body. The initially wide connection between the yolk sac and the embryo becomes the narrow vitelline duct (the omphalomesenteric duct), keeping a continuous connection to the developing gut tube. At the end of week 5 the body stalk is established. The heart tube starts to beat at 5 weeks 1 day, showing peristaltic flow at stage 11 (5 weeks 3 days).

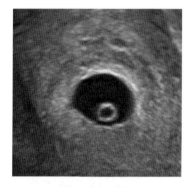

FIGURE 13.3 The yolk sac is the first structure to be seen within the gestational sac from 5 weeks of gestation

ULTRASOUND

The yolk sac becomes **sonographically** visible at the beginning of the week (Figure 13.3). The embryonic pole can be identified at the second half of the week (Figures 13.4, 13.5). The heart beat is identifiable at the end of week 5, when the heart rate is about 100 beats/minute.

Gestational age 6 weeks 0–6 days, CRL 3–8 mm

EMBRYOLOGY

At 6 weeks, the limb buds develop. At Carnegie stages 14 (around 6 weeks 3–4 days) and 15 (around 6 weeks 5 days) the forebrain divides into the telencephalon, with the cerebral hemispheres as small evaginations, and the diencephalon.[27,28] Then the ventricular system is divided into five brain regions on its cranial pole: the telencephalon (future hemispheres) and the diencephalon (future betweenbrain) derive from the prosencephalon (forebrain); the mesencephalon (midbrain) remains undivided and the metencephalon (future cerebellum and pons) and the myelencephalon (medulla oblongata) derive from the rhombencephalon (hindbrain). Successively, the brain compartments

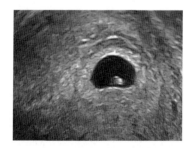

FIGURE 13.4 A small embryonic pole at the beginning of the 6th week of gestation

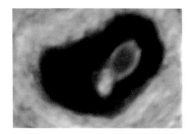

FIGURE 13.5 A three-dimensional sac at 6⁺² weeks, showing a small embryo adjacent to a yolk sac

enlarge, changing their proportions and positions to each other, and developing their specific shapes. The cerebral hemispheres develop as small evaginations from the telencephalon at about 6 weeks 4 days.

ULTRASOUND

The heart beat is always identifiable. The frequency increases from 105 beats/minute to 130 beats/minute (Figure 13.6). At the end of the week, the amniotic membrane may be seen. Not before the end of week 6 do the first brain structures become identifiable. The hypoechogenic oblong cavity of the rhombencephalon is found at the top of the embryonic head/body (Figure 13.7). Sometimes the narrow mesencephalic cavity may be detected anteriorly.[29]

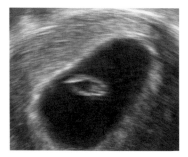

FIGURE 13.7 The embryonic brain at 6 weeks of gestation, showing a large rombencephalic cavity

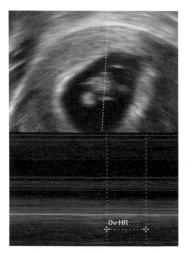

FIGURE 13.6 Measurement of embryonic heart rate using M-mode

Gestational age 7 weeks 0–6 days, CRL 9–14 mm

EMBRYOLOGY

No longitudinal fissure is found between the laterally bulging cerebral hemispheres at this Carnegie stage. At the end of the week, at Carnegie stage 17 (around 7 weeks 5 days), the interventricular foramen is delimited by the corpus striatum and the ventral thalamus. The cerebellar primordium grows, the isthmus rhombencephali is evident. At about 7.5 weeks, the primary intestinal loop can be seen projecting further into the umbilical cord as the normal umbilical hernia. The metanephros (future kidney) is now reniform.

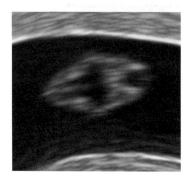

FIGURE 13.8 Frontal section through the head of an 11-mm embryo with clearly defined mesencephalic and rombencephalic cavities

ULTRASOUND

The embryonic body appears like a triangle in the sagittal section. The sides consist of the back, the roof of the rhombencephalon and the frontal part of the head, the basis of the umbilical cord and the embryonic tail. The limbs look like short hypoechogenic buds. All hypoecho-

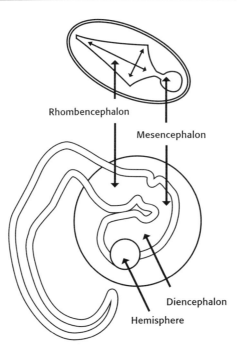

Rhombencephalon

Mesencephalon

Diencephalon

Hemisphere

FIGURE 13.9 Brain cavities of a 14-mm embryo

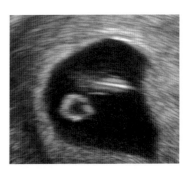

FIGURE 13.10 Longitudinal view of the embryonic spine at 7 weeks

genic brain cavities can be identified, including the separation of the cerebral hemispheres (Figure 13.8). The lateral ventricles are shaped like small round vesicles. The cavity of the diencephalon (future third ventricle) runs posteriorly. The medial telencephalon forms a continuous cavity between the lateral ventricles. The future foramina of Monro are wide during week 7. In the sagittal plane, the height of the cavity of the diencephalon (future third ventricle) is slightly greater than that of the mesencephalon (future Sylvian aqueduct). The rather broad and shallow rhombencephalic cavity is the largest cavity of the brain. It has a well-defined rhombic shape in the cranial pole of the embryo (Figure 13.9). The future spine appears as two parallel lines (Figure 13.10). The heart is large and bright, its frequency increasing from 130 beats/minute to 160 beats/minute. Details of the heart anatomy are not able to be depicted but the atrial and the ventricular compartments may be distinguished by the reciprocal movements of the walls.[18] The short umbilical cord shows a large coelomic cavity at its insertion, where the primary intestinal loop may be identified. The value of the mean diameter of the amniotic cavity is approximately identical with the corresponding crown–rump length (CRL). Blood flow can be seen in greyscale mode in the vitelline duct leading from the umbilical cord to the yolk sac.

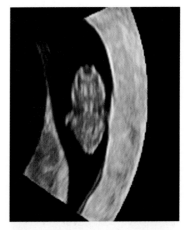

FIGURE 13.11 Coronal three-dimensional section of an embryo with 17-mm crown–rump length showing mesencephalon on the top the head with the hemispheres lateral and below

Gestational age 8 weeks 0–6 days, CRL 15–22 mm

EMBRYOLOGY

The coalescence of the maxillar, medial and lateral nasal ridge-like swellings is completed. In the heart, the membranous part of the inter-ventricular septum takes form. The septum secundum and the foramen ovale are starting to appear. The embryonic haematopoiesis shifts from the yolk sac to the liver. The cloacal membrane ruptures from urinary pressure in embryos of 16–17 mm CRL,[30] the anal membrane becomes defined. In most embryos, the choroid plexuses are present in the rhombencephalon. Half of the diencephalon is covered by the hemi-spheres. The mesencephalon is on the top of the brain.[24] The choroid plexuses of the lateral ventricles and of the fourth ventricle develop at stage 18.[7,27]

ULTRASOUND

With transvaginal ultrasound the brain cavities are easily seen as large 'holes' in the embryonic head. The hemispheres enlarge, developing a crescent shape. The choroid plexuses in the lateral ventricles become visible as tiny echogenic areas. The future foramina of Monro become more accentuated. The third ventricle is still rather wide, as is the mes-encephalic cavity. At this time, the mesencephalon lies on top of the head (Figure 13.11). The rhombencephalic cavity (future fourth ventricle) has a pyramid-like shape with the central deepening of the pontine flexure as the peak of the pyramid. The first signs of the bilateral choroid plexuses are lateral echogenic areas originating near the branches of the medulla oblongata caudal to the lateral recesses (Figure 13.12). Within a short time, the choroid plexuses traverse the roof of the fourth ventricle, meeting in the midline and dividing the roof into two portions, about two-thirds are located rostrally and one-third caudally. In the sagittal section, the choroid plexuses are identified as an echogenic fold of the roof. The back/spine can be seen as a smooth contour. The increased growth of the rostral brain structures and the deepening of the pontine flexure lead to the deflection of the brain. Slight movements of the body and some days later of the limbs are detectable (Figure 13.13). The arms and fingers are distinguishable at the end of the week. A 4-chamber view of the heart can be obtained, where the atrial compart-ment is wider than the ventricular part.[18] In some embryos the stomach becomes visible. The umbilical cord is relatively long and it can be easily traced form the embryo to the early placenta (Figure 13.14).

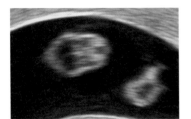

FIGURE 13.12 Section though the brain of an embryo with a crown–rump length of 18 mm showing third and fourth ventricles and choroid plexi

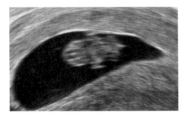

FIGURE 13.13 Limb buds are clearly visible in this embryo with a crown–rump length of 17 mm

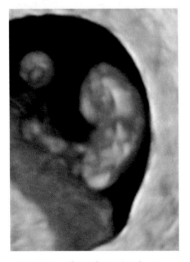

FIGURE 13.14 Three-dimensional scan at 7 weeks, showing an embryo, umbilical cord and yolk sac

Gestational age 9 weeks 0–6 days, CRL 23–31 mm

EMBRYOLOGY

The chondrocranium and the skeletogenous layer of the head become recognisable. The falx cerebri starts to develop from the skeletogenous layer. The cerebral hemispheres nearly conceal the diencephalon. Fusion of the medial walls of the hemispheres does not occur during the embryonic period. The foramina of Monro is reduced to dorsoventral slits. The insula appears. The thalami are thickening. The cavity of the mesencephalon is still wide. The rhombic lips have developed into cerebellar hemispheres. The choroid plexuses of the fourth ventricle divide the roof into a pars membranacea superior and inferior. In the columna 33–34 cartilaginous vertebrae are present. The processi spinosi have not yet developed. The truncoconal swellings grow down onto the upper ridge of the ventricular septum and onto the inferior endocardial cushion, separating the right and left ventricles. The diaphragm is established dividing the pleuroperitoneal cavity. There is still a narrow pleuroperitoneal duct connecting the pleural and peritoneal cavities. The anal membrane ruptures.[30] The kidneys ascend to level L1–3. The genital tubercle represents the indifferent phallus in both sexes.

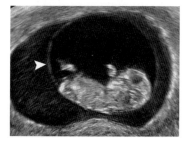

FIGURE 13.15 Section through a 9-week gestational sac demonstrating amniotic membrane separating coelomic and amniotic cavities. The embryonic limbs are fully developed and fingers and toes are clearly visible

ULTRASOUND

Fingers and toes are detectable with high frequency transducers (Figure 13.15). The movements of the arms and legs increase. The embryos often 'clap their feet'. The toes become visible. At the end of the week it is possible to obtain acceptable images of the profile, thus, it is possible to examine the mouth. The ventral body wall is well defined. The genital tubercle is relatively large. The cerebellar hemispheres are easily detectable. The choroid plexuses of the fourth ventricle are bright landmarks dividing the ventricle into a rostral and caudal compartment. During weeks 8 and 9, the rhombic fossa becomes deeper, owing to the progressive flexure of the pons. A distinct border ('isthmus prosencephali') has developed between the cavity of the mesencephalon and the third ventricle. The width of the diencephalic cavity narrows gradually while the width of the mesencephalon remains wide. The hemispheres grow fast. The lateral ventricles are always visible and their size increases rapidly (Figure 13.16). They are best seen in the parasagittal plane, where the C-shape becomes apparent. The cortex is smooth and hypoechogenic. The bright choroid plexuses of the lateral ventricles are regularly detectable at 9 weeks 4 days. They show rapid growth, similar to the hemispheres, and soon fill most of the ventricular cavities. The spine is still characterised by two echogenic parallel lines. In the

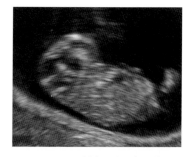

FIGURE 13.16 Sagittal section through an embryo with a crown–rump length of 22 mm, demonstrating hemispheres, third ventricle, mesencephalon, fourth ventricle and choroid plexi

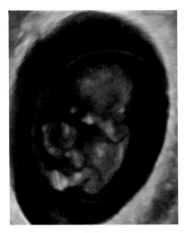

FIGURE 13.17 Three-dimensional scan of a 9-week embryo showing head, limbs and midgut physiological herniation

longitudinal section the echogenic oesophagus can be detected. The four chambers of the heart are visible in many embryos but the resolution is still too poor to enable evaluation of the heart. The heart rate has reached a maximum with a mean frequency of 175 beats/minute. The stomach is visible in about 45% of embryos. The protrusion of the midgut into the umbilical chord coelom (physiological midgut herniation) has reached its maximal extension at the end of the embryonic period (Figure 13.17).

Early post-embryonic fetal phase

While the embryologists defined the end of the embryonic period with the bone marrow formation in the humerus,[25] the knowledge of the embryological process of the midgut herniation might be used to extend the early developmental period to, at the latest, 12 weeks menstrual age, denominating it as the 'embryonic and early post-embryonic fetal period'.

___

Gestational age 10 weeks 0–6 days, CRL 32–41 mm, and 11 weeks 0–6 days, CRL 42–54 mm, 'early post-embryonic period'

EMBRYOLOGY

Among the most noticeable external changes of the brain are the union of the cerebellar hemispheres with the definition of the vermis and the increasing concealment of the diencephalon and mesencephalon by the cerebral hemispheres. The cerebellum enlarges, pulling the roof of the fourth ventricle beneath its caudal border. The development of the corpus callosum begins at 12–13 weeks. The mesencephalic cavity is still wide. After a rotation of 270 degrees, the intestine returns into the abdominal cavity during week 11 (CRL approximately 45 mm).[31] At the end of week 12 the physiological herniation is completed. The metanephros (future kidneys) becomes functional. In fetuses longer than 50 mm (embryological measurement) it is safe to make an assessment of the external gender.[24] Owing to the fixation procedures, the length of embryos, as measured in embryological studies, may be about 1–5 mm less than equivalent *in vivo* CRL measurements.[32]

ULTRASOUND

The human features of the fetus become clearer at the ultrasound examination. The head is still relatively large with a prominent forehead and a flat occiput. The limbs elongate further and the typical fetal posture appears. The future skull can be distinguished; ossification starts at

CRL (mm)	Gestational age (based on lmp)	Body (mm³)	Total brain (mm³)
10	7 weeks 2 days	96 (209; 26)	5.2 (18.2; 0.1)
15	8 weeks 0 days	402 (611; 237)	25.6 (49.4; 9.5)
20	8 weeks 5 days	918 (1222; 657)	61.3 (96.1; 34.3)
25	9 weeks 2 days	1644 (2044; 1288)	112.4 (158.1; 74.4)
30	9 weeks 6 days	2581 (3076; 2129)	178.8 (235.3; 129.9)
35	10 weeks 2 days	3727 (4318; 3180)	260.5 (328.0; 200.7)

CRL = crown–rump length | LMP = last menstrual period

TABLE 13.2 Three-dimensional ultrasound reconstructions of 34 embryos and fetuses: mean (±2 sd) volumes of embryonic body and cavities of the brain (modified from Blaas et al.) [14, 22]

about 11 weeks with the occipital bone.[33] The hemispheres occupy two-thirds of the head. The diencephalon lies between the hemispheres and the mesencephalon gradually moves towards the centre of the head. Three-dimensional ultrasound reconstructions and measurements of embryos and their brain cavities confirmed the classical descriptions of the external appearance of the embryonic body and limbs, and of the shape, size (Figure 13.18; Table 13.2) and position of the brain compartments.[27] Owing to the cerebellar growth, the choroid plexuses approach the caudal border of the cerebellum. Successively the ossification of the spine appears. The heart rate slows down to 165 beats/minute at the end of week 11. The ventricles, atria, septa, valves, veins and outflow tracts become identifiable. The stomach is usually visible at the end of week 11. The kidneys are visible; they are more echogenic than later in pregnancy. The midgut herniation has its maximal extent at the beginning of week 10; it returns into the abdominal cavity during weeks 10–11. This event marks the end of the early post-embryonic period.

Multiple pregnancy

The diagnosis of multiple pregnancy is relatively simple in the first trimester. In early pregnancy, the amnion and chorion are not fused. This enables direct visualisation of the chorionic cavity and it facilitates the diagnosis of chorionicity. The final diagnosis of twin pregnancy, however, should not be made until the 7th week of gestation, when the number of fetuses and chorionicity can be established with confidence. In higher multiples, the same principles are applied. Operators, however, should be aware of unusual findings such as dichorionic, diamniotic triplets (Figure 13.19).

In very early pregnancy, the diagnosis of monochorionic twins is difficult and it is not unusual for one of the embryos to be missed on the

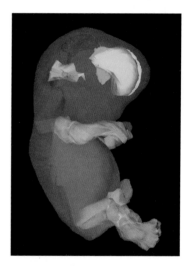

FIGURE 13.18 Three-dimensional ultrasound reconstruction of an embryo at the end of week 9, with a crown–rump length of 29 mm. The brain cavities are imaged in colours: yellow = lateral ventricles, green = 3rd ventricle, red = mesencephalic cavity, blue = 4th ventricle

Hemispheres (mm³)	Diencephalon (mm³)	Mesencephalon (mm³)	Rhombencephalon (mm³)
0.5 (2.7; 0.0)	1.7 (4.8; 0.2)	1.1 (3.3; 0.1)	7.3 (15.9; 2.0)
6.7 (15.1; 2.2)	4.4 (9.0; 1.5)	3.6 (7.1; 1.3)	13.4 (24.4; 5.7)
25.9 (44.6; 13.4)	6.7 (12.1; 2.8)	6.6 (11.2; 3.2)	18.8 (31.6; 9.4)
65.7 (98.7; 41.0)	7.5 (13.3; 3.4)	9.4 (14.7; 5.3)	22.6 (36.4; 12.0)
133.4 (184.8; 92.6)	6.7 (12.1; 2.9)	11.5 (17.3; 6.9)	23.9 (38.1; 13.0)
236.6 (310.4; 175.5)	4.5 (9.1; 1.5)	12.5 (18.6; 7.7)	22.7 (36.5; 12.1)

examination. The number of yolk sacs in monochorionic pregnancies is variable and should not be used for diagnosis.[40]

It is important not to refer to dichorionic twins as non-identical, as approximately 10% of dichorionic twins are monozygotic. Examining the ovaries for the number of corpora lutei may provide an insight into the possible zygosity (Figures 13.20, 13.21).

Unfavourable features associated with pregnancy loss in twins include a large discrepancy in CRL, oligohydramnios in one twin or smaller gestational sac diameter. Vanishing twin phenomenon, which was often described on transabdominal scan, is rarely seen transvaginally, owing to the increased ability to differentiate between intrauterine haematoma and an empty sac.[41]

Monochorionic pregnancies have much less favourable outcomes than their dichorionic counterparts and careful follow-up is necessary as early as 12–14 weeks to detect an early onset of twin-to-twin transfusion syndrome, which develops in 25% of cases.[42]

FIGURE 13.19 Principles of determining chorionicity and amnionicity in early multiple pregnancy;
○ = chorionic cavity
◐ = amniotic cavity
● = embryo

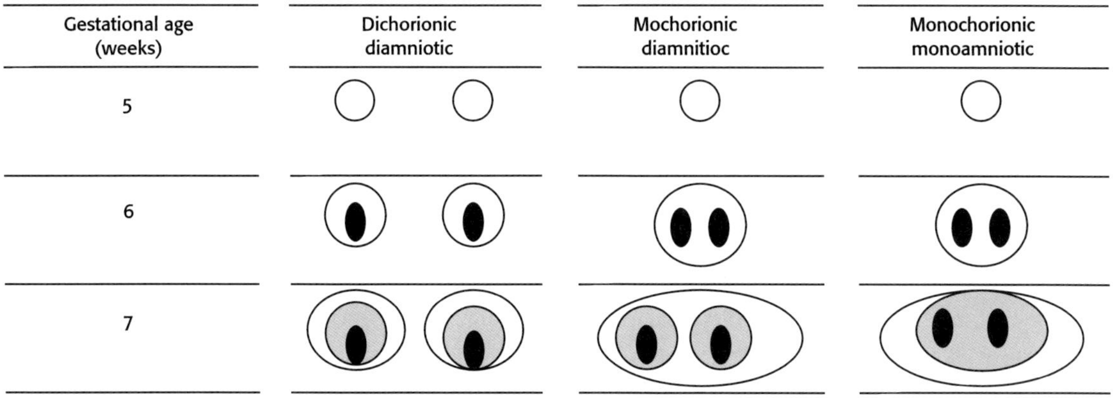

Gestational age (weeks)	Dichorionic diamniotic	Mochorionic diamnitioc	Monochorionic monoamniotic
5			
6			
7			

Ultrasound findings in abnormal pregnancies

Under optimal conditions, a 7.5 MHz frequency transvaginal transducer may have an axial resolution of 0.4 mm and a lateral resolution of 0.8 mm. Studies with such a precise device showed a uniform slow growth of the yolk sac diameter until 9 weeks from mean 4.2 mm at 7 weeks to mean 4.9 mm at 9 weeks.[15] Significant deviation from this growth pattern before 9 weeks of gestation may indicate the presence of an embryonic anomaly.[43,44] If the embryo is alive, a detailed evaluation of embryonic anatomy is advisable while later in pregnancy karyotyping may be necessary.

The mean diameter of the amniotic cavity and the mean CRL show a close correlation.[45] Significant deviation from the normal size in a viable pregnancy before 11 weeks should prompt a meticulous examination of the embryo. Though not a frequent event, the rupture of the amniotic membrane during the embryonic period may be associated with structural anomalies (Figure 13.22). The limbs may be abnormally short and craniofacial and body wall defects may also occur. The defects may be isolated or may comprise several parts of the body. Alterations of the heart rate such as irregular heart beats or bradycardia may be associated with embryonic maldevelopment.[46,47]

Diagnosis of fetal structural abnormalities is rarely made before 10 weeks of gestation, unless they cause a major disruption of embryonic anatomy. Complex body wall defects include serious anomalies that present with gross alterations in the ultrasound image. A vascular disruption during 4–6 weeks of gestation is considered as the aetiology of the limb–body wall complex (LBWC).[48] The amniotic membrane is always abnormal, continuing with the body wall to the placenta. In LBWC, persistence of the extraembryonic coelom may lead to the typical amniotic tags and adhesions.[48] In LBWC and in amniotic rupture sequence, the abnormal amniotic cavity should be detectable at 8–9 weeks. With a high-frequency transducer, details such as abnormal limbs, kyphoscoliosis and bifid spine may be identifiable if present. Large, complex defects should be relatively easy to detect, although there are only a few case reports of such conditions detected before 10 weeks of gestation; for example, amniotic rupture sequence and body stalk anomaly.[49]

Conjoined twins also cause major disruption in the embryonic body morphology and they can be diagnosed with confidence during the first trimester. Other structural anomalies are more difficult to diagnose and the potential for diagnostic errors is high. Thus, screening for structural anomalies should not be attempted before 11–14 weeks, when the fetus is large enough to be examined in sufficient detail.

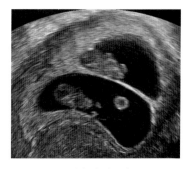

FIGURE 13.20 Dichorionic twins at 7 weeks of gestation. The embryos lie in separated gestational sacs, which are divided by a thick chorionic membrane

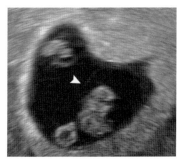

FIGURE 13.21 Monochorionic, monoamniotic twins at 7 weeks. Note the absence of any membranes separating the embryos

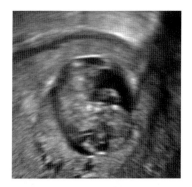

FIGURE 13.22 Severe oligohydramnios at 8 weeks of gestation

Conclusions

It has been shown that the embryonic development visualised by ultra-sound[20] was in agreement with the 'developmental time schedule' of human embryos as described in the Carnegie staging system.[24] However, without extensive knowledge of the developing anatomy of the human embryo, early pregnancy diagnosis by ultrasound is not possible. Thus, to understand the constantly changing appearance of the conceptus, we must return to the study of textbooks and literature on embryology.[24,34-37]

Three-dimensional ultrasound has now made its entry into the first trimester, giving the possibility of analysing the recorded ultrasound volume offline in any plane, including new sections through the embryo for a more precise diagnosis and the measurement of diameters and volumes of any structure of interest.[14,22,38,39] We can expect this new technology to help us to learn even more about early human development.

REFERENCES

1. MacVicar J, Donald I. Sonar in the diagnosis of early pregnancy and its complications. *J Obstet Gynæcol Br Commonw* 1963;**70**:387–95.

2. Sundén B. On the diagnostic value of ultrasound in obstetrics and gynecology. *Thesis Acta Obstet Gynecol Scand* 1964;**43 (Suppl 6)**:1–121.

3. Robinson H P. Sonar measurement of fetal crown–rump length as means of assessing maturity in first trimester of pregnancy. *Br Med J* 1973;**4**:28–31.

4. Robinson H P. 'Gestation sac' volumes as determined by sonar in the first trimester of pregnancy. *Br J Obstet Gynaecol* 1975;**82**:100–7.

5. Robinson H P, Fleming J E E. A critical evaluation of sonar 'crown–rump length' measurements. *Br J Obstet Gynaecol* 1975;**82**:702–10.

6. Robinson H P, Shaw-Dunn J. Fetal heart rates as determined by sonar in early pregnancy. *J Obstet Gynaecol Br Commonw* 1973;**80**:805–9.

7. Cyr D R, Mack LA, Nyberg D A, Shepard TH, Shuman W P. Fetal rhombencephalon: normal US findings. *Radiology* 1988;**166**:691–2.

8. Cyr D R, Mack LA, Schoenecker S A, Patten R M, Shephard TH, Shuman W P, *et al.* Bowel migration in the normal fetus: ultrasound detection. *Radiology* 1986;**161**:119–21.

9. Schmidt W, Yarkoni S, Crelin E S, Hobbins J C. Sonographic visualization of the physiologic anterior wall hernia in the first trimester. *Obstet Gynecol* 1987;**69**:911–15.

10. Green J J, Hobbins J C. Abdominal ultrasound examination of the first-trimester fetus. *Am J Obstet Gynecol* 1988;**159**:165–75.

11. Curtis J A, Watson L. Sonographic diagnosis of omphalocele in the first trimester of fetal gestation. *J Ultrasound Med* 1988;**7**:97–100.

12. Timor-Tritsch I E, Farine D, Rosen M G. A close look at the embryonic development with the high frequency transvaginal transducer. *Am J Obstet Gynecol* 1988;**159**:678–81.

13. Timor-Tritsch I E, Peisner D B, Raju S. Sonoembryology: an organ-oriented approach using a high-frequency vaginal probe. *J Clin Ultrasound* 1990;**18**:286–98.

14. Blaas H-G, Eik-Nes S H, Berg S, Torp H. In-vivo three-dimensional ultrasound reconstructions of embryos and early fetuses. *Lancet* 1998;**352**:1182–6.

15. Blaas H-G, Eik-Nes S H, Bremnes J B. Embryonic growth. A longitudinal biometric ultrasound study. *Ultrasound Obstet Gynecol* 1998;**12**:346–54.

16. BLAAS H-G, EIK-NES S H, KISERUD T, HELLEVIK LR. Early development of the forebrain and midbrain: a longitudinal ultrasound study from 7 to 12 weeks of gestation. *Ultrasound Obstet Gynecol* 1994; **4**: 183–92.

17. BLAAS H-G, EIK-NES S H, KISERUD T, HELLEVIK LR. Early development of the hindbrain: a longitudinal ultrasound study from 7 to 12 weeks of gestation. *Ultrasound Obstet Gynecol* 1995; **5**: 151–60.

18. BLAAS H-G, EIK-NES S H, KISERUD T, HELLEVIK LR. Early development of the abdominal wall, stomach and heart from 7 to 12 weeks of gestation: a longitudinal ultrasound study. *Ultrasound Obstet Gynecol* 1995; **6**: 240–49.

19. BLAAS H-G K. The examination of the embryo and early fetus: how and by whom? *Ultrasound Obstet Gynecol* 1999; **14**: 153–8.

20. BLAAS H-G K. The Embryonic Examination. Ultrasound Studies on the Development of the Human Embryo. Thesis. Trondheim: Norwegian University of Science and Technology; 1999.

21. TAKEUCHI H. Transvaginal ultrasound in the first trimester of pregnancy. *Early Hum Dev* 1992; **29**: 381–4.

22. BLAAS H-G K, EIK-NES S H. The description of the early development of the human central nervous system using two- and three-dimensional ultrasound. In: Hanson M, Lagercrantz H, editors. *The Newborn Brain: Neuroscience and Clinical Applications*. Cambridge: Cambridge University Press; 2002. p. 278–88.

23. TIMOR-TRITSCH I. Opinion: Standardization of ultrasonographic images: let's talk the same language. *Ultrasound Obstet Gynecol* 1992; **2**: 311–12.

24. O'RAHILLY R, MULLER F. *Developmental Stages in Human Embryos*. Washington, DC: Carnegie Institution Publishers; 1987.

25. STREETER G L. Developmental horizons in human embryos (fourth issue). A review of the histogenesis of cartilage and bone. *Contr Embryol* 1949; **220**: 150–73.

26. O'RAHILLY R, MÜLLER F. *Human Embryology and Teratology*. New York: Wiley-Liss; 1994.

27. O'RAHILLY R, MÜLLER F. *The Embryonic Human Brain. An Atlas of Developmental Stages*. New York: Wiley-Liss; 1994.

28. YOKOH Y. Early development of the cerebral vesicles in man. *Acta Anat* 1975; **91**: 455–61.

29. BLAAS H-G K, EIK-NES S H. Ultrasound assessment of early brain development. In: Jurkovic D, Jauniaux E, editors. *Ultrasound and Early Pregnancy*. New York: Parthenon; 1996. p. 3–18.

30. LUDWIG KS. Über die Beziehungen der Kloakenmembran zum Septum urorectale bei menschlichen Embryonen von 9 bis 33 mm SSL. *Z Anat Entwicklungsgesch* 1965; **124**: 401–13.

31. KIESSELBACH A. Der physiologische Nabelbruch. *Adv Anat Embryol Cell Biol* 1952; **34**: 83–143.

32. DRUMM J E, O'RAHILLY R. The assessment of prenatal age from the crown–rump length determined ultrasonically. *Am J Anat* 1977; **148**: 555–60.

33. ZALEN-SPROCK R, BRONS JTJ, VUGT J M G, HARTEN H J, GEIJN HP. Ultrasonographic and radiologic visualization of the developing embryonic skeleton. *Ultrasound Obstet Gynecol* 1997; **9**: 392–7.

34. CARLSON B M. *Human Embryology and Developmental Biology*. Philadelphia: Mosby; 1999.

35. LARSEN W J. *Human Embryology*. New York: Churchill Livingstone; 2001.

36. MOORE KL, PERSAUD TVN. *Before We are Born. Essentials of Embryology and Birth Defects*. Philadelphia: WB Saunders; 2003.

37. SADLER T W. *Langman's Medical Embryology*. Baltimore: Williams & Wilkins; 2000.

38. BLAAS H-G, EIK-NES S H, KISERUD T, BERG S, ANGELSEN B, OLSTAD B. Three-dimensional imaging of the brain cavities in human embryos. *Ultrasound Obstet Gynecol* 1995; **5**: 228–32.

39. BLAAS H-G K, EIK-NES S H. Chapter 4. In: Levine MI, Chervenak FA, Whittle M, editors. *Fetal and Neonatal Neurology and Neurosurgery*. London: Churchill Livingstone; 2002. p. 39–44.

40. MONTEAGUDO A, TIMOR-TRITSCH I E, SHARMA S. Early and simple determination of chorionic and amniotic type in multifetal gestations in the first fourteen weeks by high-frequency transvaginal sonography. *Am J Obstet Gynecol* 1994; **170**: 824–9.

41. JAUNIAUX E, ELKAZEN N, LEROY F, WILKIN P, RODESCH F, HUSTIN J. Clinical and morphological aspects of the vanishing twin phenomenon. *Obstet Gynecol* 1988; **72**: 577–81.

42. HECHER K, VILLE Y, SNIJDERS R, NICOLAIDES K. Doppler studies of the fetal circulation in twin-to-twin transfusion syndrome. *Ultrasound Obstet Gynecol* 1995; **5**: 318–24.

43. LINDSAY D J, LOVETT I S, LYONS EA, LEVI C S, ZHENG X-H, HOLT S C, et al. Yolk sac diameter and shape at endovaginal US: predictors of pregnancy outcome in the first trimester. *Radiology* 1992; **183**: 115–18.

44. STAMPONE C, NICOTRA M, MUTTINELLI C, COSMI EV. Transvaginal sonography of the yolk sac in normal and abnormal pregnancy. *J Clin Ultrasound* 1996; **24**: 3–9.

45. GRISIOLA G, MILANO V, PILU G, BANZI C, DAVID C, GABRIELLI S, et al. Biometry of early pregnancy with transvaginal sonography. *Ultrasound Obstet Gynecol* 1993; **3**: 403–11.

46. ACHIRON R, TADMOR O, MASHIACH S. Heart rate as a predictor of first-trimester spontaneous abortion after ultrasound-proven viability. *Obstet Gynecol* 1991; **78**: 330–4.

47. DOUBILET P M, BENSON C B, CHOW J S. Long term prognosis of pregnancies complicated by slow embryonic heart rates in the early first trimester. *J Ultrasound Med* 1999; **18**: 537–41.

48. ALLEN MIV, CURRY C, GALLAGHER L. Limb body wall complex: I. Pathogenesis. *Am J Med Genet* 1987; **28**: 529–48.

49. BECKER R, RUNKEL S, ENTEZAMI M. Prenatal diagnosis of body stalk anomaly at 9 weeks of gestation. *Fetal Diagn Ther* 2000; **15**: 301–3.

14 Diagnosis and management of miscarriage

JOHANNA TRINDER AND SANJAY VYAS

Introduction

Ultrasound examination has revolutionised the management of early pregnancy complications. In most units, this complication will account for a substantial number of the scans performed. Information about the various management options available when a miscarriage has been diagnosed is included.

Diagnosis of miscarriage

Miscarriage occurs if there is a failure of embryonic growth or if a viable fetus dies. Approximately one in seven of all pregnancies ends in spontaneous first-trimester miscarriage.[1] Although several types of miscarriage have been defined, the natural history of miscarriage is such that the type of miscarriage depends on the point in the process of miscarriage at which the woman presents and the diagnosis is made (Figure 14.1).

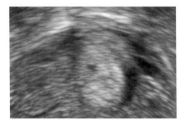

FIGURE 14.1 a

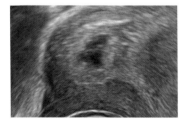

FIGURE 14.1 b

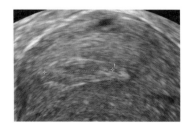

FIGURE 14.1 c

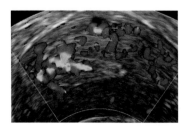

FIGURE 14.1 d

Natural history of miscarriage demonstrated on serial ultrasound scans: **a)** a gestational sac at 6 weeks of gestation, which is small for certain menstrual dates; **b)** on follow-up scan 2 weeks later, the sac has increased in size but it does not contain an embryo; **c)** at 9 weeks, the sac is not visible and only a small amount of retained products are seen within the uterine cavity; **d)** on Doppler examination the products are very vascular, which confirms the diagnosis of an incomplete miscarriage

Traditional textbooks base the diagnosis of the type of miscarriage on history and examination. A missed miscarriage is diagnosed by a history of brown discharge and examination findings of a clinically small for gestational age uterus and a closed cervical os. An incomplete miscarriage is diagnosed by history of bleeding, pain, passage of products of conception and an open internal cervical os on examination. Inevitable miscarriage is described as for incomplete miscarriage but with anticipated rather than actual passage of tissue. Complete miscarriage implies expulsion of an intact pregnancy.[2]

The traditional term 'missed miscarriage' has been criticised. Missed miscarriage implies maternal failure to recognise a non-viable pregnancy and it has been suggested that this term be replaced by 'delayed miscarriage' or 'early embryonic demise'.[3]

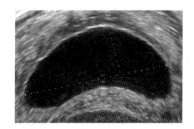

FIGURE 14.2 Ultrasound scan performed at 8 weeks of gestation showing a gestational sac measuring 32 mm in the mean diameter; there was no evidence of a yolk sac or an embryo within the gestational sac. These findings are conclusive of an early embryonic demise

Ultrasound diagnosis of miscarriage

Traditional clinical methods of diagnosing miscarriage have been largely replaced by ultrasound diagnosis. Ultrasound and, in particular, transvaginal ultrasound, has revolutionised the diagnosis of abnormal early pregnancy. Early pregnancy units have been developed to streamline the diagnosis of abnormal early pregnancy.[4] The throughput of such units and the desire to see and assess patients as rapidly as possible means that much of the assessment is protocol driven. It is now not unusual for a woman presenting with bleeding in early pregnancy to be assessed in an early pregnancy assessment unit, where an ultrasound diagnosis of miscarriage is made by an ultrasonographer and the diagnosis explained by a specialist nurse, without contact with a doctor and without a bimanual vaginal examination ever being performed.

Ultrasound definitions of early pregnancy failure have therefore become necessary. To help avoid misdiagnosis, the Royal College of Radiologists and the Royal College of Obstetricians and Gynaecologists (RCR/RCOG) issued joint guidelines on the ultrasound diagnosis of early pregnancy loss.[5] The ultrasound diagnosis of early embryonic demise requires a gestation sac size of at least 20 mm mean diameter, with no other visible internal echoes (Figure 14.2). Early fetal demise is based on the identification of a fetus with a crown–rump length (CRL) of at least 6 mm, with no fetal heart activity present (Figure 14.3). If these conditions cannot be fulfilled then the scan needs to be repeated in not less than 7 days to confirm the diagnosis of miscarriage (Table 14.1).[5]

There is no accepted ultrasound definition for the diagnosis of incomplete miscarriage (nor, therefore, complete miscarriage). Retained products of conception are visualised on ultrasound as the presence of areas of mixed echogenicity (heterogeneous areas of

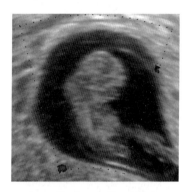

FIGURE 14.3 Sonogram of an embryo measuring 8 mm in length; there was no evidence of cardiac activity, which was conclusive of an early embryonic demise

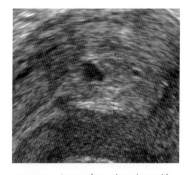

FIGURE 14.4 Incomplete miscarriage with a moderate amount of retained products within the uterine cavity. Note a disruption of the midline echo and areas of mixed echogenicity

Ultrasound findings	Action
Gestational sac < 20 mm with no embryo or yolk sac	Repeat scan in 1 week
Crown-rump length < 10 mm with no heart action	Repeat scan in 1 week
Gestational sac < 15 mm or crown–rump length < 10 mm	Repeat scan in 2 weeks

TABLE 14.1 Guidance on ultrasound diagnosis of early pregnancy loss[6]

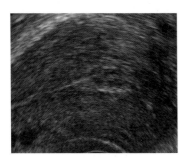

FIGURE 14.5 Longitudinal section of the uterus showing a small amount of hypoechoic tissue within the uterine cavity measuring 4 mm in anterior–posterior diameter

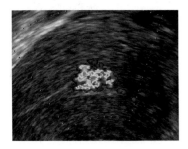

FIGURE 14.6 Colour Doppler examination showing high tissue vascularity, which confirms the diagnosis of retained products of conception

fluid mixed with solid components), with or without a disorganised gestation sac. If retained tissue or clots are present, the midline echo will be disarranged (Figure 14.4). It is usual to give an estimate of the amount of retained products by measuring this area in three dimensions. However, it is increasingly common in the literature to define incomplete miscarriage by measuring the anterior–posterior (AP) diameter or 'endometrial thickness' even though this thickness is made up of more than just endometrium (that is, blood clots and tissue). Limits of endometrial thickness between 5 mm and 15 mm have been used to define the presence of retained products.[6,7] However, chorionic villi have been obtained in most cases where endometrial thickness is greater than just 5 mm and even in some cases with as little as 2 mm (Figures 14.5, 14.6).[8] Some authors have suggested that, despite the fact that chorionic villi are still present, their presence may not be significant if endometrial thickness is less than 10 mm.[9] A study has been published which investigated the value of measuring endometrial thickness in women with suspected miscarriage undergoing dilatation and curettage because of persistent bleeding.[10] The study showed that none of the proposed cut-off points for measuring endometrial thickness is a useful test to diagnose the presence of chorionic villi within the uterine cavity. The authors concluded that subjective assessment of the intrauterine tissue on ultrasound scan was superior to the measurement of endometrial size to diagnose incomplete miscarriage.[10]

Some investigators have criticised the use of a single-dimension measurement and have instead used area or volume to define the absence of significant retained products.[11,12] Owing to the irregular shape of retained products, calculation of the volume with two-dimensional ultrasound may be difficult. However, there seems to be a good correlation between volume of retained products as measured by three-dimensional ultrasound and maximum AP diameter,[12] Thus, a measurement of the AP diameter gives a good estimate of the volume of retained products and three-dimensional ultrasound is not necessary.

ULTRASOUND FEATURES SUGGESTING EARLY EMBRYONIC/FETAL DEMISE WITHOUT A VISIBLE EMBRYO

In some failing pregnancies, the diagnosis of early embryonic demise (previously anembryonic pregnancy or blighted ovum) will be delayed if the mean gestation sac diameter is less than 20 mm, as recommended by the RCR/RCOG guidelines. This can cause distress to women, as they realise that there is a considerable chance that the final diagnosis will be that of miscarriage. A repeat scan also increases the workload and therefore costs to the unit. Thus, several investigators have attempted to identify other factors that may aid diagnosis of early embryonic demise.

The cut-off value of a mean gestation sac diameter of less than 20 mm was established in response to a national enquiry and is assumed to incorporate a wide safety margin.[13] Mean gestation sac diameters of greater than 18 mm have also been proposed to reliably identify failed pregnancy.[14] Diagnostic cut-off points of ≥17 mm mean diameter in sacs lacking an embryo and ≥13 mm in those without a visible yolk sac have been suggested as reliable predictors of non-viable gestation sacs at a single examination, with 100% specificity and 100% positive predictive value.[15] However, detailed investigation suggests that these measurements may be too low, as Elson et al.[16] have described two women with subsequently viable pregnancies presenting with empty sacs measuring more than 18 mm. With this evidence, it seems that the RCR/RCOG guideline does not incorporate a wide margin of error and operators should not be encouraged to accept lower values of mean sac diameter to diagnose early embryonic demise.

Deformed gestation sac shape (Figure 14.7), low position and thin decidual reaction can also be indicators of non-viable gestations but are not specific enough to be diagnostic.[15] Three-dimensional ultrasound theoretically has the potential to give extra information about the gestation and yolk sac shape but it has not been shown to be of any additional benefit in relation to the diagnosis of miscarriage (Figure 14.8).[17] There is, therefore, a significant proportion of empty sacs where no accurate distinction between viable and non-viable can be made according to one criterion at a single examination. In these cases, serial examinations should be carried out and the RCR/RCOG guidelines followed before any active management is advocated.

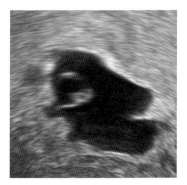

FIGURE 14.7 Early embryonic demise. A sonogram at 9 weeks of gestation shows an irregular gestational sac with a thin trophoblastic shell; a small amniotic cavity and an embryo are also visible

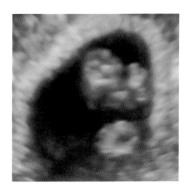

FIGURE 14.8 Three-dimensional scan of an early embryonic demise, showing an embryo measuring 7 mm with no visible cardiac activity. Note the reduced amount of coelomic fluid surrounding the embryo

Biochemical features suggesting early embryonic or fetal demise

HUMAN CHORIONIC GONADOTROPHIN

Serum human chorionic gonadotrophin (hCG) has been shown to be of value in the diagnosis of ectopic pregnancy, by determining the stage of gestation where an intrauterine gestation sac should be visible.[18] However, owing to the wide range of serum hCG levels in normal pregnancy, it is not possible to specify a useful level below which miscarriage is certain. Serial hCG levels may be of value in diagnosing miscarriage if falling levels are observed. This cannot be recommended in the usual practice of miscarriage diagnosis, as hCG levels can continue to rise even in failing pregnancies and repeated visits to the early pregnancy unit would still be necessary.

PROGESTERONE

Low levels of progesterone have long been associated with early pregnancy failure. Whereas serum hCG levels rise exponentially in early pregnancy and have a wide range, progesterone levels are relatively constant. Cut-off limits of 28 nmol/l[16,19] and 45 nmol/l[20] have been suggested to be diagnostic of early pregnancy failure (although this does not distinguish between failing intrauterine pregnancy and ectopic pregnancy). Theoretically, a low progesterone level, with a margin of error of, for example, 25 nmol/l, could be used in conjunction with an ultrasound diagnosis of an empty gestation sac to confirm a non-viable pregnancy in a single visit. This would alleviate the need for a further visit in some women and could potentially reduce distress. However, while awaiting a repeat scan for diagnosis in the absence of a progesterone level, 28% of women miscarry spontaneously and a further 28% are diagnosed with incomplete miscarriage (which resolves with expectant management in 80% of cases).[16] So women are actually undergoing expectant management by default during this diagnostic waiting period. In counselling women regarding expectant management after a single visit, a 50% failure rate may not seem an attractive option and more women may request intervention to manage their miscarriage. Thus, both diagnosis and treatment outcomes need to be considered before considering diagnostic management changes.

INHIBIN A

Inhibin A is a glycoprotein produced by the corpus luteum and the synctiotrophoblast in early pregnancy. It has a shorter half-life than hCG and progesterone and therefore theoretically may be more sensitive at identifying trophoblastic failure. In practice, the addition of inhibin A levels to serum hCG and progesterone levels does not significantly increase sensitivity in diagnosing pregnancy failure in symptomatic women.[21]

MULTIPARAMETER MODELS IN THE DIAGNOSIS OF EARLY PREGNANCY FAILURE

The combination of serum hCG and progesterone can achieve a sensitivity of 95% and a specificity of 66% in distinguishing viable from non-viable pregnancy in symptomatic women.[21]

Maternal age, gestational sac diameter and serum progesterone can be used in a logistic regression model to allow prediction of viability when an embryo cannot be visualised on ultrasound scan. With this model, at a cut-off value of 10% probability, the diagnosis of viable pregnancy can be made with a sensitivity of 99.2% and a specificity of 70.8%.[16] However, implementation of this model requires computer analysis, immediate serum progesterone levels and the accurate identification of an empty sac in an experienced unit. Caution should be exercised when applying this model to a general unit. With a sensitivity of less than 100%, active intervention for suspected miscarriage could not be undertaken. The value of these models is in counselling women as to the likelihood of a continuing viable pregnancy.

Diagnosis of miscarriage when the fetus is visible

In 5–10% of normal healthy embryos with a CRL of 2–4 mm, fetal cardiac activity cannot be demonstrated.[22] The RCR/RCOG guidelines advise that the crown–rump length should be at least 6 mm with no fetal cardiac activity, before a diagnosis of fetal demise is made (Figure 14.3).[5] If the embryo is less than 6 mm, the scan should be repeated in 7 days. These guidelines are also generally considered to incorporate a wide margin of error. Where fetal cardiac activity is absent and the crown–rump length is less than 6 mm, either an excessively large or small gestation sac size, compared with CRL, may represent early fetal demise.[12,23] This may be useful in counselling women but is not specific enough to be used diagnostically.

LOW FETAL HEART RATE AS A PREDICTOR OF MISCARRIAGE

A fetal heart rate of less than 120 beats/minute in the first trimester can be associated with increased pregnancy loss, with a sensitivity of 54% and a specificity of 95%, rising to 100% if the fetal heart rate is below 85 beats/minute.[24] However, the significance of a slow heart rate is dependent on the exact gestation, with fetuses normally having heart rates of 100 beats/minute at 6 weeks of gestation.[25] Therefore, caution is recommended before diagnosing impending early fetal demise, especially as a single glimpse of a slow heart rate does not necessarily predict subsequent embryonic death.[26]

RECURRENT MISCARRIAGE

The role of ultrasound in diagnosis of recurrent miscarriage is to help identify the point in the natural history of miscarriage at which fetal demise has occurred. Fetal demise recurrently occurring after a fetal heart beat has been identified is frequently associated with antiphospholipid syndrome,[27] whereas early embryonic demise may be due to sporadic miscarriage, probably of chromosomal aetiology.

Diagnosis of miscarriage: summary

Ultrasound has superseded clinical examination as the investigation of choice in the diagnosis of miscarriage. However, the addition of clinical examination to the ultrasound scan can add extra valuable information if the diagnosis, or best course of management is unclear. In terms of the added information that more detailed ultrasonographic examination can add, there is no diagnostic benefit in measuring fetal heart rate or mean gestation sac diameter/CRL differences or ratios, as these parameters are not sufficiently specific enough to make an accurate diagnosis of miscarriage. They may be useful in assessing risk of impending miscarriage but a further scan would still be indicated to confirm the diagnosis.

The only biochemical parameter that is of practical value is serum progesterone. A progesterone level of less than 28 nmol/ml used in conjunction with an empty sac (early embryonic demise) is diagnostic of miscarriage. If a rapid result can be obtained, this could be used with ultrasound, to diagnose miscarriage and plan subsequent treatment in a single visit, whereas a result returned a few days later would necessitate a repeat visit. The other consideration, however, is that of the natural history of early embryonic demise, as 56% of women will miscarry spontaneously by the next appointment 1 week later (28% complete and 28% incomplete). The remainder of women would have about a 50% risk of successful expectant management in the following 2 weeks. Diagnosis of failed pregnancy earlier in the natural history of miscarriage could mean the likelihood of successful expectant management will be decreased (as women may not be prepared to wait 3 weeks from diagnosis for expectant management to be successful).

Author	Miscarriage type	Inclusion criteria	Success	
			Expectant	*Surgical*
Nielsen[7]	EED and incomplete	ET 15–50 mm	81/103 (79%)	52/52 (100%)
Chipchase[31]	EED and incomplete	ET <50 mm	19/19 (100%)	16/16 (100%)
Wieringa-de-Waard[32]	EED and incomplete	ET >15 MSD >15 mm	30/64 (47%)	55/58 (98%)

EED = early embryonic demise
ET = endometrial thickness
MSD = mean gestational sac diameter

TABLE 14.2 Summary of three randomised trials comparing expectant and surgical management of miscarriage

Management of miscarriage

Traditionally, surgical curettage has been performed following the diagnosis of miscarriage, on the assumption that this prevents haemorrhage and decreases the risk of subsequent gynaecological infection. This policy is based on beliefs from half a century ago when infectious complications from illegal terminations of pregnancy led to many deaths each year in the UK. Surgical curettage, however, is not without complications. These include uterine perforation, cervical laceration and infection as a result of instrumentation of the uterus. Other management options (expectant or medical) are increasingly offered to women with a diagnosis of miscarriage. Expectant management allows spontaneous passage and medical management makes use of uterotonic agents to aid expulsion of products of conception.

Expectant management

Observational studies of expectant management indicate that up to 91–96% of women with an incomplete miscarriage will have successful resolution.[6,28] This option appears acceptable to the women who choose it.[6,28,29] However, expectant management has been found to be less acceptable[28,29] and less successful, with success rates of 25–60%[6,28,30] in the management of early fetal demise.

There have been three small randomised controlled trials of expectant versus surgical management of miscarriage (Table 14.2).[7,31,32] Expectant management was found to be successful in complete uterine evacuation in 79% of cases of incomplete miscarriage over 3 days.[7] However, efficacy was reduced to 37% when expectant management was used to treat women with miscarriage mostly diagnosed as early fetal demise.[32] No significant differences were found in these three trials with respect to the number of complications between surgical and expectant management. The trials, however, are small, with a total of 186 women allocated to expectant management, and are underpowered to detect most uncommon complications.

There is limited evidence on the prediction of the success of expectant management. Application of logistic regression to three diagnostic variables: serum progesterone, serum hCG and intrauterine diameter has been used to calculate probability of successful expectant management.[33] However, neither the presence of a gestation sac, nor the measurement of endometrial thickness appear to influence the chances of successful outcome in incomplete miscarriage[28] and the gestation sac volume as measured by three-dimensional ultrasound fails to predict the likelihood of successful outcome in early fetal demise.[34]

The length of time of vaginal bleeding is similar following expectant compared to surgical management (mean 9.9 versus 7.5 days, range 2–17 days).[35] The risk of excessive bleeding is around 3%, which is similar to that reported in surgical management.[35] The risk of infection is low. Infection rates of 0–3% have been reported.[7,32] An infection risk of 3% for expectant management has been substantiated by a large multicentre randomised controlled trial of expectant, medical and surgical management of miscarriage.[36] This trial also shows that 1/40 women randomised to expectant management required a blood transfusion because of excess haemorrhage.

There is no agreed optimal time limit for successful completion of expectant management. Based on the published evidence, it would seem reasonable to actively promote expectant management for women with incomplete miscarriage. High completion rates for incomplete miscarriage can be expected. Expectant management with as little as 5–7 days' follow-up has achieved a success rate of 83% for the management of incomplete miscarriage in routine clinical practice.[37] The success rates for expectant management are high enough that if the woman has ceased bleeding after a 14-day interval, it is unlikely that significant tissue is retained and a repeat ultrasound scan is unnecessary.

For women with early fetal (especially including embryonic) demise, expectant management may not necessarily be the most appropriate option. For a reasonable chance of success (50%), 2 weeks seems to be a reasonable length of time. To avoid the risk of extra, unplanned visits and additional scans, the woman needs to be aware that this management option involves a 14-day management course to achieve this success rate. Clear, written information needs to be given with vivid descriptions regarding the amount of bleeding and the size of clots that they may pass. Although this management option will reduce the number of planned surgical interventions by 50%, the system must be able to accommodate unplanned surgery, sometimes as an emergency, if the woman is symptomatic, which in practice occurs in 4% of women.[37]

It has been reported that many women chose expectant management through a desire for a natural approach. Many, however are unprepared for the reality of this process and in qualitative analysis some women expressed decision regret.[38] Of women who have experienced expectant management, however, 84% would undertake this management option again if they were to miscarry in the future, despite the fact that 50% received unplanned surgical treatment.[39]

Many women are concerned about the effect of the chosen management on future fertility. Compared to surgical management, expectant management does not seem to delay the onset of menstruation nor timing or likelihood of subsequent conception.[31,40]

In view of the relatively low success rate for early fetal demise, it would seem reasonable to offer either expectant or an alternative management option.

Medical management

Treatment regimens include the use of the antiprogesterone, mifepristone and a prostaglandin analogue, the most commonly used of which is misoprostol (15-deoxy, 16-hydroxy, 16-methyl analogue of prostaglandin E1). These regimens were initially devised for the management of first-trimester therapeutic abortion. When used to treat miscarriage in observational studies, success rates as high as 93% for early fetal demise[41] and 94% for incomplete miscarriage[42] were initially reported. Subsequent observational studies of inpatient medical management suggested lower success rates,[43,44] although allowing longer for the miscarriage process to complete and giving larger doses of vaginal misoprostol yielded greater success (71%, 93%, 84%, respectively).[44–46] It seems evident that success may depend upon the type of miscarriage, the use of mifepristone, the dose and route of administration of misoprostol, the time allowed for retained products to be passed and the definition of successful treatment.

The antiprogesterone, mifepristone is thought to potentiate the effects of prostaglandins and has been shown to increase the efficacy of misoprostol in management of therapeutic abortion.[47] However, failing pregnancies are associated with decreased progesterone levels and therefore the role of a progesterone antagonist is less clear. It is therefore not surprising that the use of mifepristone in addition to misoprostol has not been shown to increase the success rate of misoprostol alone in the management of early fetal demise or incomplete miscarriage.[48–50]

Misoprostol is absorbed through mucous membranes and can be administered orally, vaginally, sublingually or rectally. Misoprostol

Author	Miscarriage type	Inclusion criteria	Treatment regimen	Success Medical	Success Surgical	P value
Hinshaw[45]	EED and incomplete	Not stated	400/600/400 mg oral mifepristone 400/200 mg oral misoprostol 2 hours apart	172/186 (93%)	247/251 (98%)	0.004
Demetroulis[49]	EED and incomplete	ET >15 mm	800 mg vaginal misoprostol	33/40 (82%)	40/40 (100%)	0.005
Gronlund[50]	EED	CRL 6–20 mm MSD >15 mm	400/200 mg oral misoprostol 2 hours apart	92/127 (72%)	47/49 (96%)	—
De Jonge[52]	Incomplete	Clinical	400 mg oral misoprostol	3/23 (13%)	26/27 (96%)	<0.001
Chung[53]	EED and incomplete	Choriodecidual reaction >5 cm²	400 mg oral misoprostol 3 hours apart	159/321 (50%)	299/314 (95%)	—
Sahin[54]	Incomplete	ET <50 mm	200 mg vaginal misoprostol four times daily	37/40 (93%)	40/40 (100%)	—
Muffley[55]	EED	CRL >5 mm	800 mg vaginal misoprostol	15/25 (60%)	25/25 (100%)	—

TABLE 14.3 Summary of seven randomised trials comparing medical and surgical management of miscarriage

CRL = crown–rump length
EED = early embryonic demise
ET = endometrial thickness
MSD = mean gestational sac diameter

administered by the vaginal route has a greater bioavailability than the oral route.[51] Despite this, there does not seem to be a benefit in efficacy of using the vaginal route over the oral route. The benefit of the vaginal route however may be in the reduced incidence of gastrointestinal adverse effects and possible shorter administration-expulsion time.

Seven randomised controlled trials of medical (misoprostol) versus surgical management have been published to date (Table 14.3)[45,49,50,52–55] (although one trial[45] used a partial randomisation). Success rates as low as 13%[52] and as high as 93%[54] have been reported in small trials. However, total success was achieved in 50% of women in the largest of these trials, with a sample size of 635 women.[53] As with the observational studies, the trials have differing drug regimens and different measures of success.

The main difference between both the observational studies and the trials, in terms of clinical impact, is whether the studies or trials were conducted in an inpatient or outpatient setting. The success rates related to the type of miscarriage and dose and route of administration of the misoprostol then need to be examined and the application to a routine clinical setting explored.

INPATIENT MEDICAL MANAGEMENT

In the largest trial, 635 women were randomised to inpatient medical management (4-hourly 400 micrograms oral misoprostol – up to three doses). A medical success rate of 50% was reported. The average duration of hospital stay was 2.18 days for medical management and 1.78 days for surgical management.[53] A smaller trial reported a success rate of 82% following the administration of single vaginal dose of 800 micrograms misoprostol. 8–10 hours were allowed for completion of miscarriage. This time period was similar to the average time period (14 hours) from diagnosis to surgical management in the control group.[49] Observational studies report success rates of 84% with a median induction miscarriage interval of 8 hours (range 0.58–50.54 hours) using 800 micrograms vaginal misoprostol followed by two further 400-microgram doses at 3-hourly intervals.[46] These trials and studies of inpatient medical management indicate that with an appropriate misoprostol regimen, success, in a similar time span to that required for surgical management, can be attained.

OUTPATIENT MEDICAL MANAGEMENT

Outpatient use of misoprostol compared with surgical management has been evaluated in three trials[50,54,55] and compared with expectant management in four trials.[48,56,59,60] Efficacy of 60% after 72 hours following vaginal administration of 800 micrograms misoprostol (repeated 24 hours and 48 hours) with a mean time to expulsion of 12.6 hours, in the management of early fetal demise, has been reported.[55] Using smaller doses of misoprostol (400 micrograms then 200 micrograms 2 hours later) but allowing a longer time (8 days) for the miscarriage to complete increases the success rates in early fetal demise to 72% (96% surgical).[50]

Allowing a longer time to complete miscarriage (10 days) and small, repeated doses of misoprostol (200 micrograms four times daily for 5 days) results in rates of medical evacuation comparable to those obtained surgically (93% compared with 100%) in incomplete miscarriage.[54]

These trials confirm that medical management can be successful in managing miscarriage. When compared with surgical management, however, surgery will always have a higher success rate. It is perhaps more important in practical terms to compare outpatient medical management with expectant management, as these are the options that a woman wanting to avoid surgery will face. In the first trial of outpatient medical management of early fetal demise, no significant difference was found after 5 days following treatment with 400 micrograms of oral misoprostol or expectant management (82% compared with 76%).[7] In a subsequent randomised controlled trial of early fetal demise and incomplete miscarriage, medical management (400 micrograms misoprostol on days 1, 3 and 5) resulted in a complete miscarriage rate of 83% compared with 48% (P <0.05) in the expectant group, after 14 days.[57]

Allowing longer for the miscarriage to complete does not necessarily seem to greatly affect success rates. This is reinforced by an observational study in which successful medical management of incomplete miscarriage occurred within 10 days in 78% of women following a single oral dose of 400 micrograms misoprostol.[59]

Two randomised, double blind, placebo-controlled trials comparing medical and expectant management have been published. Management of early fetal demise has been shown to be successful in over 80% of cases following misoprostol (vaginal administration of up to two doses of 800 micrograms or 600 micrograms misoprostol 24 hours apart), compared with less than 30% receiving placebo.[56] There was no significant added benefit for misoprostol over placebo (100% misoprostol compared with 86% placebo), in management of incomplete miscarriage, although the numbers were small.[58]

COMPLICATIONS OF MEDICAL MANAGEMENT

Most published trials are underpowered to detect the infection rate following medical management. The MIST trial[36] reported an infection rate of 2% at 14 days and 3% at 8 weeks, based on clinical assessment parameters. The rate of infection was similar to that found in the expectant and surgical groups. A similar infection rate of 3% was reported in a retrospective observational study[62] and in randomised controlled trials.[50,53,54]

A meta-analysis of various doses and routes of administration of misoprostol indicates a nausea rate of 23% and diarrhoea rate of 18%.[35] Gastrointestinal adverse effects appear to be less severe if misoprostol is administered via the vaginal rather than the oral or sublingual route.[47,60,61] Interestingly, the incidence of nausea, vomiting and diarrhoea following 600 micrograms vaginally administered misoprostol has been found to be no different from those receiving vaginally administered placebo: 32%, 14% and 21%, respectively.[58] More importantly, the incidence of these gastrointestinal complications does not seem to be severe enough to dissuade women from accepting medical management. In a large randomised controlled trial, only 1% of women were unable to continue with misoprostol because of these adverse effects.[53] The number of days of vaginal bleeding following medical management is reported to be around 7–15.[37,50,57,58] The risk of heavy bleeding requiring emergency evacuation has been reported at 5%, with a significantly higher risk if the woman has been pretreated with mifepristone (11%

compared with 1% $P <$ 0.05).[50] Heavy bleeding requiring blood transfusion may occur in 1% of women pretreated with mifepristone.[37]

MEDICAL MANAGEMENT IN PRACTICE

Inpatient medical management can be difficult to organise. It is dependent on the availability of an inpatient bed, preferably in a side room to allow some degree of privacy. As both of these resources are relatively scarce, this can be hard to achieve. The alternative management option would be medical management in an outpatient setting. This appears to be successful, with few adverse effects based on low doses of misoprostol, and is acceptable to women.[58] In the management of incomplete miscarriage, there appears to be little increased efficacy over expectant management so managing these women medically may lead to unnecessary increased rates of gastrointestinal adverse effects.

The real advantage of medical management is in the outpatient management of early fetal demise, where the success rates vastly supersede those of expectant management. There appears to be no difference in the success rates of medical management with regard to gestation sac size or CRL.[50] Unlike in expectant management, the absence of vaginal bleeding does not decrease the success rates.[58]

Although still not absolutely clear, the evidence suggests that optimal management is with vaginally administered misoprostol, presumably ensuring effective blood levels with minimal adverse effects. With expectant management, women need to be clearly informed about the amount of bleeding and pain that they are likely to experience and the diarrhoea and vomiting that they may expect as adverse effects of misoprostol. If medical management fails and surgical curettage is carried out, it appears that there may be fewer surgery-related complications, probably because the softening effect on the cervix allows easier instrumentation of the uterine cavity.[35]

Surgical management

Surgical management has been the mainstay of miscarriage management for many years. Suction curettage has replaced dilatation and curettage as the usual surgical technique for the removal of retained products of conception.[62] A randomised trial comparing the two methods in the management of incomplete miscarriage concluded that suction curettage was safer and easier.[63] In a meta-analysis of women undergoing surgical curettage as the control group in randomised controlled trials of expectant and medical management of pregnancy, the rate of complete evacuation was 97%.[35] This makes it the most efficacious option in management of miscarriage.

COMPLICATIONS OF SURGICAL MANAGEMENT

Serious complications of surgery include cervical damage, perforation, intra-abdominal trauma, intrauterine adhesions, haemorrhage and potential to introduce infection as a result of uterine instrumentation. The infection risk reported by Nielsen and Hahlin[7] at 10% (5/52) for surgical management has not been reproduced in any other trial and probably reflects the low numbers in this trial. In randomised controlled trials comparing medical and surgical management, infection rates of 4–5% for the surgical group have been reported.[50,54] Infection rates of 3–4%, found in larger trials and a meta-analysis of pooled data, appear more realistic.[35,37,53]

The rate of postoperative infection with chlamydia and or gonorrhoea in women receiving suction curettage for incomplete miscarriage is around 6%.[64] The RCOG recommends that all at-risk women undergoing surgical evacuation continue to be screened for *Chlamydia trachomatis*. This particularly applies to women under the age of 25 years.[62] The number of days of reported vaginal bleeding following surgical management ranges between 3 and 9 days.[37,50]

There is evidence that significant fetomaternal haemorrhage can occur after curettage to remove products of conception but does not occur after complete spontaneous miscarriage. It is difficult to ascertain the risk incurred following medical management. The RCOG has therefore recommended that anti-D should be given to all non-sensitised Rh-negative women who miscarry after 12 weeks, whether complete or incomplete, and to those who miscarry below 12 weeks when the uterus is evacuated (either surgically or medically).[65]

MANUAL VACUUM ASPIRATION

Despite the superior success rate, up to 75% of women choose expectant as an alternative to surgical management.[28] This decision in some women is to avoid an 'operation' with its inherent risks.[38] It is usual practice in the UK to manage miscarriage by performing suction curettage under general anaesthesia.[62] In the developing world, however, manual vacuum aspiration under local anaesthesia is widely used. There is increasing experience using this technique in the UK for the management of early first-trimester termination. The procedure appears to be as safe as electric suction curettage for therapeutic abortions up to 10 weeks of gestation.[66] This technique has been evaluated for the management of incomplete miscarriage and early fetal demise, using systemic analgesia (intravenous alfentanil and midazolam) and patient-controlled analgesia (alfentanil and propofol).[67] Manual vacuum aspiration may prove to be acceptable to women who request early resolution of their miscarriage but who wish to avoid general anaesthesia. It should be possible to develop this technique to manage miscarriage in a modified outpatient setting.

HISTOLOGICAL EXAMINATION OF SURGICAL SPECIMENS

The RCOG has recommended that all women with a miscarriage should have pregnancy tissue sent for histological examination.[62] This recommendation was derived from the opinion of an expert group.[3] However, there is evidence that this does not happen in 30% of cases currently treated in hospital (surgical and medical management).[68] The purpose of the recommendation is to safeguard against the missed diagnosis of ectopic pregnancy and trophoblastic disease. There are no data on the frequency of histological examination in women undergoing expectant management but it is probably unrealistic to expect women to miscarry at home, collect tissue and return it to the early pregnancy clinic.

Management of miscarriage: summary

For women with incomplete miscarriage, expectant management should be encouraged, as at least 75% of women will be successful with no increased risk of infection. Expectant management of early fetal and embryonic demise miscarriage will be less successful, unless a long time is allowed, so women may prefer to undergo medical or surgical management. Medical management is about 80% successful in the outpatient setting for management of early fetal demise. Surgical curettage still offers the greatest success rate (97%), the least risk of requiring unplanned admission and the least duration of bleeding. It should therefore continue to be offered as a management option, particularly to those women with early fetal demise who do not wish to undergo the uncertainty of expectant, nor the procedure of expulsion of retained products, associated with medical management.

Conclusions

Diagnosis of miscarriage is straightforward in most cases. Sometimes, however, the diagnosis cannot be made after a single ultrasound assessment. In these cases the RCR/RCOG guidelines should be followed. Other parameters have been described, which may aid diagnosis but with the exception of progesterone, will not confirm the diagnosis. The value of these other parameters is in counselling women as to the likelihood of a viable pregnancy.

Subsequent management of retained products of conception following diagnosis of miscarriage has changed over the past 10 years.

Expectant, medical and surgical management options can now be offered. Each has its own benefits, complications and risks but concern regarding the risk of infection is unfounded, as it is similar in all three options. Importance needs to be placed on careful counselling, written patient information and the availability of 24-hour guidance and hospital access if the need arises.

REFERENCES

1. REGAN L, BRAUDE PB, TREMBATH PL. Influence of past reproductive performance on risk of spontaneous abortion. Br Med J 1989;299:541–5.

2. EDMONDS D K. Spontaneous and recurrent abortion. In: Shaw R, Soutter P, Stanton S, editors. Gynaecology. Edinburgh: Churchill Livingstone; 1992. p.205–18.

3. Recommendations from the 33rd RCOG study group. In: Grudzinskas J G, O'Brien P, editors. Problems in Early Pregnancy: Advances in Diagnosis and Management. London: RCOG Press; 1997. p.327–31.

4. BIGRIGG M A, READ M D. Management of women referred to an early pregnancy assessment unit: care and cost effectiveness. Br Med J 1991;302:577–9.

5. Royal College of Radiologists; Royal College Obstetricians and Gynaecologists. Guidance on Ultrasound Procedures in Early Pregnancy. Report of the RCR/RCOG Working Party. London: Royal College of Radiologists; 1995.

6 SAIRAM S, KHARE M, MICHAILIDIDIS G, THILAGANATHAN B. The role of ultrasound in the expectant management of early pregnancy loss. Ultrasound Obstet Gynecol 2001;17:506–9.

7. NIELSEN S, HAHLIN M. Expectant management of first-trimester spontaneous abortion. Lancet 1995;345:84–6.

8. KURTZ A, SHLANSKY-GOLDBERG D, CHOI H, NEEDLEMAN L, WAPNER R, GOLDBERG B. Detection of retained products of conception following spontaneous abortion in the first trimester. J Ultrasound Med 1991;10:387–95.

9. HURD W W, WHITFIELD R R, RANDOLPH J F JUNIOR, KERCHER M L. Expectant management versus elective curettage for the treatment of spontaneous abortion. Fertil Steril 1997;68:601–6.

10. SAWYER E, OFUASIA E, OFILI-YEBOVI D, HELMY S, GONZALEZ J, JURKOVIC D. The value of measuring endometrial thickness and volume on ultrasound scan for the diagnosis of incomplete miscarriage. Ultrasound Obstet Gynecol 2007;29:205–209

11. CHUNG TKH, CHEUNG LP, SAHOTA D S. Evaluation of the accuracy of transvaginal sonography for the assessment of retained products of conception after spontaneous abortion. Gynaecol Obstet Invest 1998;45:190–3.

12. ACHARYA G, MORGAN H. First-trimester, three-dimensional transvaginal ultrasound volumetry in normal pregnancies and spontaneous miscarriages. Ultrasound Obstet Gynecol 2002;19:575–9.

13. HATELY W, CASE J, CAMPBELL S. Establishing the death of an embryo by ultrasound: report of a public enquiry with recommendations. Ultrasound Obstet Gynaecol 1995;5:353–7.

14. REMPEN A. Diagnosis of viability in early pregnancy with vaginal sonography. J Ultrasound Med 1990;6:23–7.

15. TONGSONG T, WANAPIRAK C, SRISOMBOON J, SIRICHOTIYAKUL S, POLSRISUTHIKUL T, PONGSATHA S. Transvaginal ultrasound in threatened abortions with empty gestational sacs. Int J Gynecol Obstet 1994;4 6:297–301.

16. ELSON J, SALIM R, TAILOR A, BANERJEE S, ZOSMER N, JURKOVIC D. Prediction of early pregnancy viability in the absence of an ultrasonically detectable embryo. Ultrasound Obstet Gynaecol 2003;21:57–61.

17. FIGUERAS F, TORRENTS M, MUNOZ A, COMAS C, ANTOLIN E, ECHEVARRIA M, et al. Three-dimensional yolk and gestational sac volume. A prospective study of prognostic value. J Reprod Med 2003;48:252–6.

18. CACCIATORE B, STENMAN UH, YLOSTALO P. Diagnosis of ectopic pregnancy by vaginal sonography in combination with a discriminatory serum hCG level of 1000 iu/l(IRP). Br J Obstet Gynaecol 1990;97:904–8.

19. HAHLIN M, WALLIN A, SJOBLOM P, LINDBLOM B. Single progesterone assay for early recognition of abnormal pregnancy. Hum Reprod 1990;5:622–6.

20. AL-SEBAI M A H, KINGSLAND C R, DIVER M, HIPKIN L, McFADYEN I R. The role of a single progesterone measurement in the diagnosis of early pregnancy failure and the prognosis of fetal viability. Br J Obstet Gynaecol 1995;102:364–9.

21. PHIPPS M G, HOGAN J, PEIPERT J F, LAMBERT-MESSERLIAN G M, CANIK J A, SEIFER D B. Progesterone, inhibin, and hCG multiple marker strategy to differentiate viable from nonviable pregnancies. Obstet Gynecol 2000;95:2 27–31.

22. GOLDSTEIN S R. Significance of cardiac activity on endovaginal ultrasound in very early embryos. Obstet Gynecol 1992;80:670–2.

23. CHOONG S, ROMBAUTS L, UGONI A, MEAGHER S. Ultrasound prediction of risk of spontaneous miscarriage in live embryos from assisted conceptions. *Ultrasound Obstet Gynecol* 2003;**22**:571–7.

24. CHITTACHAROEN A, HERABUTYA Y. Slow fetal heart rate may predict pregnancy outcome in first-trimester threatened abortion. *Fertil Steril* 2004;**82**:227–9.

25. DOUBILET PM, BENSON CB. Embryonic heart rate in the early first trimester: what rate is normal? *J Ultrasound Med* 1995;**14**:431–4.

26. MERCHIERS EH, DHONT M, SUTTER PA, EGHIN CJ, VANDEKERCKHOVE DA. Predictive value of early embryonic cardiac activity for pregnancy outcome. *Am J Obstet Gynecol* 1991;**165**:11–14.

27. RAI RS, CLIFFORD K, COHEN H, REGAN L. High prospective fetal loss rate in untreated pregnancies of women with recurrent miscarriage and antiphospholipid antibodies. *Hum Reprod* 2005;**10**:3301–4.

28. LUISE C, JERMY K, COLLONS WP, BOURNE TH. Expectant management of incomplete, spontaneous first-trimester miscarriage: outcome according to initial ultrasound criteria and value of follow-up visits. *Ultrasound Obstet Gynecol* 2002;1 **9**:580–2.

29. MOLNAR A, OLIVER L, GEYNAM J. Patient preferences for management of first-trimester incomplete spontaneous abortion. *J Am Board Fam Pract* 2000;**13**:333–7.

30. JURKOVIC D, ROSS JA, NICOLAIDES KH. Expectant management of missed miscarriage. *Br J Obstet Gynaecol* 1998;**105**:670–1.

31. CHIPCHASE J, JAMES D. Randomised trial of expectant versus surgical management of spontaneous miscarriage. *Br J Obstet Gynaecol* 1997;**04**:840–1.

32. WIERINGA-DE WAARD M, VOS J, BONSEL GJ, BINDELS PJ, ANKUM WM. Management of miscarriage: a randomized controlled trial of expectant management versus surgical evacuation. *Hum Reprod* 2002;**17**:2445–50.

33. NIELSEN S, HAHLIN M, ODEN A. Using a logistic model to identify women with first-trimester spontaneous abortion suitable for expectant management. *Br J Obstet Gynaecol* 1996;**103**:1230–5.

34. ACHARYA G, MORGAN H. Does gestational sac volume predict the outcome of missed miscarriage managed expectantly? *J Clin Ultrasound* 2005;**3**:526–31.

35. GRAZIOSI G, MOL B, ANKUM W, BRUINSE H. Management of early pregnancy loss. *Int J Gynecol Obstet* 2004;**86**:337–46.

36. TRINDER J, BROCKLEHURST P, PORTER R, READ M, VYAS S, SMITH L. Management of miscarriage: expectant, medical, or surgical? Results of randomised controlled trial (miscarriage treatment [MIST] trial). *BMJ* 2006;**332**:1235–40.

37. BLOHM F, FRIDEN B, PLATZ-CHRISTENSEN J, MILSOM I, NIELSEN S. Expectant management of first-trimester miscarriage in clinical practice. *Acta Obstet Gynecol Scand* 2003;**82**:654–8.

38. OGDEN J, MAKER C. Expectant or surgical management of miscarriage: a qualitative study. *BJOG* 2004;**111**:463–7.

39. WIERINGA-DE WAARD M, BINDELS PJ, VOS J, BONSEL GJ, STANLEY VC, ANKUM WM. Patient preferences for expectant management compared with surgical evacuation in first-trimester uncomplicated miscarriage. *J Clin Path* 2004;**57**:167–73.

40. BLOHM F, HAHLIN M, NIELSEN S, MILSOM I. Fertility after a randomised trial of spontaneous abortion managed by surgical evacuation or expectant treatment. *Lancet* 1997;**349**:995.

41. EL REFAEY H, HINSHAW K, HENSHAW R, SMITH N, TEMPLETON A. Medical management of missed abortion and anembryonic pregnancy. *BMJ* 1992;**305**:1399.

42. HENSHAW RC, COOPER K, EL REFAEY H, SMITH NC, TEMPLETON AA. Medical management of miscarriage: non-surgical uterine evacuation of incomplete and inevitable spontaneous abortion. *BMJ* 1993;**306**:894–5.

43. CHUNG TK, CHEUNG LP, LEUNG TY, HAINES CJ, CHANG AM. Misoprostol in the management of spontaneous abortion. *Br J Obstet Gynaecol* 1995;**102**:832–5.

44. CHUNG TK, LEUNG P, CHEUNG LP, HAINES CJ, CHANG AM. A medical approach to management of spontaneous abortion using misoprostol. *Acta Obstet Gynecol Scand* 1997;**76**:248–51.

45. HINSHAW K. Medical management of miscarriage. In: Grudzinskas JG, O'Brien P, editors. *Problems in Early Pregnancy: Advances in Diagnosis and Management*. London: RCOG Press; 1997. p. 284–93.

46. WAGAARACHCHI PT, ASHOK PW, NARVEKAR N, SMITH NC, TEMPLETON A. Medical management of early fetal demise using a combination of mifepristone and misoprostol. *Hum Reprod* 2001;**16**:1849–53.

47. KULIER R, GULMEZOGLU A, HOFMEYR G, CHENG L, CAMPANA A. Medical methods for first trimester abortion. *Cochrane Database Syst Rev* 2004;(2) [CD002855].

48. NIELSEN S, HAHLIN M, PLATZ-CHRISTENSEN J. Randomised trial comparing expectant with medical management for first trimester miscarriages. *Br J Obstet Gynaecol* 1999;**106**:804–7.

49. DEMETROULIS C, SARIDOGAN E, KUNDE D, NAFTALIN A. A prospective randomised control trial comparing medical and surgical treatment for early pregnancy failure. *Hum Reprod* 2001;**16**:365–9.

50. GRONLUND A, GRONLUND L, CLEVIN L, ANDERSEN B, PALMGREN N, LIDEGAARD O. Management of missed abortion: comparison of medical treatment with either mifeprostone + misoprostol or misoprostol alone with surgical evacuation. *Acta Obstet Gynecol Scand* 2002; **81**:1060–5.

51. ZIEMAN M, FONG S, BENOWITZ N, BANSKTER D, DARNEY P. Absorption kinetics of misoprostol with oral or vaginal administration. *Obstet Gynecol* 1997;**90**:88–92.

52. DE JONGE ET, MAKIN JD, MANEFELDT E, DE WET GH, PATTINSON RC. Randomised clinical trial of medical evacuation and surgical curettage for incomplete miscarriage. *BMJ* 1995;**311**:662.

53. CHUNG TK, LEE DT, CHEUNG LP, HAINES CJ, CHANG AM. Spontaneous abortion: a randomized, controlled trial comparing surgical evacuation with conservative management using misoprostol. *Fertil Steril* 1999;**71**:1054–9.

54. SAHIN HG, SAHIN HA, KOCER M. Randomized outpatient clinical trial of medical evacuation and surgical curettage in incomplete miscarriage. *EurJ Contracept Reprod Health Care* 2001;**6**:141–4.

55. MUFFLEY PE, STITELY ML, GHERMAN RB. Early intrauterine pregnancy failure: a randomized trial of medical versus surgical treatment. *Am J Obstet Gynecol* 2002;**177**:321–6.

56. WOOD SL, BRAIN PH. Medical management of missed abortion: a randomised controlled trial. *Obstet Gynecol* 2002;**99**:563–6.

57. NGAI SW, CHAN YM, TANG OS, HO PC. Vaginal misoprostol as medical treatment for first trimester spontaneous miscarriage. *Hum Reprod* 2001;**16**:1493–6.

58. BAGRATEE J, KHULLAR V, REGAN L, MOODLEY J, KAGORO H. A randomised controlled trial comparing medical and expectant management of first trimester miscarriage. *Hum Reprod* 2004;**19**:266–71.

59. GREENLAND H, OGUNBIYI I, BUGG G, TASKER M. Medical treatment of miscarriage in a district General Hospital is safe and effective up to 12 weeks' gestation. *Curr Med Res Opin* 2005;**19**:699–701.

60. PANG MW, LEE TS, CHUNG TK. Incomplete miscarriage: a randomized controlled trial comparing oral with vaginal misoprostol for medical evacuation. *Hum Reprod* 2001;**16**:2283–7.

61. TANG OS, LAU WN, NG EH, LEE SW, HO PC. A prospective randomized study to compare the use of repeated doses of vaginal with sublingual misoprostol in the management of first trimester silent miscarriages. *Hum Reprod* 2003;**18**:176–81.

62. Royal College of Obstetricians and Gynaecologists. *The Management of Early Pregnancy Loss*. Green-top Guideline No. 25. London: RCOG;2006.

63. VERKUYL DA, CROWTHER CA. Suction conventional curettage in incomplete abortion: a randomised controlled trial. *S Afr Med J* 1993;**83**:131–15.

64. PRIETO J, ERIKSEN N, BLANCO J. A randomized trial of prophylactic doxycycline for curettage in incomplete abortion. *Obstet Gynecol* 1995;**85**:692–6.

65. Royal College of Obstetricians and Gynaecologists. *Use of Anti-D Immunoglobulin for Rh Prophylaxis*. Green-top Guideline No. 22. London: RCOG;2002.

66. GOLDBERG AB, DEAN G, KANG MS, YOUSSOF S, DARNEY PD. Manual versus electric vacuum aspiration for early first-trimester abortion: a controlled study of complication rates. *Obstet Gynecol* 2004;**103**:101–7.

67. GAZVANI R, HONEY E, MACLENNAN F, TEMPLETON A. Manual vacuum aspiration (MVA) in the management of first trimester pregnancy loss. *EurJ Obstet Gynecol Reprod Biol* 2004;**112**:197–200.

68. CAMERON MJ, PENNEY GC. Are national recommendations regarding examination and disposal of products of miscarriage being followed? A need for revised guidelines. *Hum Reprod* 2004;**20**:531–5.

15

Tubal ectopic pregnancy

DAVOR JURKOVIC

Introduction

Tubal ectopic pregnancy is an important cause of maternal morbidity and mortality worldwide. In the past three decades, the incidence of ectopic pregnancy has significantly increased in most industrialised countries to reach 100/million to 175/million women of reproductive age.[1] In recent years, the incidence of ectopics has plateaued in some Scandinavian countries.[2] The incidence in the UK has also been stable in the past decade, with the number increasing only slightly from 9.6/1000 pregnancies in 1991–1993 to 11.1/1000 pregnancies in 2003–2005.[3]

The recorded increase in the incidence of ectopic pregnancy worldwide may be attributable to a number of factors. The odds of having an ectopic pregnancy are significantly higher in women with a history of pelvic infection, women who have multiple partners and early age of intercourse. The risk of an ectopic pregnancy is particularly high in women with a history of infection with *Chlamydia trachomatis*.[4] Risk factors are shown in Box 15.1. A surge in the incidence of ectopic pregnancy was preceded by a similar peak in the incidence of acute salpingitis 15 years earlier.[5] It has also been shown that the reduction in the rate of chlamydial infection because of screening and treatment has led to a concomitant decline in the incidence of ectopic pregnancy.[2]

The incidence of ectopic pregnancy is three times higher in women aged 35–44 years in comparison with those in the age group 15–24 years.[6,7] In recent years, the age at first conception has increased, which may have contributed to an increased incidence.

The increased incidence of ectopic pregnancy may also be caused by the improved sensitivity of modern diagnostic tests. In the past, a significant number of ectopic pregnancies may have resolved spontaneously without being detected, which is less likely to occur in modern clinical practice. The increased incidence of ectopic pregnancy rate may therefore be partly explained by the increased effectiveness of screening.

- History of previous ectopic pregnancy
- Intrauterine contraceptive device or sterilisation failure
- Pelvic inflammatory disease
- Chlamydial infection
- Early age of intercourse and multiple partners
- History of infertility
- Previous pelvic surgery
- Increased maternal age
- Cigarette smoking
- Strenuous physical exercise
- In utero diethylstilbestrol exposure

BOX 15.1 Risk factors for ectopic pregnancy

Clinical presentation

Clinical presentation of ectopic pregnancy varies from mild vaginal bleeding to sudden rupture and massive intra-abdominal haemorrhage.

This is largely determined by the location of the pregnancy within the fallopian tube. In general, tubal ectopics, which are implanted closer to the uterine tubal ostium, tend to develop further and have more severe clinical presentation. Ampullary ectopics, which represent 70% of all tubal ectopic pregnancies, rarely develop beyond a very early stage.

Clinical symptoms of tubal miscarriage may be present as early as 5 weeks of gestation. On the other hand, one-third of interstitial tubal ectopics develop in a similar way to healthy intrauterine pregnancies, with evidence of a live embryo on ultrasound examination. These pregnancies tend to be clinically silent until sudden rupture occurs.[8]

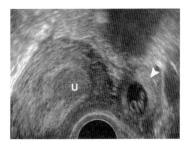

FIGURE 15.1 Transverse section through the pelvis shows an empty uterus (u) and a gestational sac in the left adnexa (arrow), which contained a live embryo and a yolk sac

Diagnosis of ectopic pregnancy

Traditionally, the diagnosis of ectopic pregnancy was made at surgery and then confirmed on histological examination following salpingectomy. At laparoscopy, an unruptured ectopic pregnancy typically presents as a well-defined swelling in the fallopian tube.[9] The diagnosis may be difficult in the presence of extensive pelvic adhesions, which impair the visualisation of the tubes. Anecdotal cases of false-positive and false-negative laparoscopic findings have been reported but no formal assessment of the accuracy of laparoscopy in the diagnosis of ectopic pregnancy has been published.

Some authors have advocated the use of dilatation and curettage in diagnosis of ectopic pregnancy. The presence of chorionic villi helps to exclude an ectopic pregnancy, as the incidence of heterotopic pregnancy is relatively low. The majority of women with absent villi on curettage, however, do not have ectopic pregnancies on subsequent laparoscopy, so the diagnostic value of curettage is very limited.[10]

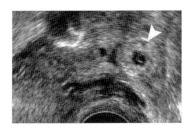

FIGURE 15.2 An ectopic gestational sac (arrow), which contains a yolk sac, is seen left to the uterus

With the advent of diagnostic ultrasound and the increasing use of conservative treatment, the diagnosis of ectopic pregnancy is routinely made without the help of surgery. The sensitivity of ultrasound examination in the diagnosis of ectopic pregnancy varies and success depends on the quality of the equipment and the experience and skill of the operator. With the use of transabdominal ultrasound, a direct visualisation of ectopic pregnancy is rarely possible.[11] The only value of transabdominal ultrasound is thus the detection of intrauterine pregnancy in women with clinical suspicion of an ectopic. Even the diagnosis of intrauterine pregnancy is difficult to make with confidence until 6–7 weeks of gestation. In addition, it is almost impossible to differentiate between interstitial ectopics and intrauterine pregnancies on transabdominal scan. For these reasons, transabdominal ultrasound should not be routinely used in women where there is a clinical suspicion of ectopic pregnancy.

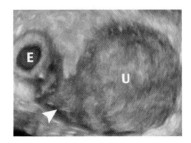

FIGURE 15.3 Three-dimensional scan demonstrating an empty uterus (U). An empty ectopic gestational sac (E) is seen within the right fallopian tube (arrow)

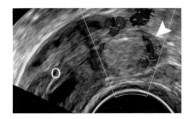

FIGURE 15.4 A scan at 7 weeks of gestation in a case of tubal miscarriage. A small solid swelling (arrow) is seen located adjacent to the right ovary (O). On colour Doppler examination, the structure was poorly vascularised

Transvaginal scanning provides much clearer images of pelvic structures in comparison with transabdominal scanning. By using a transvaginal approach, it is possible to palpate pelvic organs under visual control, which enables assessment of their mobility and helps to establish the source of pelvic pain. By applying gentle pressure with the tip of the ultrasound probe, a suspected tubal ectopic can be separated from the ovary. This 'sliding organs sign' helps to avoid a false positive diagnosis of ectopic pregnancy in women with a prominent corpus luteum on ultrasound scan.[12]

The morphology of an ectopic pregnancy can be classified into five categories:

▷ gestational sac with a live embryo (Figure 15.1)
▷ sac with an embryo but no heart rate
▷ sac containing a yolk sac (Figure 15.2)
▷ an empty gestational sac (Figure 15.3)
▷ solid tubal swelling (Figure 15.4).

The first three morphological types are very specific and they enable a conclusive ultrasound diagnosis of an ectopic to be made. The potential for a false positive diagnosis is higher when the sac is empty or in cases where there is an inhomogeneous tubal swelling.[13]

In experienced hands, transvaginal ultrasound can detect 75–80% of clinically significant tubal ectopic pregnancies at the initial examination.[14] The remaining 20–25% can be detected on follow-up visits and ultrasound should rarely fail to visualise an ectopic preoperatively. Cacciatore et al.,[15] in a study of 200 women involving 68 tubal ectopics, reported that the detection of an adnexal mass gives 99% specificity for the diagnosis of an ectopic pregnancy. Following this study, a meta-analysis published in 1994 including 2216 women, compared the various criteria for diagnosis of ectopic pregnancy.[13] The presence of an adnexal mass separate from the ovary other than a simple cyst achieved high sensitivity (84.4%) and only slightly lower specificity (98.9%) than other suggested diagnostic criteria, such as a live extrauterine pregnancy, an extrauterine gestation sac containing yolk sac and embryo or an empty tubal ring. In a later study from a single centre that included 840 women and 380 tubal ectopics, Shalev et al.[16] reported a sensitivity of 87% and specificity of 94% using as criteria for diagnosis either the presence a ring-like structure in the fallopian tube or the presence of a non-homogeneous adnexal mass.[16] The efficiency of transvaginal ultrasound for the diagnosis of tubal ectopic pregnancy was shown to be 95.6% when compared with laparoscopy in a study of 297 women who underwent laparoscopy.[17] In this study, the criterion used for diagnosis was the visualisation of a well-defined adnexal mass, separate to the ovary, in a woman with a positive pregnancy test. Similar findings are reported by others who define the adnexal mass as:

▷ an inhomogeneous mass (blob sign)
▷ a mass with hyperechoic ring around the gestation sac (bagel sign)
▷ a gestation sac with a fetal pole with or without cardiac activity.[14]

These studies indicate that, with appropriate training, a conclusive diagnosis of tubal ectopic pregnancy can be reached in most cases and that laparoscopy should be mainly used for treatment.

The presence of clear anechoic free fluid in pouch of Douglas is a frequent finding in women with normal intrauterine pregnancies and it should not be used to diagnose an ectopic (Figure 15.5). However, the presence of blood clots is important and is a common finding in ruptured ectopics. Blood clots appear hyperechoic and irregular on ultrasound scan and they may be mistaken for bowel loops (Figure 15.6). Checking for the presence of peristalsis helps in the differential diagnosis.

Slight bleeding within the uterine cavity is common in women with ectopic pregnancies and it may resemble an early intrauterine pregnancy (pseudosac). The distinction between the pseudosac and true gestational sac may be difficult on transabdominal scan. In all women at risk of ectopic pregnancy with an empty sac on transabdominal scan, a transvaginal scan should be performed to differentiate between these two conditions. An early intrauterine pregnancy is usually located eccentrically within the uterine cavity and is surrounded by an echogenic ring of trophoblast. The endometrial midline echo is intact and the pregnancy can be seen implanted below the endometrial surface (Figure 15.7). A pseudosac is surrounded by a single layer of tissue and tends to follow the contour of the cavity. In longitudinal section, the midline endometrial echo cannot be seen, which helps to confirm the presence of fluid within the uterine cavity (Figure 15.8) (Table 15.1).

Once it has been established that a gestational sac is present, it is important to ensure that the pregnancy is intrauterine. To achieve this, the uterus should be examined in the longitudinal section to demonstrate continuity between the gestational sac and the cervical canal (Figure 15.9).

In normal uteri, problems can also occur when an early pregnancy is located in the upper lateral aspect of the uterine cavity. This may raise suspicion of an interstitial tubal pregnancy. In pregnancies of less than 7 weeks it is possible to visualise both interstitial portions of the fallopian tubes. If the gestational sac is located medially to the interstitial part of

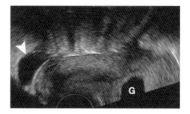

FIGURE 15.5 Longitudinal section through a uterus at 6 weeks of gestation showing an early intrauterine gestational sac (G). Note the presence of a small amount of clear fluid in the pouch of Douglas (arrow), which is a normal finding in early pregnancy

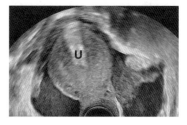

FIGURE 15.6 Longitudinal section through the pelvis in a case of ruptured tubal ectopic pregnancy. The uterus (U) is empty and it is surrounded by a large amount of blood and clots, which appear hyperechoic on ultrasound scan

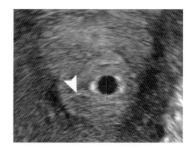

FIGURE 15.7 A 4-week intrauterine gestational sac measuring 5mm in size is seen embedded into endometrium of the central posterior aspect of the uterine cavity. The endometrial echo is clearly visible (arrow) anterior to the sac

	Early gestational sac	Pseudosac
Location	Below the midline echo buried into the endometrium	Along the cavity line, between endometrial layers
Shape	Steady, usually round	May change during scan, usually ovoid
Borders	Double ring	Single layer
Colour flow pattern	High peripheral flow	Avascular

TABLE 15.1 Differential diagnosis between early intrauterine gestational sac and pseudosac

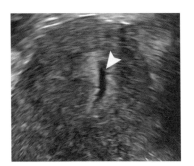

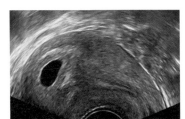

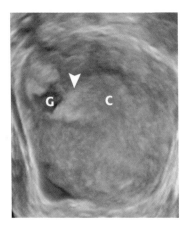

FIGURE 15.8 Longitudinal section of the uterus in an ectopic pregnancy. The uterine cavity is filled with fluid, which resembles an early collapsed intrauterine sac (arrow). On closer inspection, however, it is clear that the fluid is surrounded by a single layer of tissue and the midline echo is not visible. These features are typical of pseudosac and they facilitate differential diagnosis from an early intrauterine pregnancy

FIGURE 15.9 Longitudinal section through the uterus showing a continuity between the cervix and the gestational sac located at the fundal aspect of the uterine cavity

FIGURE 15.10 An early intrauterine pregnancy (G), which is located high in the right lateral aspect of the uterine cavity (c). Note the presence of a wide communication between the gestational sac and the cavity (arrow), which facilitate differential diagnosis between intrauterine pregnancy and interstitial ectopic

the tubes, the pregnancy is intrauterine. If the interstitial portions of the fallopian tubes cannot be seen, than it is important to examine the area medial to the sac. In intrauterine pregnancies, it is possible to visualise a continuum of the endometrial contours embracing the gestational sac. In addition, the communication between the sac and the uterine cavity is wide, which is not the case in interstitial pregnancies (Figure 15.10).

Some authors use the term 'angular' pregnancy to describe pregnancies located in the lateral aspect of the uterine cavity close to the tubal ostium.[18] On laparoscopy, an 'angular' pregnancy is distinguished from an interstitial pregnancy by being located medially to the round ligament. It has even been suggested in the past that differential diagnosis between interstitial and 'angular' pregnancy is difficult and that a term 'pregnancy in cornus' should be used to describe them. However, with the use of modern ultrasound equipment, it should always be possible to differentiate between an intrauterine and ectopic pregnancy.

The term 'angular pregnancy' is therefore probably obsolete, as it simply refers to a normal intrauterine pregnancy, which happens to be located laterally within the uterine cavity.

The diagnosis of intrauterine pregnancy becomes more difficult if the uterus is enlarged by fibroids. Fibroids often distort the shape of the endometrial cavity and prevent the operator from visualising in a single plane the continuity between the gestation sac and the cervical canal. In such cases, it is best to identify the cervix first and then follow the cervical canal into the endometrial cavity until the gestation sac is encountered, which would confirm an intrauterine pregnancy. Occasionally, the uterus becomes so enlarged that it is impossible to visualise the whole of the uterine cavity transvaginally. In these cases, a transabdominal scan is helpful to identify intrauterine pregnancy, which could not be seen using the transvaginal route (Figure 15.11).

In cases of suspected congenital uterine anomalies, a careful examination of the fundal region may reveal a variety of myometrial and cavity abnormalities. A precise description of the uterine anomaly is often difficult and three-dimensional scanning is usually necessary to achieve this.[19] In anomalous uteri, the gestational sac is often found laterally in the uterus and this may give rise to suspicion of an interstitial pregnancy (Figure 15.12). The diagnosis of intrauterine pregnancy should be based on the same criteria that are used in women with normal uteri. It is useful to remember that bleeding often occurs in the empty part of the anomalous uterus, which may create the picture of a 'pseudosac' adjacent to a normal pregnancy.

In women with intrauterine pregnancy on scanning, a possibility of heterotopic pregnancy should be excluded. This is particularly important in those who conceived after stimulation of ovulation or *in vitro* fertilisation. In symptomatic women with spontaneous pregnancies, it is helpful to examine the number of corpora lutea. If more than one corpus is present, a concomitant ectopic needs to be excluded (Figure 15.13).

Pregnancies of unknown location

Women who present with mild clinical symptoms and in whom an ultrasound scan fails to identify a location for the pregnancy are diagnosed with pregnancies of unknown location. The majority of these women have either had a complete miscarriage or a normal early pregnancy which is too small to be visualised on the scan. A small number of these women have tubal ectopics, which are not seen on the scan because they are too small or because they were not detected on examination. To facilitate differentiation between women who are at no risk of complications from those with a potentially significant ectopic

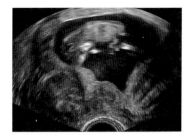

FIGURE 15.11 A 9-week pregnancy in a large fibroid uterus. The uterine anatomy is severely distorted, which makes it difficult to identify landmarks used for the diagnosis of a normal intrauterine pregnancy

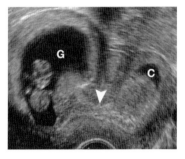

FIGURE 15.12 An 8-week pregnancy (G) in the right cornu of a bicornuate uterus. Note a wide communication (arrow) between the right cornu containing the pregnancy and the empty left uterine cornu (C)

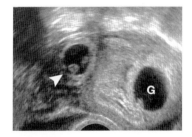

FIGURE 15.13 Heterotopic pregnancy. An intrauterine pregnancy (G) is seen on the left surrounded by a thick myometrial layer. A smaller ectopic sac (arrow) is seen in the right adnexa

pregnancy, many clinical units offer measurements of serum human chorionic gonadotrophin (hCG) and progesterone.[20]

Serum human chorionic gonadotrophin

Serum hCG measurements are routinely used to assess the risk of ectopic pregnancy when ultrasound examination fails to identify a pregnancy in women with a positive urine pregnancy test. Using transabdominal ultrasound, a normal pregnancy could be seen in most cases when serum hCG exceeded 6500 iu/l (Third International Reference 75/537, World Health Organization).[21] With transvaginal ultrasound this threshold is much lower and a normal pregnancy is usually seen with serum hCG greater than 1000 iu/l.[15] These observations have helped to introduce the concept of a 'discriminatory hCG zone' above which a normal intrauterine pregnancy should be detectable on ultrasound scan. However, the concept of the discriminatory zone is often misinterpreted in clinical practice. There are many clinicians who assume that, in the absence of a visible intrauterine pregnancy on ultrasound scan, a serum hCG reading below a predefined level equals normal intrauterine pregnancy and that the reading above is diagnostic of an ectopic.[22] This is clearly not the case, as hCG levels are often high in the aftermath of a complete miscarriage because of its long half life of 24–36 hours. It has also been shown that more than 50% of ectopic pregnancies which are detectable on the scan present with hCG levels of less than 1000 iu/l.[23] In view of this fact, the concept of the discriminatory zone is of limited value in clinical practice and it is only useful in assessing asymptomatic women with uncertain menstrual dates.

An abnormally slow rise in serum hCG has also been used to diagnose ectopic pregnancy. In normal early pregnancy, the hCG doubling time is 1.4 days up to 4 weeks and 6 days of gestation, then 2.4 days until the 7th week of gestation. A prolonged hCG doubling time is an indicator of an abnormal pregnancy. However, it cannot discriminate between intrauterine miscarriages and ectopics. It has also been shown that, in about 10% of ectopic pregnancies, serum hCG shows a normal rate of increase.[24] In the context of inconclusive scans, decline of serum hCG is equally or even more important, because it facilitates the detection of spontaneously resolving pregnancies, which do not require any medical intervention. It has been shown that, when the ratio of the initial serum hCG measurement to another taken 48 hours later is less than 0.87, this is an accurate test to diagnose spontaneous resolution of pregnancy.[25] The use of hCG to select women for expectant, medical and surgical management of ectopic pregnancy and to assess the efficacy of treatment at follow-up visits will be discussed later.

Progesterone

Progesterone production from the corpus luteum is dependent upon the slope of hCG increase in early pregnancy. The half-life of progesterone clearance is only 2 hours compared with 24–36 hours for serum hCG.[26] As a result, serum progesterone levels respond quickly to any decrease in hCG production. The progesterone measurement can therefore be used as a bioassay of early pregnancy viability. Serum progesterone levels of less than 20 nmol/l reflect fast decreasing hCG levels and can be used to diagnose spontaneously resolving pregnancies with a sensitivity of 94% and specificity of 91%.[23] Progesterone levels greater than 60 nmol/l indicate normal increase in hCG levels and those of 20–60 nmol/l are strongly associated with abnormal pregnancies. In clinical practice, serum progesterone measurements are particularly useful in women whose ultrasound scan is non-diagnostic. Although the majority of these women have failed intrauterine pregnancies, they are usually followed up with serial hCG measurement because of the fear of missing potentially significant ectopic pregnancies. The routine measurement of serum progesterone can reliably diagnose pregnancies in regression and can reduce by 50–60% the need for follow-up scans and serial hCG measurements in pregnant women with non-diagnostic scan findings.[23]

Management of tubal ectopic pregnancy

Surgical management

Surgery remains the main therapeutic option for the treatment of tubal ectopic pregnancy. With recent advances in operative laparoscopy, minimally invasive surgery has become accepted as the method of choice to treat most tubal ectopic pregnancies. There are important advantages of laparoscopic over open surgery, such as less postoperative pain, shorter hospital stay and faster resumption of social activity.[27] However, the future reproductive outcomes following laparoscopic or open surgery are not significantly different. Although recurrent ectopic rates are slightly lower following laparoscopic surgery, the rates of subsequent intrauterine pregnancies appear to be similar.[28]

It remains unclear whether laparoscopic salpingotomy with tubal conservation offers any advantages over salpingectomy. A large international multicentre trial is currently under way, which aims to answer this question.[29] At present, there is a consensus that tubal conservation should be attempted if the woman desires further pregnancies and there is evidence of contralateral tubal damage at laparoscopy. In the presence of a healthy contralateral tube, salpingectomy may be performed with the woman's consent.[28]

Medical management

Medical management of ectopic pregnancy has grown in popularity following several observational studies which reported success rates in excess of 90% with single-dose systemic methotrexate.[30] However, the diagnosis of ectopic pregnancy was based in many cases on monitoring the dynamics of serum hCG and progesterone, rather than on direct visualisation of the ectopic on ultrasound scan or at laparoscopy. It is therefore possible that, in a significant number of cases, intrauterine miscarriages were misdiagnosed as ectopics, contributing to the high success rates. Nevertheless, there are some obvious attractions of medical treatment, such as the possibility for management on an outpatient basis and avoidance of surgery. Owing to the need for prolonged follow-up and increased failure rate in women presenting with higher initial hCG measurements, medical treatment is only cost effective in ectopics with serum hCG levels of less than 1500 iu/l.[31] Selection criteria for treatment with methotrexate include:

▷ minimal clinical symptoms
▷ no evidence of embryonic cardiac activity
▷ diameter less than 5 cm
▷ no evidence of haematoperitoneum on ultrasound scan
▷ initial serum hCG levels of less than 3000 iu/l
▷ normal liver and renal function tests.

Two randomised trials which compared methotrexate and surgery showed that only one-third of all tubal ectopics satisfied these criteria and were suitable for medical treatment, with success rates between 65% and 82%.[32,33] The overall contribution of medical management to the successful treatment of tubal ectopic was between 23% and 30%, while all other women required surgery. The other problem with methotrexate is the risk of tubal rupture and blood transfusion, which occurred significantly more often in women receiving methotrexate when compared with those who had surgery, emphasising the need for close follow-up.[32]

There is also a risk of adverse effects, including gastritis, stomatitis, alopecia, headaches, nausea and vomiting. Disturbances in hepatic and renal function and leucopenia or thrombocytopenia may also occur.

In view of all these factors, the overall role of methotrexate in the management of ectopic pregnancy is limited but it may be offered on an individual basis to highly motivated women with small unruptured ectopics and serum hCG levels of 1500–3000 iu/l who are likely to comply with a well-organised follow up.

Expectant management

Expectant management has important advantages over medical treatment, as it follows the natural history of the condition and is free from the serious adverse effects of methotrexate. Expectant management requires prolonged follow-up, which may cause anxiety to both women and their carers. However, the main reason limiting the use of expectant management is its relatively high failure rate and the inability to identify with accuracy women who are likely to fail expectant management. To minimise the risk of failure, many authors have used very strict selection criteria for expectant management, such as the initial hCG levels of less than 250 iu/l.[34] The use of strict selection criteria has resulted in relatively high success rates for expectant management, sometimes reaching 70–80%.[35,36] However, only a small minority of ectopics were considered suitable for expectant management, resulting in a low overall contribution to successful management of tubal ectopic of only between 7% and 25%. Recent studies have shown that by using more liberal selection criteria for expectant management, up to 40% of all tubal ectopics may resolve spontaneously on expectant treatment.[37] This observation reflects the increased sensitivity of modern ultrasound equipment which enables the detection of very small ectopics. It is likely that a large proportion of these small ectopics were undiagnosed in the past and were treated as early intrauterine miscarriages.

According to the current literature the success of expectant management may be determined by the serum hCG levels at the initial presentation. In general, if hCG levels are less that 1500 iu/l and the ectopic pregnancy is clearly visible on ultrasound scan, the success of expectant management is 60–70%.[37] The addition of serum progesterone levels and morphological features of ectopics on ultrasound scan will refine further the prediction of the likely success of expectant management.

Fertility after ectopic pregnancy

Intrauterine pregnancy rates following ectopic pregnancy range between 50% and 70%.[38] Recurrent ectopic pregnancies occur in 6–16% of women with a previous history of ectopics.[39] There is some evidence to suggest that intrauterine pregnancy rates may be better following salpingotomy than salpingectomy but this issue has not yet been addressed in a prospective randomised trial. Subsequent intrauterine and recurrent ectopic pregnancy rates are not significantly different among women who underwent either surgical or medical treatment of ectopic pregnancy with methotrexate.[32]

Long-term fertility outcomes in women treated expectantly have not been extensively reported. Several authors have reported no significant differences in the ipsilateral tubal patency rates and the rates of subsequent intrauterine and extrauterine pregnancies after successful expectant management compared with ectopics managed surgically.[40] One study, however, has shown that expectant management was associated with a significantly higher rate of subsequent intrauterine pregnancies in comparison with surgical treatment.[41] The rate of recurrent ectopics, however, was similar. These studies indicate that the avoidance of any intervention remains the main advantage of expectant management, while the possible improvements in subsequent fertility outcomes need to be assessed further. Whatever management strategy has been used in women with a history of previous ectopic pregnancy, they should all be offered early scans in all their future pregnancies to detect recurrent ectopics before complications can occur.

Conclusion

Modern ultrasound equipment enables an accurate diagnosis of tubal ectopic pregnancy to be made in the majority of cases. This has transformed the care of women with tubal ectopics and has facilitated the use of non-surgical treatment. More effective screening for tubal ectopics has led to the detection of many cases of tubal miscarriages which are destined to resolve spontaneously without any intervention. Such cases can be managed expectantly with a low risk of complications. Continuous improvements in the quality of ultrasound equipment will further increase our ability to detect small tubal miscarriages. One of the major challenges for the future clinical practice will be the development of clinical algorithms that can reliably separate clinically significant ectopics, which may cause harm, from spontaneously resolving cases, which can be managed expectantly.

REFERENCES

1. COSTE J, BOUYER J, UGHETTO S, GERBAUD L, FERNANDEZ H, POULY J, et al. Ectopic pregnancy is again on the increase. Recent trends in the incidence of ectopic pregnancies in France (1992–2002). *Hum Reprod* 2004; **19**: 2014–18.

2. EGGER M, LOW N, DAVEY SMITH G, LINDBLOM B, HERRMANN B. Screening for chlamydial infections and the risk of ectopic pregnancy in a county in Sweden: ecological analysis. *BMJ* 1998; **316**: 1776–80.

3. Confidential Enquiry into Maternal and Child Health. *Saving Mothers' Lives: Reviewing Maternal Deaths to Make Motherhood Safer 2003–2005. The Seventh Report of the Confidential Enquiries into Maternal Deaths in the United Kingdom.* London: CEMACH; 2007.

4. ANKUM W M, MOL B W J, VAN DER VEEN F, BOSSUYT P M M. Risk-factors for ectopic pregnancy: a meta-analysis. *Fertil Steril* 1996; **65**: 1093–9.

5. BJARTLING C, OSSER S, PERSSON K. The frequency of salpingitis and ectopic pregnancy as epidemiologic markers of Chlamydia trachomatis. *Acta Obstet Gynecol Scand* 2000; **79**: 123–8.

6. GOLDNER T, LAWSON H, XIA Z, ATRASH H. Surveillance for ectopic pregnancy: United States, 1970–1989. *MMWR CDC Surveill Summ* 1993; **42**: 73–85.

7. WESTROM L, BENGTSSON L P H, MARDH P A. Incidence, trends and risks of ectopic pregnancy in a population of women. *Br Med J* 1981; **282**: 15–18.

8. HAFNER T, ASLAM N, ROSS J A, ZOSMER N, JURKOVIC D. The effectiveness of non-surgical management of early interstitial pregnancy: a report of ten cases and review of the literature. *Ultrasound Obstet Gynecol* 1999; **13**: 131–6.

9. GARRY R. Laparoscopic surgery. *Best Pract Res Clin Obstet Gynaecol* 2006; **20**: 89–104.

10. LINDAHL B, AHLGREN M. Identification of chorion villi in abortion specimens. *Obstet Gynecol* 1986; **67**: 79–81.

11. ATHEY P A, LAMKI N, MATYAS M A, WATSON A B JR. Comparison of transvaginal and transabdominal ultrasonography in ectopic pregnancy. *Can Assoc Radiol J* 1991; **42**: 349–52.

12. TIMOR-TRITSCH I E, ROTTEM S. Transvaginal ultrasonographic study of the Fallopian tube. *Obstet Gynecol* 1987; **70**: 424-8

13. BROWN D L, DOUBILET P M. Transvaginal sonography for diagnosing ectopic pregnancy. *J Ultrasound Med* 1994; **13**: 259–66.

14. CONDOUS G, OKARO E, KHALID A, LU C, VAN HUFFEL S, TIMMERMAN D, et al. The accuracy of transvaginal sonography for the diagnosis of ectopic pregnancy prior to surgery. *Hum Reprod* 2005; **20**: 1404–9.

15. CACCIATORE B, STENMAN U H, YLOSTALO P. Diagnosis of ectopic pregnancy by vaginal ultrasonography in combination with a discriminatory serum hCG level of 1000 IU/L (IRP). *BJOG* 1990; **97**: 904–8.

16. SHALEV E, YAROM I, BUSTAN M, WEINER E, BEN-SHLOMO I. Transvaginal sonography as the ultimate diagnostic tool for the management of ectopic pregnancy: experience with 840 cases. *Fertil Steril* 1998; **69**: 62–5.

17. OFILI-YEBOVI D, CASSIK P, LEE C, ELSON J, HILLABY K, JURKOVIC D. The efficacy of ultrasound-based protocol for the diagnosis of tubal ectopic pregnancy. *Ultrasound Obstet Gynecol* 2003; **22 (Suppl. 1)**: 1–69.

18. JANSEN R P, ELLIOTT P M. Angular intrauterine pregnancy. *Obstet Gynecol* 1981; **58**: 167–75.

19. SALIM R, REGAN L, WOELFER B, BACKOS M, JURKOVIC D. A comparative study of the morphology of congenital uterine anomalies in women with and without a history of recurrent first trimester miscarriage. *Hum Reprod* 2003; **18**: 162–6.

20. CONDOUS G, TIMMERMAN D, GOLDSTEIN S, VALENTIN L, JURKOVIC D, BOURNE T. Pregnancies of unknown location: consensus statement. *Ultrasound Obstet Gynecol* 2006; **28**: 121–2.

21. KADAR N, DEVORE G, ROMERO R. Discriminatory hCG zone: its use in the sonographic evaluation for ectopic pregnancy. *Obstet Gynecol* 1981; **58**: 156–61.

22. PISARSKA M D, CARSON S A, BUSTER J E. Ectopic pregnancy. *Lancet* 1998; **351**: 1115–20.

23. BANERJEE S, ASLAM N, WOELFER B, LAWRENCE A, ELSON J, JURKOVIC D. Expectant management of early pregnancies of unknown location: a prospective evaluation of methods to predict spontaneous resolution of pregnancy. *BJOG* 2001; **108**: 158–63.

24. FRIDSTROM M, GAROFF L, SJOBLOM P, HILLENS T. Human chorionic gonadotropin patterns in early pregnancy after assisted conception. *Acta Obstet Gynecol Scand* 1995; **74**: 534–8.

25. KIRK E, CONDOUS G, VAN CALSTER B, VAN HUFFEL S, TIMMERMAN D, BOURNE T. Rationalizing the follow-up of pregnancies of unknown location. *Hum Reprod* 2007; **22**: 1744–50.

26. HAHLIN M, THORBURN J, BRYMAN I. The expectant management of early pregnancies of uncertain site. *Hum Reprod* 1995; **10**: 1223–7.

27. GRAY D, THORBURN J, LUNDORFF P, STRANDELL A, Lindblom B. A cost-effectiveness study of a randomised trial of laparoscopy versus laparotomy for ectopic pregnancy. *Lancet* 1995; **345**: 1139–43.

28. Royal College of Obstetricians and Gynaecologists. *The Management of Tubal Pregnancy.* Green-top Guideline 21. London: RCOG; 2004.

29. MOL F, STRANDELL A, JURKOVIC D, YALCINKAYA T, VERHOEVE H R, KOKS C A, et al. The ESEP study: salpingostomy versus salpingectomy for tubal ectopic pregnancy; the impact on future fertility: a randomised controlled trial. *BMC Womens Health* 2008; **8**: 11.

30. STOVALL T G, LING FW. Single-dose methotrexate: an expanded clinical trial. *Am J Obstet Gynecol* 1993; **168**: 1759–65.

31. SOWTER M, FARQUHAR C, GUDEX G. An economic evaluation of single dose methotrexate and laparoscopic surgery for the treatment of unruptured ectopic pregnancy. *BJOG* 2001; **108**: 204–12.

32. HAJENIUS PJ, ENGELSBEL S, MOL B W, VAN DER VEEN F, ANKUM W M, BOSSUYT PM M, *et al*. Randomised trial of systemic methotrexate versus laparoscopic salpingostomy in tubal pregnancy. *Lancet* 1997; **350**: 774–9.

33. SOWTER M C, FARQUHAR C M, PETRIE KJ, GUDEX G. A randomised trial comparing single dose systemic methotrexate and laparoscopic surgery for the treatment of unruptured tubal pregnancy. *BJOG* 2001; **108**: 192–203.

34. CACCIATORE B, KORHONEN J, STENMAN U-H, YLOSTALO P. Transvaginal sonography and serum hCG in monitoring of presumed ectopic pregnancies selected for expectant management. *Ultrasound Obstet Gynecol* 1995; **5**: 297–3.

35. YLOSTALO P, CACCIATORE B, SJOBERG J, KAARAIANEN M, TENHUNEN A, STENMAN UH. Expectant management of ectopic pregnancy. *Obstet Gynecol* 1992; **80**: 345–8.

36. MAKINEN J I, KIVIJARVI A K, IRJALA KM A. Success of non-surgical management of ectopic pregnancy. *Lancet* 1990; **335**: 1099.

37. ELSON J, TAILOR A, BANERJEE S, SALIM R, HILLABY K, JURKOVIC D. Expectant management of tubal ectopic pregnancy: prediction of successful outcome using decision tree analysis. *Ultrasound Obstet Gynecol* 2004; **23**: 552–6.

38. STROBELT N, MARIANI E, FERRARI L, TRIO D, TIEZZI A, GHIDINI A. Fertility after ectopic pregnancy. *J Reprod Med* 2000; **45**: 803–7.

39. DUBUISSON J B, AUBRIOT F X, FOULOT H. Reproductive outcome after laparoscopic salpingectomy for tubal ectopic pregnancy. *Fertil Steril* 1990; **53**: 1004–7.

40. OLOFSSON J I, POROMAA I S, OTTANDER U, KJELLBERG L, DAMBER M G. Clinical and pregnancy outcome following ectopic pregnancy; a prospective study comparing expectancy, surgery and systemic methotrexate treatment. *Acta Obstet Gynecol Scand* 2001; **80**: 744–9.

41. HELMY S, SAWYER E, OFILI-YEBOVI D, YAZBEK J, BEN NAGI J, JURKOVIC D. Fertility outcomes following expectant management of tubal ectopic pregnancy. *Ultrasound Obstet Gynecol* 2007; **30**: 988–93.

16 Non-tubal ectopic pregnancies

Joseph Yazbek and Davor Jurkovic

Introduction

Ectopic pregnancy is a significant health problem in the developed world, which affects 1–2% of women of reproductive age, causing significant morbidity and mortality. Most ectopic pregnancies are located in the ampullary, fimbrial or isthmic parts of the fallopian tube. However, approximately 7% of ectopic pregnancies are not located within these parts of the tube[1] and they are classified as non-tubal ectopics. Each of these rare forms of ectopic pregnancies often represents a diagnostic and therapeutic challenge because of their atypical location and paucity of experience in their management.

In this chapter, we will provide a summary of each type of non-tubal ectopic pregnancy, with particular emphasis on the ultrasound diagnosis and management options.

Interstitial pregnancy

Interstitial pregnancy is characterised by the implantation of the conceptus in the interstitial portion of the fallopian tube, which is surrounded by the muscular wall of the uterus.[2] Interstitial pregnancy is sometimes referred to as cornual pregnancy. However, the term cornual pregnancy is more appropriately used to describe implantation of pregnancy in the rudimentary or atretic cornu of a congenitally abnormal uterus.

Incidence and predisposing factors

Interstitial pregnancy rates are increasing steadily, mirroring the increase in ectopic pregnancy rates. Interstitial pregnancy complicates between 2% and 6% of all ectopic pregnancies or 1 in 2500–5000 live births.[1,3] Risk factors predisposing to an interstitial pregnancy include previous tubal ectopic pregnancy, previous ipsilateral salpingectomy, assisted reproductive technology and sexually transmitted infections.[2,4] The maternal morbidity associated with interstitial pregnancy is still high, and the maternal mortality rate of this form of ectopic pregnancy is 2% to 2.5%.[1,5–7]

Diagnosis

Interstitial pregnancy remains the most difficult type of ectopic pregnancies to be diagnosed preoperatively.[8] In the past, the diagnosis used to be made at laparotomy following rupture, or during histological examination of the uterus following an emergency hysterectomy. The classic triad of amenorrhoea, abnormal vaginal bleeding and abdominal pain, is only present in 40% of patients.[8] These symptoms are not specific to interstitial pregnancy as they are also present in other forms of early pregnancy disorders.

ULTRASOUND

The advances in high-resolution transvaginal ultrasonography and the establishment of early pregnancy units have facilitated the early non-invasive diagnosis of most cases of interstitial pregnancy well before serious complications occur. This has opened the door for more conservative management options such as medical treatment with methotrexate. The ultrasound appearance of an interstitial pregnancy varies and ranges from a viable pregnancy to a solid inhomogeneous mass.[9]

Different ultrasound criteria for the diagnosis of interstitial pregnancy have been suggested by various authors,[9-14] but most use the following criteria: an empty uterine cavity and a gestational sac seen adjacent to the lateral aspect of the uterine cavity surrounded by a thin myometrial layer. A particularly useful observation was made by Ackerman et al.,[14] who described the 'interstitial line sign'. This refers to the proximal part of the interstitial tube, which joins the lateral aspect of the uterine cavity and the ectopic gestational sac (Figures 16.1, 16.2). The 'interstitial line sign' is reported to have a sensitivity of 80% and specificity of 98% in the diagnosis of interstitial pregnancy.[14] This sign is particularly helpful for differential diagnosis between small intramural fibroids affecting the lateral aspect of the uterus close to the origin of the fallopian tube and small solid interstitial pregnancies. In the case of intramural fibroids, the interstitial part of the tube is displaced and can be seen bypassing the mass.

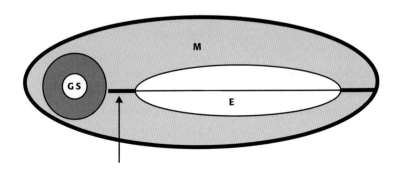

FIGURE 16.1 The ultrasound criteria to diagnose an interstitial pregnancy; M = myometrium, E = endometrium, GS = gestational sac, arrow = interstitial tube

It may be difficult to differentiate between an interstitial pregnancy and an intrauterine pregnancy that is implanted high in the lateral aspect of the uterine cavity. Some authors classify these pregnancies as angular pregnancy,[15] although their clinical course is no different from other normally implanted intrauterine gestations. Three-dimensional ultrasound can also be helpful to differentiate between intrauterine and interstitial pregnancies.[16,17] Three-dimensional ultrasound facilitates both the examination of the myometrial mantle and the visualisation of the interstitial tube, so the diagnosis can be made with more confidence (Figure 16.3).

Despite the published diagnostic criteria, diagnostic errors are not uncommon and they may occur in up to 42% of surgically proven cases of interstitial pregnancies.[18]

OTHER DIAGNOSTIC METHODS

The use of magnetic resonance imaging (MRI) in the diagnosis of interstitial pregnancy has been reported.[19] However, the use of this complex and expensive technique will inevitably be limited to the few cases in which ultrasound diagnosis cannot be made with certainty. In modern clinical practice laparoscopy should rarely be used to diagnose an interstitial pregnancy. Laparoscopic diagnosis is based on the visualisation of a swelling that is lateral to the uterine insertion of the round ligament and it involves the origin of the fallopian tube.[15] Hysteroscopic diagnosis of interstitial pregnancy has been reported in isolated case reports.[20,21] However, hysteroscopy should not be used in the routine investigation of a suspected ectopic pregnancies as it could lead to the loss of a normal intrauterine pregnancy. Furthermore, interstitial pregnancies, by definition, are located outside the uterine cavity and therefore it is not clear how they could be seen at hysteroscopy.

Management

SURGICAL MANAGEMENT

Traditionally, the management of interstitial pregnancy was surgical, in the form of cornual resection or hysterectomy.[3] The reason for this was the late detection of this condition, which used to be diagnosed at laparotomy following tubal rupture.

Rupture typically occurs later than in cases of tubal pregnancy, owing to the increased blood supply and the presence of thick myometrium covering the interstitial portion of the tube.[2]

In 1988, Reich *et al.*[22] were the first to describe the laparoscopic treatment of an interstitial pregnancy. The techniques described involved laparoscopic cornual resection using either unipolar knife or bipolar

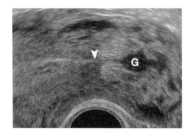

FIGURE 16.2 Transverse view through the uterine fundus showing a 9-week, non-viable, left interstitial pregnancy. Note the continuity of myometrial mantle surrounding the gestational sac (G) and the interstitial tube (arrow) adjoining the uterine cavity and the gestational sac

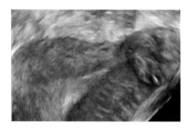

FIGURE 16.3 Three-dimensional scan clearly showing a small, solid, left interstitial pregnancy

forceps and scissors.[22] Lau and Tulandi[5] analysed 22 cases reported in the literature involving the use of laparoscopic cornual resection, cornuostomy or salpingotomy. Most of the authors injected vasopressin intramyometrially at the start of the operation, to minimise blood loss and improve visibility. To minimise blood loss, some authors have used a suture-loop tourniquet applied through the avascular area of the broad ligament.[23,24] The success of laparoscopic surgery seems to be high in skilled hands but there is also a risk of failure owing to uncontrollable bleeding and the risk of incomplete excision of pregnancy, which may require further treatment.

MEDICAL MANAGEMENT

Medical management using methotrexate, a folate antagonist, has been increasingly used in the treatment of women identified as having an unruptured interstitial pregnancy, who are haemodynamically stable, had normal hepatorenal function and a normal full blood count.

Methotrexate can be administered systemically or locally. Systemic methotrexate has been used with different dosing regimens. A multi-dose regimen of 1 mg/kg intramuscularly, with 0.1 mg/kg of folinic acid (calcium folinate) rescue on alternate days has been used in a number of reports. The first case of interstitial pregnancy treated successfully with multiple doses of methotrexate was reported in 1982 by Tanaka et al.[25] Alternatively, a single-dose regimen, which is based on body surface area, may be administered at 50 mg/m^2 intramuscularly without the need for folinic acid rescue.[5,26]

Methotrexate may also be administered locally into the gestational sac under transvaginal ultrasound guidance. The vagina is cleansed using an antiseptic and prophylactic antibiotic cover is usually given. A thin, long needle is placed into a needle guide and advanced through the vaginal fornix and uterine wall into the gestational sac; 25 mg of methotrexate is then injected directly into the coelomic sac or amniotic cavity. In viable pregnancies, an embryocide is first performed with an intracardiac injection of 0.2–0.4 mEq of potassium chloride.[27] In a literature review, Lau and Tulandi[5] identified 41 women with interstitial pregnancy treated with methotrexate systemically, locally or in combination, and found an overall success rate of 83%. They also found that local methotrexate (91% success) may be slightly more effective than systemic methotrexate (79% success). The β-hCG resolution time was three times faster in the local treatment group compared to those who received systemic methotrexate. This may be due to a higher concentration of the drug at the trophoblastic site with local treatment. They also speculated that folinic acid may prolong the β-hCG resolution time, as

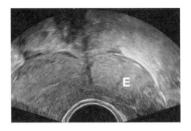

FIGURE 16.4 Moderately large, solid, left interstitial ectopic pregnancy (E) in an asymptomatic woman. The initial serum hCG was 855iu/l and the pregnancy was managed expectantly

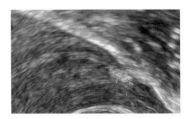

FIGURE 16.5 Sonogram of the same woman 9 months later, showing that the pregnancy has been fully absorbed and only small amount of fibrosis is still visible

women who received local methotrexate did not receive folinic acid.[5]

Similar results have also been reported by others.[9,28] The main factor determining the success of conservative treatment is the initial serum hCG measurement. High readings, greater than 10 000 iu/l, seem to be associated with an increased risk of failure of conservative management.[27]

EXPECTANT MANAGEMENT

When no intervention is carried out to actively treat the ectopic pregnancy, the management is called expectant. This management option should only be used when good follow-up arrangements are available. Expectant management is usually offered to women who are clinically stable with non-viable interstitial pregnancies and declining or plateauing serum β-hCG measurements. Serial β-hCG measurements are required, until β-hCG becomes undetectable. It usually takes between 4–9 months for ectopic pregnancy to become completely absorbed when managed expectantly or medically, if monitored by ultrasound (Figures 16.4, 16.5).[29]

The main benefit of expectant management is the avoidance of adverse effects associated with medical treatment.[27] Expectant management may be suitable for up to 20% of interstitial ectopics and the success rate can be as high as 70%.[27] However, experience with expectant management is limited and further work is necessary to define its role in the management of interstitial pregnancy.

UTERINE ARTERY EMBOLISATION

Uterine artery embolisation has been described for control of various bleeding conditions in obstetrics and gynaecology.[30] Ophir et al.[31] described the use of selective uterine artery embolisation in the treatment of interstitial pregnancy, after failure of systemic methotrexate treatment. They concluded that this treatment modality may be effective for the conservative management of interstitial pregnancy, and as a prophylactic measure before surgical intervention to prevent major bleeding.[30,31]

Fertility after interstitial pregnancy

There is little information about fertility following interstitial pregnancy. One study included a total of 24 women who were followed up for a period of 7 years. The majority of women who tried for another pregnancy had a successful spontaneous conception. The rate of recurrent ectopic pregnancy was 23%, which is similar to fertility outcomes following successful conservative treatment of tubal ectopics. The majority of recurrent ectopics were located in the ipsilateral interstitial tube.[32]

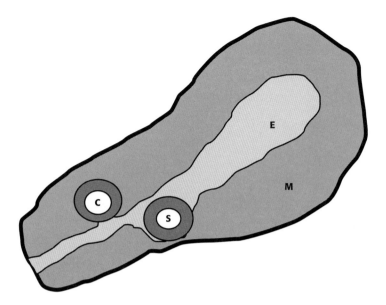

FIGURE 16.6 Typical locations of cervical (c) and caesarean scar (s) ectopic pregnancies. Cervical pregnancies are located below the internal os and they tend to penetrate into the myometrium. Caesarean-scar ectopics are typically located within a deficient lower-segment caesarean section scar at the level of the internal os

There are few case reports of uterine rupture during pregnancy in women who had a previous interstitial pregnancy following both surgical resection of the uterine cornu and conservative treatment.[33,34] However, the overall risk of rupture appears to be low.

Cervical pregnancy

Cervical pregnancy is defined as the implantation of the conceptus within the cervix, below the level of the internal os. Cervical pregnancy is associated with high morbidity, as it often leads to severe haemorrhage, which sometimes requires a life-saving emergency hysterectomy.[35]

Cervical pregnancy should be distinguished from a caesarean scar pregnancy, which is also located close to the internal os but it is implanted into a deficient caesarean section scar, rather than the cervix. It is important to differentiate between these two types of ectopic pregnancy as they have different clinical and diagnostic features and they require different management approaches (Figure 16.6).

Incidence and predisposing factors

Cervical pregnancy is an unusual form of ectopic pregnancy, accounting for fewer than 1% of all ectopic pregnancies or approximately 1/8628 deliveries.[36] Predisposing factors for cervical pregnancy include previous curettage, previous caesarean delivery, prior cervical surgery, infertility and IVF treatment.[37,38] However, in a literature review of all reported cases of cervical pregnancy between 1978 and 1994, Ushakov et al.[36]

found that 11.8% of the women diagnosed with a cervical pregnancy had no detectable risk factors.

Diagnosis

In the past, the diagnosis of cervical pregnancy was made histologically after hysterectomy, which was usually performed to control severe bleeding and save the woman's life.[39] Painless vaginal bleeding is the most common presenting feature in women with cervical pregnancy. Urinary frequency or dysuria have been reported as a presenting complaint in women with more advanced pregnancies.[40]

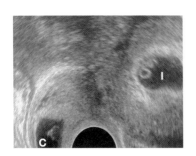

FIGURE 16.7 Heterotopic intrauterine (I) and cervical pregnancy (C) diagnosed at 12 weeks of gestation

Intracervical localisation of an ectopic gestational sac or trophoblastic mass is the cornerstone for the ultrasound diagnosis of cervical pregnancy (Figure 16.7).[36] The ultrasound criteria for the diagnosis of cervical pregnancy have been described by Timor-Tritsch et al.,[41] who suggested that the finding of a gestational sac, which contains an embryo with visible heart activity within the cervical canal, gives a definitive diagnosis of cervical pregnancy. It can be difficult to distinguish a cervical implantation from the cervical phase of intrauterine miscarriage. Oval or round sacs and those containing a yolk sac are more likely to represent cervical implantation, while collapsed, irregular sacs may represent miscarriage (Figure 16.8).[35] The diagnosis of cervical pregnancy can be made on follow-up scan if there has been interim development of an embryo or growth in the size of the gestational sac.[42]

To differentiate a spontaneous miscarriage in progress from a continuing cervical pregnancy, the authors have described the use of the 'sliding organs sign', where gentle pressure of the endovaginal probe on the cervix causes sliding of the gestational sac within the cervical canal in case of spontaneous miscarriage.[43] Doppler examination may also be used to examine for the presence of peritrophoblastic blood flow, which is not visible in cases of incomplete miscarriage.

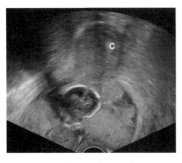

FIGURE 16.8 Advanced cervical pregnancy diagnosed at 15 weeks of gestation. Note an empty uterine cavity and very thin endometrium (C). The cervix is distended and it contained a fetus and placenta. The membranes were ruptured and amniotic fluid is absent

Ushakov et al.,[36] in their literature review, found that the correct ultrasound diagnosis was made in 81.1% of women. They divided cervical pregnancy into four morphological types: viable cervical pregnancy (61.5%), missed (miscarriage) cervical pregnancy (13.8%), cervical mass (13.8%) and early cervical pregnancy (10.8%).[36] Miscarriage and Nabothian cysts are the common diagnostic pitfalls for early cervical pregnancy.

Management

The lack of contractile myometrium within the cervix is the main cause of severe haemorrhage in cases of cervical pregnancy. The bleeding tends to occur during surgical evacuation of cervical pregnancy, which has prompted interest in conservative management options. Conservative treatment has evolved in recent years and has replaced hysterectomy, which used to be the traditional method to stop severe bleeding in advanced cervical pregnancy. Conservative management is the preferred treatment option in all women who are haemodynamically stable with a certain diagnosis of cervical pregnancy.

SURGICAL MANAGEMENT

In the past, the only surgical method used to treat cervical pregnancy was total abdominal hysterectomy. In modern clinical practice, hysterectomy is usually only performed as a life-saving operation in cases of uncontrollable haemorrhage and not as a first-line management option. However, in cases of advanced cervical pregnancies over 16 weeks of gestation, hysterectomy is often the only available management option. Ushakov et al.[36] reported that, between 1960 and 1980, the rate of hysterectomy in women with cervical pregnancy was 49–68%. A literature review by Jurkovic et al.[43] showed that, in the 1980s and 1990s, with the improved ultrasound detection of early cervical pregnancy hysterectomy was performed on only 6/40 (15%) women with cervical pregnancy.

An attempt to remove cervical pregnancy by dilatation and curettage (D&C) without additional procedures to contain blood loss carries a risk of hysterectomy of 40%.[43] As a result, a number of perioperative methods aimed at reducing the bleeding from the uterine cervix have been developed to be used in conjunction with D&C.[33,43,44] These methods include the insertion of a Foley catheter into the cervix, intracervical vasopressin injection, cervical Shirodkar cerclage, transvaginal ligation of the cervical branches of uterine arteries and angiographic uterine artery embolisation.

The insertion of a Foley catheter is a simple procedure that can be successfully performed by most trained gynaecologists. The catheter is placed within the cervical canal and the tip of the catheter is passed through the internal os following dilatation and curettage. The balloon, which is placed within the dilated cervical canal, is inflated with 20–70 ml of sterile water to control bleeding by compressing the cervical blood vessels. The catheter is usually left in place for 24–48 hours and then gradually deflated until final removal.

The insertion of Shirodkar cervical suture can also be used in conjunction with D&C to prevent haemorrhage. Cerclage has also been used as a primary treatment modality in the management of cervical pregnancy, which can avoid hysterectomy as well as the adverse effects of methotrexate.[45]

Angiographic uterine artery embolisation appears to be a successful method for massive haemorrhage control, which can be used alone or in conjunction with methotrexate or D&C in the treatment of cervical pregnancy.[44,46,47] The reported success of embolisation in the treatment of cervical pregnancy has been as high as 89%.[43,44,46,47]

MEDICAL MANAGEMENT

Methotrexate administered systemically or locally has become a popular option for the management of cervical pregnancy.[35] The use of methotrexate in the treatment of cervical pregnancy was first reported in 1983 by Farabow et al.[48]

The reported success rate of systemic methotrexate in the treatment of cervical pregnancy is around 81%.[32,33] However, almost 50% of the women treated with systemic methotrexate suffered systemic adverse effects, including stomatitis and abnormal liver function.[35,43]

Local injection of methotrexate in cervical pregnancy requires a much lower dose than systemic therapy. The therapeutic effectiveness of local injection is high and adverse effects are rare, which makes it more acceptable to patients than systemic methotrexate.

Fertility after cervical pregnancy

The reported recurrence rate of cervical pregnancy was only 3% following successful conservative treatment with uterine preservation. However, the risks of preterm delivery and tubal ectopic pregnancy were significantly increased.[36] More than 50% of women with a history of cervical pregnancy had normal full-term pregnancies, which justifies the use of conservative management in all cases of early cervical pregnancy.[36]

Caesarean-scar pregnancy

The implantation of the conceptus into a deficient uterine caesarean section scar is termed caesarean-scar pregnancy. The caesarean-scar pregnancy is considered to represent a form of ectopic pregnancy because of its location outside the uterine cavity and because of the myometrial involvement, which is classified as intramural pregnancy (Figure 16.6).

Incidence and predisposing factors

The reported incidence of caesarean-scar pregnancy varies between 1/1800 to 1/2216.[49,50] The rise in the number of reported cases in recent years is likely to be explained by the increased rate of caesarean sections and improvements in early diagnosis. The risk is particularly high in women with multiple previous caesarean sections.[49] Many hypotheses have been suggested as to why and how caesarean-scar pregnancy occurs but the most logical explanation is that the conceptus enters the myometrium through a microscopic or visible defect in the caesarean section scar.[51]

Diagnosis

Women usually present with non-specific symptoms such as vaginal bleeding, which is occasionally accompanied by mild to moderate uterine contractions. Women with this form of ectopic pregnancy usually have less bleeding and cramping pain than those with a spontaneous or inevitable miscarriage.[50]

Ultrasound is by far the best tool for the diagnosis of caesarean-scar pregnancy. To improve the detection rate, clinicians should always take a careful medical history before examination and maintain a high index of suspicion by attempting to visualise the caesarean section scar on ultrasound and determining its relation to the pregnancy. The ultrasound diagnosis is based on the visualisation of the gestational sac, which is located at the level of the internal os and penetrating the anterior uterine wall approaching the bladder.[52] The use of Doppler helps to confirm that the implantation has occurred within the myometrial defect (Figures 16.9, 16.10).[49]

The diagnosis of caesarean pregnancy is most accurate in the early first trimester and becomes more difficult as the pregnancy progresses.

Management

SURGICAL MANAGEMENT

Different surgical methods have been used with various degrees of success in the treatment of caesarean-scar pregnancy. These include D&C[50] in combination with insertion of cervical suture, Foley catheter or uterine artery embolisation to decrease perioperative blood loss.[49,50] Other surgical options include laparoscopic resection of pregnancy, hysterotomy and hysterectomy.[53]

Seow et al.[50] have successfully treated eight caesarean-scar pregnancies with simple D&C. However, three women required insertion of a Foley catheter into the cervix to control blood loss, which ranged between 500 ml and 1000 ml. A large series of caesarean scar pregnancies, treated surgically, showed that the insertion of Shirodkar cervical suture may be an effective way to secure haemostasis following evacuation of caesarean scar pregnancy (Figures 16.11, 16.12, 16.13). In all 22 women, the uterus was successfully preserved and the median blood

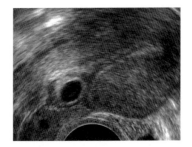

FIGURE 16.9 Caesarean-scar pregnancy diagnosed at 5 weeks of gestation. Note the position of the sac deep in the myometrium within the anterior uterine wall

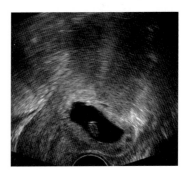

FIGURE 16.10 A 7-week caesarean-scar pregnancy; the gestational sac is herniating through the deficient myometrium of the anterior uterine wall

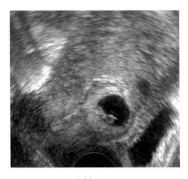

FIGURE 16.11 A viable caesarean scar pregnancy before surgical evacuation

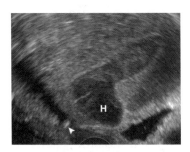

FIGURE 16.12 Another image of the same pregnancy following surgical evacuation and insertion of a Shirodkar cervical suture. Note a large haematoma (H) in the anterior uterine wall, which is herniating towards the bladder. The suture is seen as a bright linear echo (arrow), which is located below the internal os and the haematoma

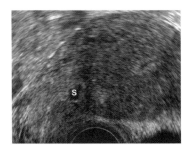

FIGURE 16.13 The same woman 2 months after evacuation of caesarean-scar pregnancy. Deficient lower-segment caesarean section scar (s) is clearly visible

loss was only 300 ml. Only 9% of the women required blood transfusion, which was significantly lower in comparison with other methods of haemostasis.[54]

Lee *et al.*[53] performed the first laparoscopic resection of a caesarean-scar pregnancy. The procedure involved incising the mass and removing dark-reddish tissue, later confirmed pathologically to represent necrotic chorionic villi. Haemostasis was achieved with bipolar cautery and endoscopic suturing was used to close the uterine defect.[53]

MEDICAL MANAGEMENT

The use of systemic methotrexate in the management of caesarean-scar pregnancy has been reported with various degrees of success.[49,51,55–57] Other treatment options include the use of ultrasound-guided local injection of methotrexate, potassium chloride or hyperosmolar glucose.[49–51] The transvaginal approach is preferable over the transabdominal approach because it is simpler and safer.[49] The dose of methotrexate for systemic and local treatment is the same as in other ectopics. The success rates of conservative treatment ranges between 71% and 100%.[49,50] However, an important drawback of medical treatment is the long time required for the elimination of non-viable trophoblast. Being located deep within a deficient myometrium, the pregnancy cannot be spontaneously expelled by uterine contractions. The process of pregnancy clearance is further hampered by decreased vascularity of the deficient and scarred myometrium. It is therefore not unusual to see women with residual trophoblast many months after 'successful' medical treatment with methotrexate.

EXPECTANT MANAGEMENT

Expectant management of viable caesarean-scar pregnancy is likely to lead to emergency hysterectomy if the pregnancy progresses beyond 14 weeks of gestation, owing to the risk of placenta accreta or percreta and the risk of rupture in the second trimester.[58] However, expectant management may be suitable for small non-viable caesarean scar pregnancies with declining serum hCG. Similar to medical treatment, expectant management is also associated with prolonged time required for the complete absorption of non-viable trophoblast.

Future fertility

The risk of recurrent caesarean-scar pregnancy following successful conservative treatment appears to be low. In a series of 46 women with a caesarean scar pregnancy who desired future pregnancies, 86% were able to achieve a spontaneous conception.[59] Only one woman suffered a recurrent scar ectopic pregnancy. The first-trimester miscarriage rate was 35%, which could be explained by a relatively high maternal age in this group of women. None of the women suffered a scar rupture during pregnancy. However, they were all delivered by elective caesarean section and therefore the risk of scar rupture in labour is unknown.[59] Seow et al.[50] suggested that a subsequent pregnancy should be avoided for 3 months after successful treatment of a caesarean-scar pregnancy to facilitate scar healing. They also suggested that an elective caesarean section is the best option for future deliveries.

Fylstra[60] stated that a definitive treatment of a caesarean-scar pregnancy is by laparotomy and hysterotomy, with repair of the accompanying uterine scar. However, in view of the low risk of recurrence, this option should be considered only in rare cases of repeated scar pregnancies.

Ovarian pregnancy

Ovarian pregnancy is defined as implantation of the conceptus on the surface or inside the ovary.

Incidence and predisposing factors

The reported incidence of ovarian pregnancy after spontaneous conception ranges between 1/712 to 1/60 000 deliveries, accounting for 0.5–6.0% of all ectopic pregnancies.[1,60–64] There are no direct risk factors associated with primary ovarian pregnancy; however, there are reports of associations with the use of an intrauterine contraceptive device, pelvic inflammatory disease and assisted conception.[60–64]

Diagnosis

The clinical presentation of ovarian pregnancy is similar to tubal ectopics. At surgery, ovarian pregnancy is suspected in women with normal tubes and swelling in the ovary separate from corpus luteum. The diagnosis is usually confirmed at histology by showing the presence of ovarian tissue attached to the gestational sac in the specimen.

There are no set ultrasonic criteria for the diagnosis of ovarian pregnancy. Various findings have been reported in individual case reports; most of them included the description of a cystic structure surrounded by an echogenic ring and healthy ovarian tissue (Figure 16.14). When the gestational sac within the ovary contains a live embryo, the ultrasound diagnosis of ovarian pregnancy becomes simpler. However, in most cases, women with ovarian pregnancy present earlier in pregnancy where these features might still have not developed.[60,65] The use

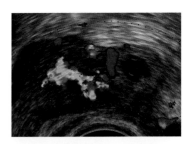

FIGURE 16.14 An ovarian ectopic pregnancy. A small gestational sac with a yolk sac is seen in the left-lateral pole of the ovary. A solid corpus luteum is identified by an area of high vascularity in the opposite pole of the ovary

of Doppler to distinguish a gestational sac from a corpus luteum is not always helpful.[66]

Management

Traditionally, ovarian pregnancy was managed by laparotomy and ovariectomy or, at least, a wedge resection.[67] The early detection of ovarian pregnancy has allowed the use of more conservative surgical techniques, preserving ovarian tissue and future fertility. Laparoscopy has recently emerged as a best method for the management of ovarian pregnancies.[62,63,68] The technique of laparoscopic removal depends on the size and location of the pregnancy within the ovary, as well as the woman's haemodynamic status. The described surgical approaches include ovarian resection, aspiration of the ovum combined with coagulation of the implantation site and removal of the products of conception using biopsy forceps and hydrodissection.[63,68,69]

The use of intraoperative ultrasound has also been proposed to facilitate identification of gestational sac within the ovary.[70]

The role of medical management in the treatment of ovarian pregnancy has not been determined. Only few cases have been reported in the literature, using methotrexate.[71,72] However, it is unknown whether methotrexate offers an advantage over expectant management in these cases, some of which could have resolved spontaneously.[62]

Abdominal pregnancy

The implantation of the conceptus within the peritoneal cavity excluding the uterus, ovaries or fallopian tubes is referred to as abdominal pregnancy. Abdominal pregnancy is divided into primary and secondary relating to the primary site of implantation, or early and late based on the gestational age.

In 1942, Studdiford[73] set the following surgical criteria to diagnose primary abdominal pregnancy which include normal ovaries and fallopian tubes, no evidence of uterine rupture and pregnancy adherent exclusively to the peritoneal surface early enough in gestation to eliminate the possibility of secondary implantation after a primary nidation elsewhere.[73]

Incidence and predisposing factors

Abdominal pregnancy is rare and constitutes approximately 1% of ectopic pregnancies.[74] It has a reported incidence of 1/2200 to 1/10 200 pregnancies and 1/6000–1/9000 births.[74,75] The maternal mortality of abdominal pregnancy is 7.7 times that of a tubal ectopic pregnancy and 89.8 times that of an intrauterine pregnancy.[74] Fetal survival varies between 20% and 40% in cases of advanced abdominal pregnancies[76] and perinatal mortality rates may reach 95%.[77] Fetal malformations are found in 20–40% of living infants,[77] which may be attributed to oligo-hydramnios and compression or vascular interruption.

Risk factors associated with abdominal pregnancy include pelvic inflammatory disease, intrauterine contraceptive device, history of ectopic pregnancy, endometriosis, congenital uterine anomalies and use of assisted reproductive technology.[78]

Diagnosis

A high index of suspicion has to be maintained, as the early diagnosis of abdominal pregnancy is a difficult task. Women with this form of ectopic pregnancy present with non-specific symptoms such as abdominal pain and vaginal bleeding. Ultrasound is the method of choice for the diagnosis of abdominal pregnancy. Ultrasound detection is easier in early pregnancy but the differential diagnosis between tubal ectopic and abdominal pregnancy is difficult. In late pregnancy, an abdominal pregnancy is characterised by an empty uterus, abnormal fetal lie, oligo-hydramnios and poor placental definition.[79] However, differentiating an abdominal pregnancy from a tubal ectopic pregnancy might be difficult in early pregnancy. An empty uterus and the presence of a gestational sac or a mass separate from the uterus, adnexa and ovaries should raise the degree of suspicion of an early abdominal pregnancy.

Laparoscopy seems to play an important role in the diagnosis and treatment of early abdominal pregnancies.[76,79] MRI may also help to aid the diagnosis.

Management

The traditional management of abdominal pregnancy is by laparotomy. However, the early diagnosis of this condition allowed the use of minimally invasive surgery such as laparoscopy to be used. Usually, the operative approach involves removal of the fetus after carefully removing it from the sac and tying off the cord close to the placenta,[79] which is left in place. This is because of the invasion of placental tissue into surrounding organs, potentially causing severe torrential haemorrhage if removal is attempted. However, leaving the placenta in place is associated with postoperative complications such as sepsis, secondary haemorrhage, abscess formation and wound dehiscence.[77] Reabsorption of the placenta is slow and may take up to 5.5 years.[76]

Laparoscopic removal has been attempted at various stages of pregnancy. Rahaman et al.[76] reported a successful laparoscopic removal of a 21-week embryo. Preoperative arterial embolisation was carried out to reduce the bleeding. They also used four cycles of methotrexate administered intramuscularly at 50 mg/m² every 3 weeks.[76] However, laparoscopic removal of these pregnancies is subject to case reports and its role in abdominal pregnancy has yet to be defined.

Conclusion

Many non-tubal ectopic pregnancies are caused by previous surgical interventions and therefore it is not surprising that their incidence is rising. Although they are relatively rare in comparison with tubal pregnancies, they are associated with much higher maternal morbidity and mortality. It is therefore imperative that all sonographers are trained in the diagnosis of different forms of non-tubal ectopic pregnancy. Thus, a high index of suspicion should always be maintained. Once the diagnosis is established, it is important to treat non-tubal ectopics as soon as possible. Any delay in terminating these pregnancies makes further management more complicated and could have detrimental effects on the patient due to the associated severe morbidity, with the loss of reproductive potential as well as the negative impact on the survival rates.

Improvement in early diagnosis of non-tubal ectopic pregnancies would promote the use of more conservative treatment options such as laparoscopic surgery or methotrexate. This should result in less morbidity and mortality, and it may improve the chances of future fertility.

REFERENCES

1. BOUYER J, COSTE J, FERNANDEZ H, POULY J L, JOB-SPIRA N. Sites of ectopic pregnancy: a 10 year population-based study of 1800 cases. *Hum Reprod* 2002; **17**: 3224–30.

2. TULANDI T, AL-JAROUDI D. Interstitial pregnancy: results generated from the society of reproductive surgeons registry. *Obstet Gynecol* 2004; **103**: 47–50.

3. FELMUS LB, PEDOWITZ P. Interstitial pregnancy; a survey of 45 cases. *Am J Obstet Gynecol* 1953; **66**: 1271–9.

4. SIMPSON J W, ALFORD C D, MILLER A C. Interstitial pregnancy following homolateral salpingectomy. A report of 6 new cases and review of the literature. *Am J Obstet Gynecol* 1961; **82**: 1173–9.

5. LAU S, TULANDI T. Conservative and surgical management of interstitial ectopic pregnancy. *Fertil Steril* 1999; **72**: 207–15.

6. LURIE S. The history of the diagnosis and treatment of ectopic pregnancy: a medical adventure. *Eur J Obstet Gynecol Reprod Biol* 1992; **43**: 1–7.

7. LEWIS G, DRIFE J, editors. *Why Mothers Die 1997–1999. Fifth Report of The Confidential Enquiries into Maternal Deaths in the United Kingdom*. London: RCOG Press; 2001.

8. KUN W M, TUNG W K. On the look out for a rarity: interstitial/cornual pregnancy. *Eur J Emerg Med* 2001; **8**: 147–50.

9. HAFNER T, ASLAM N, ROSS JA, ZOSMER N, JURKOVIC D. The effectiveness of non-surgical management of early interstitial pregnancy: a report of ten cases and review of the literature. *Ultrasound Obstet Gynecol* 1999; **13**: 131–6.

10. GRAHAM M, COOPERBERG PL. Ultrasound diagnosis of interstitial pregnancy: findings and pitfalls. *J Clin Ultrasound* 1979; **7**: 433–7.

11. JAFRI SZ, LOGINSKY SJ, BOUFFARD JA, SELIS JE. Sonographic detection of interstitial pregnancy. *J Clin Ultrasound* 1987; **15**: 253–7.

12. DE BOER CN, VAN DONGEN PW, WILLEMSEN WN, KLAPWIJK CW. Ultrasound diagnosis of interstitial pregnancy. *Eur J Obstet Gynecol Reprod Biol* 1992; **47**: 164–6.

13. TIMOR-TRITSCH IE, MONTEAGUDO A, MATERA C. VEIT CR. Sonographic evolution of cornual pregnancies treated without surgery. *Obstet Gynecol* 1992; **79**: 1044–9.

14. ACKERMAN TE, LEVI CS, DASHEFSKY SM, HOLT SC, LINDSAY DJ. Interstitial line: sonographic finding in interstitial (cornual) ectopic pregnancy. *Radiology* 1993; **189**: 83–7.

15. JANSEN RPS, ELLIOTT PM. Angular intrauterine pregnancy. *Obstet Gynecol* 1981; **58**: 167–75.

16. ANANDAKUMAR C, MOHAMMED NB. Three-dimensional transvaginal sonographic diagnosis of asymptomatic interstitial pregnancy at 6 weeks of gestation. *Acta Obstet Gynecol Scand* 2004; **83**: 408–10.

17. IZQUIERDO LA, NICHOLAS MC. Three-dimensional transvaginal sonography of interstitial pregnancy. *J Clin Ultrasound* 2003; **31**: 484–7.

18. CHAN LYS, FOK WY, YUEN PM. Pitfalls in diagnosis of interstitial pregnancy. *Acta Obstet Gynecol Scand* 2003; **82**: 867–70.

19. KUCERA E, HELBICH TH, KLEM I, SCHURZ B, SLIUTZ G, LEODOLTER S, et al. Systemic methotrexate treatment of interstitial pregnancy–magnetic resonance imaging (MRI) as a valuable tool for monitoring treatment. *Wien Klin Wochenschr* 2000; **112**: 772–5.

20. KABUKOBA JJ, DE COURCY-WHEELER RH. Hysteroscopy in the diagnosis of suspected interstitial pregnancy. *Int J Gynaecol Obstet* 1992; **37**: 121–6.

21. REID P, BUDDHA LL. Hysteroscopic diagnosis of interstitial pregnancy. *BJOG* 2004; **111**: 89–90.

22. REICH H, JOHNS DA, DECAPRIO J, McGLYNN F, REICH E. Laparoscopic treatment of 109 consecutive ectopic pregnancies. *J Reprod Med* 1988; **33**: 885–90.

23. OSTRZENSKI A. A new laparoscopic technique for interstitial pregnancy resection. *J Reprod Med* 1997; **42**: 363–6.

24. MOON HS, CHOI YJ, PARK YH, KIM SG. New simple endoscopic operations for interstitial pregnancies. *Am J Obstet Gynecol* 2000; **182**: 114–21.

25. TANAKA T, HAYASHI H, KUTSUZAWA T, FUJIMOTO S, ICHINOE K. Treatment of interstitial ectopic pregnancy with methotrexate: report of a successful case. *Fertil Steril* 1982; **37**: 851–2.

26. BARNHART KT, GOSMAN G, ASHBY R, SAMMEL M. The medical management of ectopic pregnancy: a meta-analysis comparing 'single dose' and 'multidose' regimens. *Obstet Gynecol* 2003; **101**: 778–84.

27. CASSIK P, OFILI-YEBOVI D, YAZBEK J, LEE C, ELSON J, JURKOVIC D. Factors influencing success of conservative treatment of interstitial pregnancy. *Ultrasound Obstet Gynecol* 2005; **26**: 279–82.

28. JERMY K, THOMAS J, DOO A, BOURNE T. The conservative management of interstitial pregnancy. *BJOG* 2004; **111**: 1283–8.

29. CHEN CL, WANG PH, CHIU LM, YANG ML, HUNG JH. Successful conservative treatment for advanced interstitial pregnancy. A case report. *J Reprod Med* 2002; **47**: 424–6.

30. BADAWY SZ, ETMAN A, MANVINDER S, MURPHY K, MAYELLI T, PHILADELPHIA M. Uterine artery embolization: the role in obstetrics and gynecology. *Clin Imaging* 2001; **25**: 288–95.

31. OPHIR E, SINGER-JORDAN J, OETTINGER M, ODEH M, TENDLER R, FELDMAN Y, FAIT V, BORNSTEIN J. Uterine artery embolization for management of interstitial twin ectopic pregnancy. *Hum Reprod* 2004; **19**: 1774–7.

32. SAWYER E, HELMY S, BEN NAGI J, DAY A, YAZBEK J, JURKOVIC D. Fertility outcomes following expectant management of tubal ectopic pregnancy. *Ultrasound Obstet Gynecol* 2007; **30**: 988–93.

33. DOWNEY GP, TUCK SM. Spontaneous uterine rupture during subsequent pregnancy following non-excision of an interstitial ectopic gestation. *Br J Obstet Gynaecol* 1994; **101**: 162–3.

34. WEISSMAN A, FISHMAN A. Uterine rupture following conservative surgery for interstitial pregnancy. *Eur J Obstet Gynecol Reprod Biol* 1992; **44**: 237–9.

35. BENSON CB, DOUBILET PM. Strategies for conservative treatment of cervical ectopic pregnancy. *Ultrasound Obstet Gynecol* 1996; **8**: 371–2.

36. USHAKOV FB, ELCHALAL U, ACEMAN PJ, SCHENKER JG. Cervical pregnancy: past and future. *Obstet Gynecol Surv* 1996; **52**: 45–57.

37. SHINAGAWA S, NAGAYAMA M. Cervical pregnancy as a possible sequela of induced abortion. Report of 19 cases. *Am J Obstet Gynecol* 1969; **105**: 282–4.

38. JAUCHLER GW, BAKER RL. Cervical pregnancy: review of literature and a case report. *Obstet Gynecol* 1970; **35**: 870–4.

39. STUDDIFORD WE. Cervical pregnancy: a partial review of the literature and a report of two probable cases. *Am J Obstet Gynecol* 1945; **49**: 169–73.

40. COPAS P, SEMMER J. Cervical ectopic pregnancy: sonographic demonstration at 28 weeks' gestation. *J Clin Ultrasound* 1983; **11**: 328–30.

41. TIMOR-TRITSCH IE, MONTEAGUDO A, MANDEVILLE EO, PEISNER DB, ANAYA GP, PIRRONE EC. Successful management of viable cervical pregnancy by local injection of methotrexate guided by transvaginal ultrasonography. *Am J Obstet Gynecol* 1994; **170**: 737–9.

42. FRATES M C, BENSON C B, DOUBILET P M, SALVO D N, BROWN D L, LAING F C, REIN M S, OSATHANONDH R. Cervical ectopic pregnancy: results of conservative treatment. *Radiology* 1994;**191**:773–5.

43. JURKOVIC D, HACKET E, CAMPBELL S. Diagnosis and treatment of early cervical pregnancy: a review and a report of two cases treated conservatively. *Ultrasound Obstet Gynecol* 1996;**8**:373–80.

44. LOBEL S M, MEYEROVITZ M F, BENSON C C, GOFF B, BENGTSON J M. Preoperative angiographic uterine artery embolization in the management of cervical pregnancy. *Obstet Gynecol* 1990;**76**:938–41.

45. MASHIACH S, ADMON D, OELSNER G, PAZ B, ACHIRON R, ZALEL Y. Cervical Shirodkar cerclage may be the treatment modality of choice for cervical pregnancy. *Hum Reprod* 2002;**17**:493–6.

46. COSIN J A, BEAN M, GROW D, WICZYK H. The use of methotrexate and arterial embolization to avoid surgery in a case of cervical pregnancy. *Fertil Steril* 1997;**67**:1169–71.

47. SUZUMORI N, KATANO K, SATO T, OKADA J, NAKANISHI T, MUTO D, *et al*. Conservative treatment by angiographic artery embolization of an 11-week cervical pregnancy after a period of heavy bleeding. *Fertil Steril* 2003;**80**:617–9.

48. FARABOW W S, FULTON J W, FLETCHER V, VELAT C A, WHITE J T. Cervical pregnancy treated with methotrexate. *N C Med J* 1983;**44**:91–3.

49. JURKOVIC D, HILLABY K, WOELFER B, LAWRENCE A, SALIM R, ELSON CJ. First-trimester diagnosis and management of pregnancies implanted into the lower uterine segment Cesarean section scar. *Ultrasound Obstet Gynecol* 2003;**21**:220–7.

50. SEOW K M, HUANG L W, LIN Y H, LIN M Y, TSAI Y L. Cesarean scar pregnancy: issues in management. *Ultrasound Obstet Gynecol* 2004;**23**:247–53.

51. GODIN P A, BASSIL S, DONNEZ J. An ectopic pregnancy developing in a previous caesarean section scar. *Fertil Steril* 1997;**67**:398–400.

52. VIAL Y, PETIGNAT P, HOHLFELD P. Pregnancy in a cesarean scar. *Ultrasound Obstet Gynecol* 2000;**16**:592–3.

53. LEE C L, WANG C J, CHAO A, YEN C F, SOONG Y K. Laparoscopic management of an ectopic pregnancy in a previous Caesarean section scar. *Hum Reprod* 1999;**14**:1234–6.

54. JURKOVIC D, BEN-NAGI J, OFILLI-YEBOVI D, SAWYER E, HELMY S, YAZBEK J. The efficacy of Shirodkar cervical suture in securing haemostasis following surgical evacuation of Cesarean scar ectopic pregnancy. *Ultrasound Obstet Gynecol* 2007;**30**:95–100.

55. AYOUBI J M, FANCHIN R, MEDDOUN M, FERNANDEZ H, PONS J C. Conservative treatment of complicated cesarean scar pregnancy. *Acta Obstet Gynecol Scand* 2001;**80**:469–70.

56. LAM P M, LO K W K, LAU T K. Unsuccessful medical treatment of cesarean scar ectopic pregnancy with systemic methotrexate: a report of two cases. *Acta Obstet Gynecol Scand* 2004;**83**:108–16.

57. HAIMOV-KOCHMAN R, SCIAKY-TAMIR Y, YANAI N, YAGEL S. Conservative management of two ectopic pregnancies implanted in previous uterine scars. *Ultrasound Obstet Gynecol* 2002;**19**:616–19.

58. BEN-NAGI J, OFILI-YEBOVI D, MARSH M, JURKOVIC D. First-trimester cesarean scar pregnancy evolving into placenta previa/accreta at term. *J Ultrasound Med* 2005;**24**:1569–73.

59. BEN-NAGI J, HELMY S, OFILI-YEBOVI D, YAZBEK J, SAWYER E, JURKOVIC D. Reproductive outcomes of women with a previous history of Caesarean scar ectopic pregnancies. *Hum Reprod* 2007;**22**:2012–15.

60. FYLSTRA D. Ectopic pregnancy within a cesarean scar: a review. *Obstet Gynecol Surv* 2002;**57**:537–43.

61. GRIMES H G, NOSAL R A, GALLAGHER J C. Ovarian pregnancy: a series of 24 cases. *Obstet Gynecol* 1983;**61**:174–80.

62. GAUDOIN M R, COULTER K L, ROBINS A M, VERGHESE A, HANRETTY K P. Is the incidence of ovarian ectopic pregnancy increasing? *Eur J Obstet Gynecol Reprod Biol* 1996;**70**:141–3.

63. SEINERA P, DI GREGORIO A, ARISIO R, DECKO A, CRANA F. Ovarian pregnancy and operative laparoscopy: a report of eight cases. *Hum Reprod* 1997;**12**:608–10.

64. RAZIEL A, SCHACHTER M, MORDECHAI E, FRIEDLER S, PANSKI M. RON-EL R. Ovarian pregnancy: a 12-year experience of 19 cases in one institution. *Eur J Obstet Gynecol Reprod Biol* 2004;**114**:92–6.

65. COMSTOCK C, HUSTON K, LEE W. The ultrasonographic appearance of ovarian ectopic pregnancies. *Obstet Gynecol* 2005;**105**:42–5.

66. STEIN M W, RICCI Z J, NOVAK L, ROBERTS J H, KOENIGSBERG M. Sonographic comparison of tubal ring of ectopic pregnancy with the corpus luteum. *J Ultrasound Med* 2004;**23**:57–62.

67. RAZIEL A, GOLAN A, PANSKY M, RON-EL R, BUKOVSKY I, CASPI E. Ovarian pregnancy: a report of twenty cases in one institution. *Am J Obstet Gynecol* 1990;**163**:1182–5.

68. MORICE P, DUBUISSON J B, CHAPRON C, DE GAYFFIER A, MOUELHI T. Laparoscopic treatment of ovarian pregnancy. *Gynaecol Endosc* 1996;**5**:247–9.

69. NADARAJAH S, SIM LN, LOH S F. Laparoscopic management of an ovarian pregnancy. *Singapore Med J* 2002;**43**:95–6.

70. EINENKEL J, BAIER D, HORN L C, ALEXANDER H. Laparoscopic therapy of an intact primary ovarian pregnancy with ovarian hyperstimulation syndrome. *Hum Reprod* 2000;**15**:2037–40.

71. SHAMMA FN, SCHWARTZ LB. Primary ovarian pregnancy successfully treated with methotrexate. *Am J Obstet Gynecol* 1992;**167**:1307–8.

72. CHELMOW D, GATES E, PENZIAS AS. Laparoscopic diagnosis and methotrexate treatment of an ovarian pregnancy: a case report. *Fertil Steril* 1994;**62**:879–81.

73. STUDDIFORD WE. Primary peritoneal pregnancy. *Am J Obstet Gynecol* 1942;**44**:487.

74. ATRASH HK, FRIEDE A, HOGUE CJ. Abdominal pregnancy in the United States: frequency and maternal mortality. *Obstet Gynecol* 1987;**69**:333–7.

75. ALTO WA. Abdominal pregnancy. *Am Fam Physician* 1990;**41**:209–14.

76. RAHAMAN J, BERKOWITZ R, MITTY H, GADDIPATI S, BROWN B, NEZHAT F. Minimally invasive management of an advanced abdominal pregnancy. *Obstet Gynecol* 2004;**103**:1064–8.

77. ATTAPATTU JAF, MENON S. Abdominal pregnancy. *Int J Gynecol Obstet* 1993;**43**:51–5.

78. MARTIN JN, JUNIOR, SESSUMS JK, MARTIN RW, PRYOR JA, MORRISON JC. Abdominal pregnancy: current concepts of management. *Obstet Gynecol* 1988;**71**:549–57.

79. KWOK A, CHIA KKM, FORD R, LAM A. Laparoscopic management of a case of abdominal ectopic pregnancy. *Aust N Z J Obstet Gynaecol* 2002;**42**:300–2.

Ovarian cysts in pregnancy

JOSEPH YAZBEK, CHRISTOPHER LEE AND DAVOR JURKOVIC

Introduction

In the past, ovarian cysts coincidental with pregnancy were considered to be rare. However, the reported prevalence of ovarian cysts detected antenatally has significantly increased in recent years.[1,2] A likely cause of this trend is the increasing use of ultrasound examination in pregnancy. In addition to the traditional 20-week anomaly scan, many women are now also being offered ultrasound scans in the first trimester of pregnancy. The indications for this include pregnancy dating, suspected early pregnancy failure and first-trimester screening for chromosomal abnormalities. A routine examination of the adnexa is a standard part of ultrasound examination in obstetrics and gynaecology. This practice has introduced an informal 'screening process' whereby a large number of asymptomatic pregnant patients are screened for adnexal pathology.

The presence of an ovarian cyst is traditionally considered to be an indication for operative intervention for fear of ovarian cancer and acute complications of ovarian cysts, such as torsion, rupture and obstruction of labour. However, these risks are difficult to quantify and it is possible that many asymptomatic women with ovarian cysts are being overtreated. This is of particular concern in pregnancy, when the risks of operative complications are increased.

Epidemiology

The prevalence of ovarian cysts in pregnancy depends on the sensitivity of the screening test, the diagnostic criteria defining an ovarian cyst and the timing of the examination in pregnancy. Two studies described the prevalence of ovarian cysts in pregnancy before the routine use of ultrasound, when the diagnosis was based on clinical examination of women with symptoms suggestive of an adnexal mass.[2,3] These studies reported the prevalence of ovarian tumours to be approximately 1/1000.

With the introduction of routine second-trimester obstetric ultrasound examination, the reported prevalence of ovarian cysts has increased. Hogston and Lilford[4] reviewed the results of 26 110 routine ultrasound scans and found 137 adnexal cysts, giving a prevalence of 1/190. Only 45% of these cysts could be detected on clinical examination.[4]

A more recent study by Hill et al.[5] included 7996 women, 55% of whom were examined before 20 weeks of gestation. A total of 335 adnexal cysts were found. The prevalence of cysts was 1/24 (4%), which is ten times higher than the findings of Hogston and Lilford.[4] Another screening study was conducted at the time of the 11–14 week nuchal translucency scan. A total of 728 cysts were found in 2925 women – a prevalence of 24.9%.[1] The increased prevalence in the latter studies may be partly attributable to the improved resolution of modern ultrasound machines. However, it is more likely that it is due to the more liberal use of ultrasound in early pregnancy. During the first trimester, it is much easier to visualise the ovaries than later in gestation and the prevalence of functional ovarian cysts is much higher earlier in pregnancy.

A cross-sectional study by Hill showed that the prevalence of ovarian cysts is four times higher at 13–15 weeks when compared with 34–39 weeks of gestation.[5] A longitudinal study[1] showed that 85% of cysts detected during the first trimester spontaneously resolved during pregnancy. The resolution rates were observed even in cases of large complex cysts. Similar findings were also reported by Condous et al.[6] These results indicate that the majority of ovarian cysts are functional in nature and that their reported prevalence is likely to increase in the future with the widespread use of transvaginal scanning in very early pregnancy in women with suspected early pregnancy failure.

Pathological characteristics

Functional cysts

The vast majority of adnexal cystic masses detected in early pregnancy are functional cysts, such as corpus luteum cysts or follicular cysts. Kobayashi, et al.[7] performed a study designed to follow changes in size of the functional cyst observed on ultrasonography during early pregnancy.[8] The study retrospectively examined results of 6357 first-trimester ultrasound reports and identified 250 women with adnexal masses. Functional cyst was classified as being smooth, round and thin-walled, with no evidence of internal echoes or nodularity on ultrasonography. Maximum functional cyst size was reached at about 7 weeks of gestation, with gradual diminution thereafter. There was a wide variation in the way that functional cysts behaved and they could not be defined in terms of a maximum cyst diameter or of persistence beyond a certain gestation, as has previously been described (Figure 17.1).

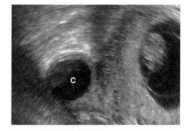

FIGURE 17.1 Ultrasound scan performed at 12 weeks of gestation, showing a normal intrauterine pregnancy and a small simple cyst in the right ovary (c)

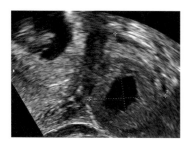

FIGURE 17.2 A haemorrhagic corpus luteum in the left ovary at 7 weeks of gestation

Corpus luteum cysts, however, are not uncommonly observed to contain areas of mixed internal echoes representing haemorrhage within the cyst. The cyst may have a fine 'web-like' appearance, may form a 'jelly-like' area across the cyst (Figure 17.2) or have a ground-glass appearance like an endometrioma, depending on how organised the blood in the cyst cavity has become. It appears, therefore, that the most important feature in confirming diagnosis of functional cysts is the transient nature of these structures. Thus, the diagnosis is normally confirmed at follow up scan 4–6 weeks after the initial scan, upon noting spontaneous resolution.

Physiological cysts are typically detected incidentally and they rarely cause any complications. However, a large haemorrhagic corpus luteum may cause pain. Rupture of the corpus luteum may also occur and it can cause severe abdominal pain mimicking an ectopic pregnancy. Functional cysts in pregnancy are rarely associated with torsion, unless they reach a very large size.

Dermoid cysts

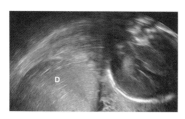

FIGURE 17.3 A large dermoid cyst (D) at 26 weeks of gestation, located in the pouch of Douglas below the presenting part. A large dermoid in this location may obstruct labour and lead to caesarean section

Dermoid cysts or mature cystic teratomas are the most common complex ovarian masses encountered in pregnancy, making up 24–40% of all ovarian tumours.[8] On ultrasound examination, they appear as predominantly cystic masses containing areas of hyperechogenicity and acoustic shadowing owing to the presence of hair and bone (see also Chapter 6) (Figure 17.3). Their ultrasound appearance is fairly typical and in most cases they can be accurately diagnosed on the scan.[9–13]

Although uncommon, dermoid cysts have associated complications such as rupture and torsion. In addition, during pregnancy and because of their dense content, benign cystic teratomas could be a cause of labour dystocia, depending on their size and location in relation to the birth canal.

Caspi, et al.[14] followed 49 women with ultrasonically diagnosed ovarian dermoid cysts smaller than 6 cm for assessment of possible complications during pregnancy and labour in 68 pregnancies. They performed serial ultrasound scans before, during pregnancy and after delivery to detect changes in the size of the dermoid cyst. None of the women included in the study suffered any of the classical complications attributable to dermoid cysts in pregnancy such as torsion, rupture and dystocia. The authors concluded that ovarian dermoid cysts smaller than 6 cm in diameter could be conservatively followed during pregnancy and labour. The study also showed no evidence of growth of any dermoid cysts throughout pregnancy.[14]

In the authors' study,[1] 18 dermoid cysts were managed expectantly with no adverse outcomes. These constituted 6.1% of the total cysts included in the study and 40% of persistent cysts. These results indicate that expectant management is appropriate for most dermoid cysts detected in pregnancy.

Endometrioma

The ovarian endometrioma represents an advanced stage of endometriosis. Although many reports describe them as having typical ultrasound features, they are a common source of false-positive diagnosis of malignancy. They are typically seen on ultrasound examination as well-circumscribed, thick-walled cysts that contain homogeneous low-level internal echoes. Their so-called 'ground glass' appearance is due to altered blood. The fluid is often hypoechoic so, in some cases, it may be necessary to increase the gain setting to detect the low-level echogenicity.[15] Internal septations have been described in 10–30% of all endometriotic cysts seen, which may cause diagnostic difficulties.[16–18] In addition, ovarian endometriomas may undergo decidualisation in pregnancy, which sometimes creates confusing morphological and Doppler features (Figure 17.4).[19]

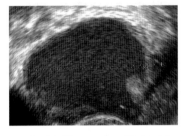

FIGURE 17.4 A large endometrioma at 12 weeks of gestation. The cyst contains focal deposits of hyperechoic material typical of a decidualised endometrioma

Although, endometriomas are considered to be rare in pregnancy,[20] in the authors' screening study,[1] they were found to be the second most common persistent benign ovarian cyst diagnosed in pregnancy, constituting 3% of the total number of cysts included in the study and 20% of persistent cysts.[3]

There are variable reports on the behaviour of endometriosis in pregnancy. Some women show marked progression of endometriosis or significant increase in the size of their endometriomas during pregnancy.[21,22] In animal models, such as rats and mice, pregnancy has been shown to confer a beneficial effect on endometriosis.[23] It has also been observed that pregnancy provides subjective and objective improvements in many women with extensive pelvic endometriosis and this has become the basis for some forms of medical treatment.

Benign epithelial ovarian tumours

Benign ovarian cystadenomas are usually seen in women over the age of 40 years.[24] They are less common in pregnancy than dermoid cysts and endometriomas and account for 1.5% of ovarian cysts diagnosed during pregnancy and 10% of ovarian cysts persisting throughout pregnancy.

Serous cystadenomas are more common than mucinous and they are bilateral in approximately 10% of cases. They are usually unilocular,

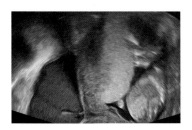

FIGURE 17.5 a

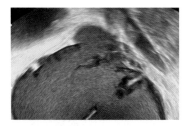

FIGURE 17.5 b

a) A large cyst is seen adjacent to the cervix at 16 weeks of gestation. The cyst contains hyperechoic material and **b)** incomplete septations. These appearances are typical of a benign mucinous cystadenoma

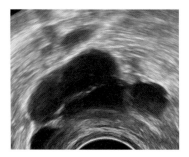

FIGURE 17.6 A large hydrosalpinx adjacent to a normal right ovary

papillary processes are often seen projecting from the internal capsule into the cyst cavity.

Mucinous cystadenomas tend to occur in older women. Typically, they are large, unilateral and multilocular with a smooth internal capsule. The cyst fluid is generally thick and gelatinous (Figure 17.5).[25]

Tubal pathology

Fimbrial cysts are usually seen on ultrasound examination as thin-walled, anechoic, unilocular adnexal masses. They have a smooth internal capsule and minimal blood flow revealed by colour flow Doppler interrogation. Importantly, from a diagnostic viewpoint, they can be identified separately from the ovary on ultrasound examination. This observation may be facilitated by gentle pressure applied with the tip of the ultrasound probe while visualising both ovary and cyst.

Hydrosalpinx is caused by fluid accumulation within the fallopian tube, owing to occlusion of the distal fimbrial portion of the tube. The most common aetiology of tubal occlusion is previous salpingitis. Prevalence varies with geographical location and population studied. In the authors' screening study,[1] tubal pathology was the cause of 1.2% of adnexal masses detected in pregnancy and 12.1% of persistent adnexal masses requiring surgical intervention.

Ultrasound examination reveals a tubular anechoic structure with thickened mucosal folds (incomplete septations) and nodular projections into the lumen (Figure 17.6). The structure may be thin or thick walled and these have been described as different pathological entities.[15,26] The appearance of internal echoes in the distended lumen with the absence of blood flow suggests pyosalpinx. However, acute pelvic infection in pregnancy is exceedingly rare.

Malignant ovarian tumours

Although rare, ovarian cancer is the second most common gynaecological cancer diagnosed during pregnancy, after cervical carcinoma.[27] The incidence of ovarian cancer associated with pregnancy is estimated as 1/12 000 to 1/25 000 births.[28] Earlier reports suggested that 2–5% of ovarian cysts in pregnancy are malignant but that the prognosis is relatively good.[29–32] It is unclear whether the prognosis is good because of earlier diagnosis by antenatal ultrasound screening or because ovarian malignancy in pregnancy is of lower grade than in nonpregnant women, or a combination of both.[33] The distribution of ovarian tumour subtypes in pregnancy is different from that seen in the general population. This is not surprising, as pregnant women comprise a relatively young segment of the population. It seems that, in general, the incidence of ovarian cancer in pregnancy parallels that in women of childbearing age.[34,28] Consequently, one would expect a greater proportion of germ-cell tumours than in the general population and this indeed proves to be the case. Copeland *et al.*[35] reviewed the literature on ovarian cancer occurring during pregnancy and found that 45% are germ-cell tumours (dysgerminomas in particular) and only 37.5% are epithelial.[35] This contrasts with figures for the general population, where epithelial tumours constitute approximately 90% of all ovarian cancers.[24]

Borderline ovarian tumours (or tumours of low malignant potential) have been shown to constitute 33–50% of ovarian cancers in pregnancy (Figure 17.7).[35,36]

Ovarian cancers diagnosed during pregnancy seem to be associated with a better maternal prognosis because they are more likely to be of lower stage at diagnosis. However, stage for stage, the prognosis appears to be the same as for nonpregnant women.[34,36]

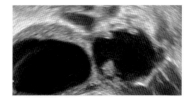

FIGURE 17.7 A small mucinous borderline tumour and the lateral aspect of the left ovary, which was detected on a routine 14-week nuchal scan

Differential diagnosis of adnexal masses

Ultrasound diagnosis

The ability of ultrasound examination to discriminate between benign and malignant ovarian tumours varies between different reports. The main factor determining the success of ultrasound diagnosis appears to be the experience of the operator.[37] Several scoring systems and multiparameter diagnostic tests have been proposed in an attempt to standardise the assessment of ovarian tumours and reduce the operator dependence on the quality of ultrasound diagnosis.[38–40] Although the initial reports were encouraging, the prospective assessment of the proposed models showed much lower diagnostic accuracy that expected.[41,42] It has also been shown that the models are less accurate than an experienced ultrasound operator in detecting ovarian malignancy. It is important to stress that none of the models has been developed for this use in pregnancy, which affects morphological characteristics of the cyst and significantly increases vascularity of pelvic tumours.

Subjective assessment can be used to exclude ovarian malignancy in a vast majority of women with simple unilocular cysts, dermoid cysts, endometrioma and tubal pathology,[43] which account for most persistent cysts in pregnancy. In cases of persistent cysts with uncertain morphology, a referral for an expert examination should be considered.

Magnetic resonance imaging

Magnetic resonance imaging (MRI) gives no radiation exposure and is a useful adjunct in the evaluation of adnexal masses. It provides clear anatomical delineation of masses because of its multiplanar imaging capability and excellent spatial resolution. There is no impediment by bowel gas or bone as there is with ultrasound. It may be beneficial as an adjunct to ultrasound in selected cases where diagnostic need sufficiently warrants such an intervention.[44] Shetty and Lamki[44] advocate the use of MRI in all cases in which ultrasound demonstrates a solid suspicious mass or is unable to adequately define the site of origin of a mass. However, no randomised controlled trial comparing ultrasound with MRI for the diagnosis of pelvic abnormalities has ever been published and it is likely that the accuracy of MRI will also be largely determined by the experience of the operator in interpreting its findings. Clearly, requirements for such intervention will vary depending on the ability and experience of the ultrasound operator.

Biochemical indices

Measurement of serum CA125 levels has been widely used as a second-line investigation of persistent ovarian cysts detected on ultrasound. This is because elevated serum CA125 levels are observed in more than 80% of women with ovarian cancer. It has been noted, however, that serum CA125 levels are altered in pregnancy.[45] Aslam *et al*.[46] measured maternal serum CA125 in 188 women with uncomplicated pregnancies between 11 and 14 weeks of gestation at the routine nuchal translucency screening visit. All women included in the study had morphologically normal ovaries observed on ultrasound examination. The study showed that 20% of pregnant women with morphologically normal ovaries exceed a serum CA125 level of 35 iu/ml, which corresponds to the 99th centile in the nonpregnant population. They therefore concluded that the serum CA125 level is physiologically increased at 11–14 weeks of gestation and that cut-off values used to assess the nature of ovarian cysts in nonpregnant women cannot be applied to pregnant women at this gestation. A new cut-off level for maternal serum CA125 at 11–14 weeks of gestation of 112 iu/ml was proposed to achieve a discriminatory power similar to that in nonpregnant women, as this value corresponded to the 99th centile in the study.[46]

Complications

Adnexal torsion

Adnexal torsion is one of the few causes of acute abdomen that is more common in pregnancy than in the non-pregnant state.[47] The potential danger of adnexal torsion is permanent destruction of the organs exposed to a prolonged ischaemic insult. Presentation is typically with unilateral lower quadrant pain, often acute in onset. Nausea, vomiting, fever and leucocytosis are all common features, although their specificity is low, particularly in pregnancy. Ultrasound examination is usually helpful, considered in conjunction with the clinical picture. Typical scan findings include visualisation of a tender adnexal mass. Ovarian stromal volume is normally increased, owing to interstitial oedema secondary to impaired venous return. Colour flow Doppler interrogation may reveal absence of ovarian blood flow if torsion is complete.[47]

Traditional management of adnexal torsion without pregnancy has been moulded by the belief that untwisting of the adnexa and conservation of the involved ovary would be likely to precipitate acute thrombotic events such as pulmonary embolism. This has meant that the accepted treatment has been salpingo-oophorectomy. Zweizig *et al.*[48] retrospectively reviewed 94 cases of ovarian torsion between 1989 and 1991, 65% of which were treated by untwisting of potentially viable adnexa and ovarian cystectomy (termed conservative management) and 35% of which were treated by the more traditional approach of salpingo-oophorectomy. They reported no thromboembolic complications or increase in postoperative morbidity, although they did comment that their sample size was too small to demonstrate a lack of increased morbidity from pulmonary embolus when adnexa are untwisted in appropriate cases.[48] A literature review failed to find any cases of thromboembolic morbidity associated with the practice of untwisting of the adnexa as treatment of adnexal torsion.[47] In a series of 54 women with black–bluish ovaries, all underwent detorsion with sparing of the affected ovary; 93% were documented on follow-up to have normal ovarian volume with follicular development. The authors concluded that ovarian torsion should be treated by untwisting, regardless of colour, and that cystectomy should be performed instead of oophorectomy.[49]

Dystocia

Labour dystocia is a rare complication associated with ovarian cysts in pregnancy. The main risk factors appear to be large cyst size (typically over 10 cm in diameter) and cysts located low in the pelvis. Obstetricians are alerted to the requirement for intervention by failure of engagement of the fetal head in the pelvis in late gestation.

When intervention is deemed necessary, the decision on the nature of intervention is based on morphological characteristics of the cyst. If the cyst is simple, anechoic, with no solid component and no increased vascularity demonstrable on colour flow Doppler examination, ultrasound-guided fine-needle aspiration is the treatment of choice for prevention and treatment of labour dystocia. However, if the cyst displays complex morphology on ultrasound examination, prevention and treatment of labour dystocia is achieved through delivery by caesarean section. Ovarian cystectomy may be performed at the same time.

Management

There are several key questions that need to be addressed when considering how best to manage adnexal masses detected during pregnancy:

▷ Is intervention warranted or is expectant management possible?
▷ What type of intervention is most appropriate?
▷ When should intervention take place?

Platek et al.[50] carried out a retrospective study evaluating pathological features and outcome of pregnancy complicated by a persistent adnexal mass that was managed conservatively or with surgical intervention. They examined the records of 43 372 women who delivered between January 1988 and June 1994. Only women with adnexal masses 6 cm in diameter or above were included in the study, irrespective of morphological characteristics or symptomatology. Women with cysts that resolved during pregnancy before delivery were not included. Women with a cyst diagnosed incidentally at delivery (at caesarean section) were also not included. Of the 43 372 records examined, persistent ovarian cysts meeting the above criteria were identified in 31 women (0.07%). Of these, 19 (59%) had an operative intervention at a mean gestational age of 18.6 weeks (range 15–22 weeks). Of those operated on during pregnancy, all had laparotomies (74% by low transverse incision, 26% by midline incision). Histology revealed that of these 19, nine were functional cysts, six were dermoid cysts, two were paratubal cysts, one was an endometrioma and one was luteal hyperplasia. There were adverse outcomes in two of the 19 women operated on (10.6%). One had a spontaneous miscarriage at 17 weeks of gestation within 24 hours of the operation to remove a paratubal cyst. The other had spontaneous rupture of the membranes at 20 weeks of gestation at the time of extubation from anaesthesia, following bilateral ovarian cystectomy for endometriomas. She did, however, go on to have a normal delivery of a healthy baby at term.

The management approach in this study[50] was that all women with complex adnexal tumours of 6 cm or more persisting beyond 16 weeks of gestation should be treated by surgical intervention in pregnancy, even if women were entirely asymptomatic. As a result, 45% of women with persistent cysts underwent surgical intervention in pregnancy. This is of concern because operating in pregnancy may have adverse effects on both mother and fetus.

Reedy *et al.*[51] compared fetal outcome variables between laparoscopy and laparotomy performed during pregnancy with use of the Swedish Health Registries from 1973 to 1993. When they compared infants born after maternal laparoscopy or laparotomy during pregnancy with all infants born, they found a significant increase in low-birth-weight infants, delivery before 37 weeks and an increase in growth-restricted infants.[51]

In a prospective study[1] at King's College Hospital, London, women were screened for ovarian pathology at the time of nuchal translucency scan at 11–14 weeks; 2925 women were scanned, 24.9% of whom had ovarian cysts. Simple cysts (defined as anechoic, unilocular with a smooth internal capsule with no papillary projections) less than 5 cm in diameter were detected in 13.7% of women scanned. Complex cysts or simple cysts greater than 5 cm in diameter were detected in 11.2% of women.

Women found to have a simple cyst less than 5 cm in diameter were not followed up. Management of complex and large simple cysts was based mainly on clinical rather than ultrasound findings. There were 328 large simple and complex cysts. 90% were managed expectantly and 10% underwent surgical intervention; 84% of cysts managed expectantly resolved spontaneously, either during pregnancy between 14 and 34 weeks (82%) or by the time of the postpartum follow-up scan (18%). Surgical intervention during pregnancy was performed in only two (0.6%) cases and four (1.2%) further cysts were removed at caesarean section. There were no cases of ovarian cancer among the 2925 women scanned. This study concluded that expectant management is suitable for most women found to have an ovarian cyst in pregnancy and that surgery should be performed only if clinically indicated or if the cyst shows rapid growth on follow up scan 4–6 weeks after the initial scan. Furthermore, the study demonstrated that subjective assessment on ultrasound scan would correctly classify most cysts.

Following this study, the authors designed a model for the management of ovarian cysts detected in pregnancy, which is currently used at King's College Hospital (Figure 17.8).

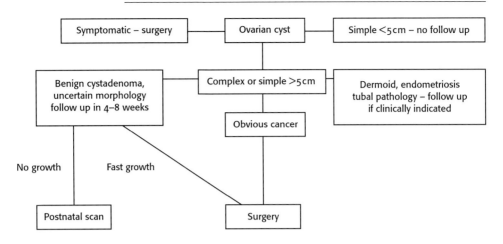

FIGURE 17.8 Flow chart for the management of ovarian cysts in pregnancy developed at King's College Hospital, London

There are several advantages of this approach compared with that proposed by Platek et al.[50] Management decisions are centred around clinical indications in conjunction with ultrasound findings, rather than being based primarily on ultrasound findings. Interventions are therefore rarely required in asymptomatic women. This results in a significant reduction in the rate of surgical interventions and the associated risks.

Surgical management

The traditional detection of ovarian cysts in pregnancy was by symptoms and clinical examination followed by operation. Before the advent of diagnostic ultrasound and acceptance of laparoscopy, women with symptoms with a clinically detectable adnexal mass were diagnosed and treated at laparotomy. Treatment would have been by oophorectomy or ovarian cystectomy.

LAPAROTOMY

Traditionally, most adnexal masses in pregnancy were treated by surgical extirpation. Suspected malignant tumours and occasionally some cases of very large complex cysts are inevitably removed via a laparotomy, as laparoscopic removal might be practically difficult in achieving the aims of the operation. In late pregnancy, as the gravid uterus enlarges and occupies a large proportion of the abdominal cavity, laparoscopic surgery becomes less safe, as there is an increased risk of injury to visceral organs with the insertion of the trocars. Although laparotomy can be performed in a shorter time, it has a longer postoperative recovery time and hospital stay.

Regional anaesthesia is preferable to general and tocolysis should usually be administered before commencement of the procedure.

A midline incision is usually necessary to afford sufficient access in cases warranting laparotomy; the alternative is transverse incision above the cyst itself.

LAPAROSCOPY

The use of laparoscopic surgery during pregnancy is on the increase; as most adnexal tumours or ectopic pregnancies are removed laparoscopically, most gynaecologists are becoming more familiar with this technique.

Laparoscopic surgery has several advantages over laparotomy, including shorter hospitalisation, shorter recovery period and return to normal activity, early mobilisation, early return of bowel function, lower rate of wound infection and hernia and less postoperative pain.[52] Furthermore, because of the minimal manipulation of the uterus while obtaining adequate exposure, there is less uterine irritability and fewer incidences of miscarriage, preterm labour and premature delivery.[53]

Laparoscopy during pregnancy is not without disadvantages. The presence of an enlarged gravid uterus is technically more challenging, with the possibility of injury to the uterus during Verres needle or trocar insertion. The gravid uterus also displaces the intestines out of the pelvis, increasing the risk of bowel injury. Thus, the use of laparoscopic surgery could be limited to the first half of the second trimester. Furthermore, the effect of carbon dioxide pneumoperitoneum on fetal physiologic characteristics and its teratogenic effects remain uncertain. This problem could be overcome by using gasless laparoscopic ovarian cystectomy, with mechanical abdominal wall lifting. Using this method, the ovarian cyst is punctured with an 18-gauge needle and its contents aspirated, then the ovarian cyst is pulled through a small transverse incision (2–3 cm in length) and an extra-abdominal cystectomy is performed.[54]

Laparoscopy during pregnancy should be performed with a great degree of caution. The following steps are advisable[52]:

▷ The woman can be placed in the dorsal lithotomy position in the first half of pregnancy. In the second half of pregnancy, slight left-lateral positioning is desirable to alleviate impaired venous return.
▷ No instrument should be applied to the cervix or inserted into the uterine cavity.
▷ Because of the enlarged gravid uterus, care should be taken with trocar insertion. The primary trocar should be inserted after determining the height of the uterine fundus. The trocar may be inserted by open technique or alternatively at supraumbilical, subxiphoid midline or left upper quadrant (Palmer's point).

▷ Depending on the height of the uterus, the second trocars are inserted higher than in the nonpregnant condition and they should be inserted under direct vision.

▷ Maintaining the intra-abdominal pressure to less than 12mmHg and minimising the length of operative time will decrease the possible risk of maternal hypercapnia and fetal acidosis.[52]

Prophylactic tocolysis is not usually needed but it can be administered if the woman experiences uterine irritability or contraction. Some clinicians administer glucocorticoids in the late second trimester or in the third trimester of pregnancy to enhance lung maturity.

Risks of surgery in pregnancy

There are several studies that have shown significant rates of adverse pregnancy outcomes associated with surgery for removal of adnexal masses during pregnancy. Usui *et al.*[55] reviewed 69 cases of women in Japan diagnosed with adnexal masses during pregnancy that required surgery. Sixty-eight of these underwent laparotomy for treatment and one had ultrasound-guided fine needle aspiration; 12% of these had preterm deliveries and 3% experienced miscarriages. There were three perinatal deaths (two of these were because of major anomalies).[55]

Whitecar *et al.*[13] reviewed 130 cases of women undergoing surgical intervention during pregnancy. Of these, 86 underwent exploratory laparotomy before delivery and 43 underwent extirpation of the mass at the time of caesarean section. One woman underwent ultrasound-guided cyst aspiration. There were adverse pregnancy outcomes (defined as perinatal death or preterm delivery) in 14 of the 56 (25%) women who underwent laparotomy for whom fetal records were available.[13]

It has been well documented in the nonpregnant population that laparoscopic surgery has the potential to reduce both postoperative morbidity and recovery time and unnecessary bed occupancy compared with open abdominal surgery. These features, in turn, may reduce the danger of thromboembolism.

Concerns expressed regarding the use of laparoscopic surgery during pregnancy have included potential direct trauma to the uterus or fetus, compromise of the uteroplacental perfusion owing to increased intra-abdominal pressure associated with carbon dioxide insufflation and carbon monoxide poisoning because of exposure to smoke generated by thermal energy in the form of laser surgery or bipolar diathermy.[56]

Moore and Smith[57] reported on 14 cases of adnexal masses diagnosed during the second trimester of pregnancy and managed laparoscopically. The average gestational age was 16 weeks, with an average operating time of 84 minutes and a hospital stay of 2 days. There were no postoperative complications or episodes of preterm labour associated with surgery. The authors concluded that laparoscopic surgery during pregnancy could be performed for significant adnexal masses.[57]

A possible impact of laparoscopic surgery on fetal or neonatal outcome was evaluated by analysing the Swedish Health Registry from 1973 to 1993.[51] The authors compared the fetal outcome of 2233 laparoscopies and 2491 laparotomies performed in women with a singleton pregnancy of between 4 and 20 weeks of gestation. There were no significant differences in birth weight, gestational duration, intrauterine growth restriction, infant death or fetal malformation. However, there was a significant increase in low-birth-weight infants (less than 2500 g), delivery before 37 weeks of gestation and an increase in growth-restriction, when comparing infants born after laparoscopy or laparotomy with all infants born.

When to intervene

In most cases, surgery can be safely postponed until after delivery. Indications for surgery during pregnancy include rapid growth of an ovarian cyst noted on follow-up scan 4–6 weeks after the initial diagnosis; high index of suspicion for malignancy based on morphological features and severe symptoms warranting intervention. Advantages of repeating the scan 4–6 weeks after the initial diagnosis include avoiding operating on functional cysts that would otherwise resolve spontaneously, assessing whether a cyst is growing rapidly and waiting until the second trimester, which is generally considered to be the safest time in pregnancy to intervene.

Whitecar et al.[13] reviewed 130 cases of women undergoing surgical intervention during pregnancy.[13] They found that there were significantly fewer adverse pregnancy outcomes (defined as perinatal death or preterm delivery) in those women who underwent laparotomy before 23 weeks of gestation than in those who underwent laparotomy after 23 weeks of gestation. Lavie et al.,[58] however, reported that when surgical intervention is indicated, diagnostic and therapeutic laparoscopy should be considered as an elective first-line modality as far as the 16th week of gestation. Beyond this gestational age, the size of the gravid uterus is a technical obstacle forcing the use of laparotomy as the primary surgical procedure.[58]

The second trimester is considered to be the safest time to perform laparoscopic surgery for several reasons[52]:

▷ the miscarriage rate attributable to surgery is 5.6% in the second trimester compared with 12.0% in the first trimester

▷ the rate of preterm labour in the second trimester is low

▷ the uterus is still of such proportion that it does not obliterate the operative field compared with the uterus in the third trimester

▷ the theoretical risk of teratogenesis in the second trimester is low.

Ultrasound-guided fine needle aspiration

Ultrasound-guided cyst aspiration offers a less invasive alternative to the traditional techniques employed for surgical management of ovarian cysts in pregnancy. It is particularly useful for symptomatic cysts, which are shown on ultrasound to be simple benign-appearing cysts. As mentioned above, the use of high-resolution ultrasound to distinguish benign from malignant disease is remarkably effective.[43] There are several features that make this an attractive management option. The procedure can be performed in an outpatient setting with no requirement for general anaesthesia; the reported procedure-related complication rate is extremely low[59] and symptom relief is prompt in most cases.

The main limitation of the procedure is that a high proportion of women managed in this way will require further intervention at later dates. Caspi et al.[59] reported a recurrence rate of 40% in their series of ten women. Two required laparotomies during pregnancy and two underwent laparotomies in the postpartum period.[59] Guariglia et al.[60] reported a 33.3% recurrence rate after one aspiration and 11.1% after two aspirations.[60]

Ultrasound-guided cyst aspiration therefore may be thought of as a minimally invasive safe and effective means of symptom control in selected women, with the added benefit of deferring definitive treatment (when required) until the postpartum period.

Conclusion

The prevalence of ovarian cysts detected during pregnancy is increasing and will continue to do so as first-trimester scanning becomes available to a wider section of the pregnant population and the sensitivity of ultrasound to detect ovarian cysts continues to improve.

All patients with cysts other than simple unilocular cysts less than 5 cm in diameter should be offered a rescan 4–6 weeks later. Most cysts detected are asymptomatic and expectant management is appropriate. Intervention should be limited to cases where the risk of complication may be high, as with very large cysts, cysts located very low in the pelvis and cysts with a large solid component. Intervention may be indicated for treatment of symptoms.

In cases where there is a high index of suspicion for malignancy, women should be referred to centres with expertise in gynaecology ultrasound, where a multidisciplinary approach to care should be implemented.

REFERENCES

1. YAZBEK J, SALIM R, WOELFER B, ASLAM N, LEE CT, JURKOVIC D. The value of ultrasound visualization of the ovaries during the routine 11–14 weeks nuchal translucency scan. *Eur J Obstet Gynecol Reprod Biol* 2007; **132**: 154-8.

2. BEISCHER N A, BUTTERY B W, FORTUNE D W, MACAFEE C A. Growth and malignancy of ovarian tumours in pregnancy. *Aus N Z J Obstet Gynaecol* 1971; **11**: 208–20.

3. WHITE K C. Ovarian tumours in pregnancy. A private hospital ten-year survey. *Am J Obstet Gynecol* 1973; **116**: 544–50.

4. HOGSTON P, LILFORD R J. Ultrasound study of ovarian cysts in pregnancy: prevalence and significance. *Br J Obstet Gynaecol* 1986; **93**: 625–8.

5. HILL L M, CONNORS-BEATTY D J, NOWAK A, TUSH B. The role of ultrasonography in the detection and management of adnexal masses during the second and third trimesters of pregnancy. *Am J Obstet Gynecol* 1998; **179**: 703–7.

6. CONDOUS G, KHALID A, OKARO E, BOURNE T. Should we be examining the ovaries in pregnancy? Prevalence and natural history of adnexal pathology detected at first-trimester sonography. *Ultrasound Obstet Gynecol* 2004; **1**: 62–6.

7. KOBAYASHI H. YOSHIDA, A, KOBAYASHI M, YAMADA T. Changes in size of the functional cyst on ultrasonography during early pregnancy. *Am J Perinatol* 1997; **14**: 1–4.

8. TEMPLEMAN C L, FALLAT M E, LAM, AM PERLMAN S E, HERTWECK S P, O'CONNOR D M. Managing mature cystic teratomas of the ovary. *Obstet Gynecol Surv* 2000; **33**: 738–45.

9. JERMY K, LUISE C, BOURNE T. The characterisation of common ovarian cysts in pre-menopausal women. *Ultrasound Obstet Gynecol* 2001; **17**: 140–4.

10. TEKAY A, JOUPILLA P. Validity of pulsatility and resistance index in classification of adnexal tumours with transvaginal color Doppler ultrasound. *Ultrasound Obstet Gynaecol* 1992; **2**: 338–4.

11. ZANETTA G, VERGANI P, LISSONI A. Colour Doppler ultrasound in the preoperative assessment of adnexal masses. *Acta Obstet Gynecol Scand* 1994; **73**: 637–41.

12. CHOU C, CHANG C H, YAO B, KUO H. Colour Doppler ultrasound and serum CA 125 in the differentiation of benign and malignant ovarian tumours. *J Clin Ultrasound* 1994; **22**: 491–6.

13. WHITECAR P, TURNER S, HIGBY K. Adnexal masses in pregnancy: a review of 130 cases undergoing surgical management. *Am J Obstet Gynecol* 1999; **181**: 19–24.

14. CASPI B, LEVI R, APPELMAN Z, RABINERSON D, GOLDMAN G, HAGAY Z. Conservative management of ovarian cystic teratoma during pregnancy and labor. *Am J Obstet Gynecol* 2000; **182**: 503–5.

15. TAILOR A, HACKET E, BOURNE T. Ultrasonography of the ovary. In: Anderson JC, editor. *Gynaecological Imaging*. London: Churchill Livingstone; 1999. p. 332–3.

16. ATHEY P A, DIMENT D D. The spectrum of sonographic findings in endometriomas. *J Ultrasound Med* 1989; **8**: 487–91.

17. KUPFER M C, SCHWIMER S R, LEBOVIC J. Transvaginal sonographic appearance of endometriomata: spectrum of findings. *J Ultrasound Med* 1992; **11**: 129–33.

18. VOLPI E, DE GRANDIS T, ZUCCARO G, LA VISTA A, SIMONDI P. Role of transvaginal sonography in the detection of endometriomata. *J Clin Ultrasound* 1995; **23**: 163–7.

19. FRUSCELLA E, TESTA A C, FERRANDINA G, MANFRED R, ZANNONI G F, LUDOVISI M, MALAGGESE M, SCAMBIA G. Sonographic features of decidualized ovarian endometriosis suspicious for malignancy. *Ultrasound Obstet Gynecol* 2004; **24**: 578–80.

20. GREGORA M, HIGGS P. Endometriomas in pregnancy. *Aust N Z J Obstet Gynaecol* 1998; **38**: 106–9.

21. JOHNSON T, WOODRUFF J. Surgical emergencies of the uterine adnexae during pregnancy. *Int J Gynaecol Obstet* 1986; **24**: 331–5.

22. VERCELLINI P, FERRARI A, VENDOLA N, CARINELLI S G. Growth and rupture of ovarian endometrioma in pregnancy. *Int J Gynaecol Obstet* 1992; **37**: 203–5.

23. CUMMINGS A M, METCALF J L. Effects of surgically induced endometriosis on pregnancy and effect of pregnancy and lactation on endometriosis in mice. *Proc Soc Exp Biol Med* 1996; **212**: 332–7.

24. GIRLING J C, SOUTTER W P. Benign tumours of the ovary. In: Shaw R W, Soutter W P, Stanton S L, editors. *Gynaecology*, 2nd ed. Edinburgh: Churchill Livingstone; 1997. p. 615–25.

25. HERRMANN U J. Sonographic patterns of ovarian tumours. *Clin Obstet Gynecol* 1993;**36**:375–83.

26. BROSENS I A, GORDON A G. *Tubal Infertility*. Philadelphia, PA: Lippincott; 1989. p. 26–9.

27. JOLLES C J. Gynecologic cancer associated with pregnancy. *Semin Oncol* 1989;**16**:417–24.

28. ANTONELLI N, DOTTERS D J, KATZ V L, KULLER J A. Cancer in pregnancy: a review of the literature. Part 1. *Obstet Gynecol Surv* 1996;**51**:125–34.

29. JUBBE E D. Primary ovarian carcinoma in pregnancy. *Am J Obstet Gynecol* 1963;**8**:345.

30. CREASMAN W T, RUTLEDGE F, SMITH J P. Carcinoma of the ovary associated with pregnancy. *Obstet Gynecol* 1971;**38**:111–16.

31. CHUNG A, BIRNBAUM S J. Ovarian cancer associated with pregnancy. *Obstet Gynecol* 1973;**41**:211–14.

32. LUTZ M H, UNDERWOOD P B, ROZIER J C, PUTNEY F W. Genital malignancy in pregnancy. *Am J Obstet Gynecol* 1977;**129**:536–42.

33. THORNTON J G, WELLS M. Ovarian cysts in pregnancy: does ultrasound make traditional management inappropriate? *Obstet Gynecol* 1987;**69**:717–20.

34. BOULAY R, PODCZASKI E. Ovarian cancer complicating pregnancy. *Obstet Gynecol Clin North Am* 1998;**25**:385–99.

35. COPELAND L J, LANDON M B. Malignant disease in pregnancy. In: Gabbe S G, Niebyl J R, Simpson J L, editors. *Obstetrics: Normal and Problem Pregnancies*, 3rd ed. New York: Churchill Livingstone; 1996. p. 1155–81.

36. OTTON G, HIGGINS S, PHILLIPS K, QUINN M. A case of early-stage epithelial ovarian cancer in pregnancy. *Int J Gynecol Cancer* 2001;**11**:413–17.

37. TIMMERMAN D, SCHWARZLER P, COLLINS W P, CLAERBOUT F, COENEN M, AMANT F, et al. Subjective assessment of adnexal masses with the use of ultrasonography: an analysis of interobserver variability and experience. *Ultrasound Obstet Gynecol* 1999;**13**:11–16.

38. SASSONE A M, TIMOR-TRITSCH I E, ARTNER A, WESTHOFF C, WARREN W B. Transvaginal sonographic characterization of ovarian disease: evaluation of a new scoring system to predict ovarian malignancy. *Obstet Gynecol* 1991;**78**:70–6.

39. TAILOR A, JURKOVIC D, BOURNE T H, COLLINS W P, CAMPBELL S. Sonographic prediction of malignancy in adnexal masses using multivariate logistic regression analysis. *Ultrasound Obstet Gynecol* 1997;**10**:41–7.

40. JACOBS I, ORAM D, FAIRBANKS J, TURNER J, FROST C, GRUDZINSKAS J G. A risk of malignancy index incorporating CA125, ultrasound and menopausal status for the accurate pre-operative diagnosis of ovarian cancer. *Br J Obstet Gynaecol* 1990;**97**:922–9.

41. ASLAM N, TAILOR A, LAWTON F, CARR J, SAVVAS M, JURKOVIC D. Prospective evaluation of three different models for the preoperative diagnosis of ovarian cancer. *BJOG* 2000;**107**:1347–53.

42. ASLAM N, BANERJEE S, CARR J V, SAVVAS M, HOOPER R, JURKOVIC D. Prospective evaluation of logistic regression models for the diagnosis of ovarian cancer. *Obstet Gynecol* 2000;**96**:75–80.

43. VALENTIN L, HAGEN B, TINGULSTAD S, EIK-NES S. Comparison of 'pattern recognition' and logistic regression models for discrimination between benign and malignant pelvic masses: a prospective cross validation. *Ultrasound Obstet Gynecol* 2001;**18**:357–65.

44. SHETTY M K, LAMKI N. Imaging of pelvic masses during pregnancy. *Journal of Women's Imaging* 2001;**3**:63–8.

45. KOBAYASHI F, SAGAWA N, NAKAMURA K, NONOGAKI M, BAN C, FUJII S, et al. Mechanism and clinical significance of elevated CA125 levels sera in the sera of pregnant women. *Am J Obstet Gynecol* 1989;**160**:563–6.

46. ASLAM N, TAILOR A, LAWTON F, CARR J, SAVVAS M, JURKOVIC D. Serum CA125 at 11–14 weeks gestation in women with morphologically normal ovaries. *BJOG* 2000;**107**:689–90.

47. SHARP H T. The acute abdomen during pregnancy. *Clin Obstet Gynecol* 2002;**45**:405–13.

48. ZWEIZIG S, PERRON J, GRUBB D, MISHELL D. Conservative management of adnexal torsion. *Am J Obstet Gynecol* 1993;**168**:1791–5.

49. COHEN S B, OELSNER G, SEIDMAN D S, ADMON D, MASHIACH S, GOLDENBERG M. Laparoscopic detorsion allows sparing of the twisted ischaemic adnexa. *J Am Assoc Gynecol Laparosc* 1999;**6**:139–43.

50. PLATEK D N, HENDERSON C E, GOLDBERG G L. The management of a persistent adnexal mass in pregnancy. *Am J Obstet Gynecol* 1995;**173**:1236–40.

51. REEDY M B, KALLEN B, KUEHL T J. Laparoscopy during pregnancy: a study of fetal outcome parameters with use of the Swedish Health Registry. *Am J Obstet Gynecol* 1997;**177**:673–9.

52. AL-FOZAN H, TULANDI T. Safety and risks of laparoscopy in pregnancy. *Curr Opin Obstet Gynecol* 2002;**14**:375–9.

53. CURET M J. Special problems in laparoscopic surgery. Previous abdominal surgery, obesity, and pregnancy. *Surg Clin North Am* 2000;**80**:1093–110.

54. AKIRA S, YAMANAKA A, ISHIHARA T, TAKESHITA T, ARAKI T. Gasless laparoscopic ovarian cystectomy during pregnancy: comparison with laparotomy. *Am J Obstet Gynecol* 1999;**180**:554–7.

55. USUI R, MINAKAMI H, KOSUGE S, IWASAKI R, OHWADA M, SATO I. A retrospective survey of clinical, pathologic and prognostic features of adnexal masses operated on during pregnancy. *J Obstet Gynaecol Res* 2000;**26**:89–93.

56. SEIDMAN D S, NEZHAT C H, NEZHAT F, YUVAL Y, OELSNER G, *et al.* Is laparoscopic surgery safe during pregnancy? Abstracts of the American Pediatric Society for Pediatric Research. 6–10 May 1996, Washington DC. *Pediatr Res* 1996;**39 Suppl 2**:112. Abstract 657.

57. MOORE R D, SMITH W G. Laparoscopic management of adnexal masses in pregnant women. *J Reprod Med* 1999;**44**:97–100.

58. LAVIE O, NEUMAN M, BELLER U. The management of a persistent adnexal mass in pregnancy. *Am J Obstet Gynecol* 1996;**175**:750.

59. CASPI B, BEN-ARIE A, APPELMAN Z, OR Y, HAGAY Z. Aspiration of simple pelvic cysts during pregnancy. *Gynecol Obstet Invest* 2000;**49**:102–5.

60. GUARIGLIA L, CONTE M, ARE P, ROSATI P. Ultrasound-guided fine needle aspiration of ovarian cysts during pregnancy. *Eur J Obstet Gynecol Reprod Biol* 1999;**82**:5–9.

Index

Note: page numbers in *italics* refer to figures and tables